CONSCIOUS EATING

By
Gabriel Cousens, M.D.

Conscious Eating

Printed in the United States of America
First Printing 1992
Second Edition 1993
Third Edition 1995

Library of Congress Cataloging-in-Publication Data

   Cousens, Gabriel, 1943-
   Conscious Eating
   p. cm.
   Includes bibliographical references and index.
   ISBN 0-9644584-0-3 pbk. (previously ISBN 1-56550-014-8)
   1. Nutrition   2. Health I. Title.
   Library of Congress Catalog Card Number: 92-62432

Cover art: Renee'
Cover graphics and design: Ken Alexander
Cover photo: John Burgess, Press Democrat
Illustration art: Ruben Lovato
Supplemental illustrations: Stephen Grettenberg
Managing Editor: Bob Warden
Copy Editor: Suzanne Stasa
Consultant: Bethany S. ArgIsle

Paperback ISBN 0-9644584-0-3

Essene Vision Books
PO Box 1080
Patagonia, AZ 85624
800-754-2440
602-394-2060

Dedication

To the service of God who inspired me to write this book and to carry on the teaching of *Genesis 1:29** – as the spiritual nutritional blueprint for humanity's preparation for the golden age of peace.

* "See, I give you every seed-bearing plant that is upon all the earth, and every tree that has seed-bearing fruit; they shall be yours for food."

Acknowledgements

This book, inspired by the Divine, has manifested with the help of many people whom I most gratefully acknowledge:

Nora Cousens, my mate of 23 years and co-director of Tree of Life Seminars who patiently supported me with her love and thoughtful feedback on every aspect of the book.
Eliot Jay Rosen, M.S.W., an expert in the field of nutrition who spent many hours doing the initial editing and giving inspirational support.
Wind D' Golds, who teaches Lving foods and who reviewed the recipe section.
Joanna Brick, nutripath and writer who helped to edit the book.
Pat Furger, our Spiritual Nutrition Workshop food preparer who helped develop some of the recipes and who is working on her own recipe book.
Bobbie Spurr, N.D., who reviewed my Ayurvedic work and the recipe section.
Steven Schechter, N.D., author of *Fighting Radiation and Chemical Pollutants with Foods, Herbs, and Vitamins—Documented Natural Remedies that Boost Your Immunity and Detoxify* who went over the Radiation Protection Chapter.
Carol Meer, my office manager, who spent hours of computer time on the book and shared her insights and a quote.
Irv Neuman, a Jewish scholar who reviewed my section on Judaism and Vegetarianism.
Father Dunstan Morissey, a Benedictine monk, and **Brother David Owen,** Archbishop of the Essene Church of Christ, who reviewed the chapter on the Vegetarianism of Jesus.
Pastor Terry Swanson, who reviewed the section on the Seventh Day Adventists.
Drs. Harold Kristal, Howard Loomis, James Barody and Ted Morter, Jr., who gave valuable information and feedback on the acid-base chapter.
Hal and Linda Kramer of Kramer Publishing who supported the early development of this book and gave valuable feedback.
The Bawa Muhaiyaddeen Fellowship for translating an interview for me and letting me use it.
Beth Hamilton, C.A., David Walker, C.A, and Isaac Elias, M.D., who reviewed the acupuncture section.
Patricia and Tom Lee of Enzyme Express in Anchorage Alaska, who organized my Alaskan raw food study.
Dr. Patrick and Gael Crystal Flanagan, authors of *Crystal Energy*, and **Duane Taylor**, a certified water specialist, Northcoast Waterworks, Inc. for reviewing the water chapter.
Suzanne M. Stasa, M.A., for the love she put into editing the second and third editions.

And to the many others who helped create this book—**thank you.**

RECYCLED PAPER

Table of Contents

Foreward

I believe the great American painter, Frederick Remington, would have appreciated Dr. Gabriel Cousens, and this book, *Conscious Eating.* Remington was a gifted and courageous frontier artist, who went to the American West in the mid-1800s to see and survey this new territory and then reported to us by painting vivid and insightful pictures. Gabriel Cousens is also surveying a most important and exciting frontier—*optimal care and feeding of the total human being.*

Gabriel Cousens, M.D., is a physician, teacher, nutritionist, artist, scientist, visionary, and spiritually awakened man, with something very important to tell us. Daily in his medical practice and research, he sees what our food choices do to us to create glowing health or to promote dread disease. In *Conscious Eating,* Dr. Cousens has not so much written a valuable nutritional guide, as painted a most remarkable picture.

Gabriel uses his many insights into the effects of food on the human body as "colors" on his palette—rich textures of nutritional science, brilliant flashes of spiritual insight, and deep shades of intuitive logic and common sense—to outline and illustrate the rich landscapes of applied nutrition. His years of clinical experience and research, as well as his personal depth and awareness, combine in his snapshots, portraits, and ultimately, murals, that illustrate how what we eat, think, and do determines who we become—and how we can optimize the process.

Yet, Dr. Cousens is wise enough to know that each person must find their own way to their optimal health program. He clearly describes and maps the nutritional territory, from the wellsprings of the religious origins of conscious food choices, through the thickets of myths surrounding vegetarian nutrition, to the vantage points of wise shopping and food preparation—all along encouraging us to determine our own course according to the truths of our own body.

Dr. Gabriel Cousens is a nutritional pioneer who sees the larger picture of food and health and who cares enough to report back to us so we may make the wisest choices. As a student of nutrition, as well as a teacher, I know I learned a great deal from *Conscious Eating.* The nutritional frontier makes more sense to me now, and I'm sure it will enlarge your world, too—not to mention making you a much healthier "explorer" in the process.

Conscious Eating will vastly expand your understanding of the role of optimal nutrition in creating true health. This book will be seen as a pillar in the growing body of foundation work on vegetarianism. You are in the h   ds of a most capable nutritional guide—Dr. Gabriel Cousens—enjoy the journey!

Michael Klaper, M.D.

Author's Update

There has been an increasing demand by *Conscious Eating* readers to have a center to transition into a 'conscious eating' lifestyle. In response to this growing need, we have begun the development of a residential center where we have expanded the vision from 'conscious eating' to conscious living. The Tree of Life Rejuvenation Center is located on 166 acres on a beautiful Arizona mesa, surrounded by a magnificent 360-degree view, and nestled in the Patagonia mountains.

A general lifestyle program, called "Living the Good Life," will offer training in: preparing and eating organic, vegetarian, 80%-live food diet; 'conscious eating' lectures; sprouting and organic gardening; ecological thinking; permaculture (sustainable living design); hatha yoga; breathing exercises; meditation; sunrise and sunset meditations; expressive arts; and meadow and mountain hikes.

Following this initial week, there will be a series of week-long, self-healing empowerment courses including: Relationship Intimacy; Family Dynamics (including a children's Tree of Life Course; Spiritual Juice Fasting; Hands-on Healing for Self and Others (Reiki); and a psycho-spiritual, self-development course called Zero Point Process.

The center plans to open in September 1996. A spa will be available offering a variety of massages, constitutional hydrotherapy, outdoor and indoor hot and cold soaking baths, and hyperbaric oxygen treatments.

Presently, I am offering optimal health and Ayurvedic evaluations and treatment programs on an individual basis. Medical supervision is now available for long-term juice fasting, weight loss programs, harmful health habits, and Pancha Karma, an Ayurvedic detoxification program.

The Tree of Life is a unique concept for a health vacation. We want to empower you to succeed in your efforts to create a more healthy lifestyle and have a good time while doing it. The key to changing to a more healthy lifestyle is inspiration for the commitment to change, rather than simply more education. This is where the real secret to healing happens. This inspiration we call the *Tree of Life Experience.*

We have designed a rejuvenation environment to empower people with skills to change lifestyle and provide on site and home support to help individuals, couples, and whole families make the transition into joyous health.

You are welcome to write Tree of Life Rejuvenation Center at PO Box 1080, Patagonia, AZ 85624 for additional information or reservations.

We hope to empower people with skills to change lifestyle and provide on-site and home support to help individuals, couples, and whole families make the transition into joyous health. You are welcome to call 602-394-2060 for additional information or reservations.

Blessings for joyous health on every level.
Gabriel Cousens, M.D.

Introduction

The time for a new beginning is dawning. *Conscious Eating* is a self-help book written to help bring about, and prepare for, this new day. ***Conscious Eating* is the awareness of how the food we eat affects our body, emotions, mind, and spiritual life. It is understanding how what we eat directly affects the planetary ecology and the degree of peace we have with the human and animal life on this planet, and even who lives or starves to death on this planet.** It is my hope that this expanded approach to nutrition prepares and inspires the reader to increase awareness of the Divine and to participate in this dawning of the golden age of peace.

Our diet and the way we lead our lives are both the cause and effect of our diet and lifestyle. Our food choices reflect the ongoing harmony with ourself, the world, all of creation, and the Divine. This synergistic view of nutrition is part of a core understanding of what it means to live an integrated, harmonious, and peaceful life on this planet. In this book, the reader will begin to understand:

1. How the spirit, mind, emotions, and body are affected by the food we eat. Foods have unique energies that interact with our psychophysiological constitutions which in turn affect our physical, emotional, mental, and spiritual states.
2. How to develop an individualized diet.
3. A new paradigm of nutrition and assimilation.
4. How to decide what is your own psychophysiological constitution and how to eat to enhance this specific constitution.
5. How to balance one's individual acid-base balance or pH. Some of my original, clinical, acid-base research in relationship to diet will be presented for the first time.
6. An in depth approach to the psychological and spiritual aspects of developing an optimal individualized diet.
7. Four transition phases to conscious eating and the transition to a vegetarian way of life from a biological, emotional, psychological, and spiritual perspective. This includes practical ways of making and sustaining this metamorphosis, even when traveling.
8. A wholeness approach to diet which will explore the larger planetary implications of what we eat, including its effect on the ecology, conserving natural resources, world hunger, world peace, and ethical and moral issues regarding cruelty to animals. You will see how a vegetarian diet, and particularly a nondairy vegetarian diet, creates the preconditions for making the shift from hoarding of natural resources to sharing of these resources. This is because a nondairy vegetarian diet consumes from one tenth to one

twentieth of the energy and natural resources of a flesh food diet and therefore can potentially create an abundance for the needy millions of God's children. When we care more about creating harmony within ourselves, with nature, and with God than we care about our short-term "greed needs," the soul of the planet will have a chance to be healed; and so will we.

9. Vegetarianism as the dietary part of the blueprint for enhancing our communion with the Divine and ushering in the age of peace.

10. The role of vegetarianism in different spiritual and religious traditions. You will be introduced to how vegetarianism has been recognized as an important part of most world religions and spiritual practices, when they are carefully examined at their core level.

11. A new concept in the art of live food cuisine that shows how to prepare food to enhance your awareness of conscious assimilation and match your psychophysiological constitution and your acid/base balance. Recipes are designed to help us eat our food in a way to experience the food's full energy on the most subtle levels.

12. Considerations of many of the issues, concerns, and questions raised about the adequacies and advantages of a vegetarian and live food diet.

One cannot eat one's way to God, but a vegetarian diet, and particularly a high-percentage, live-food diet, is a powerful aid in the process of spiritual evolution. However, alone, without the context of right livelihood, right association, love, and connection with God through meditation and/or prayer, the practice of vegetarianism may result in an unbalanced ego state. A vegetarian diet is a true blueprint and a preparatory precondition for the golden age that is about to dawn. How else could the lamb lie with the wolf/lion?

Conscious Eating **is a comprehensive effort to bring clarity and light to the most essential questions regarding our food choices and the process of living healthfully, happily, and in increased harmony with the Divine. After reading this book, one can no longer claim ignorance concerning the effects of diet on personal and world health.** You, the reader, will have been sufficiently informed, coached, and alerted to these most important issues.

It is my hope that when God calls, those who have read this book will be prepared to not turn their back and reach for another plate of spare ribs or dish of chocolate ice cream. May all be blessed with the inspired will to make the changes in diet that are needed to enhance their communion with the Divine. In *Revelations* 2:7 it says:

> "He (she) who has ears, let him (her) hear what the spirit says to the churches: To him (her) who overcomes, I will give to eat of the Tree of Life, which is in the midst of the paradise of my God."

Part I

Principles of Individualizing the Diet

There are a great many diets offered to the public. A major point of this book is to give you, the reader, some basic guidelines on how to develop a diet that is individualized to your specific needs rather than trying to fit yourself into a general, prescribed diet. This section empowers the reader with a new set of conceptual tools and whole new approach to diet by presenting a more complete theory of nutrition and assimilation, and considering one's particular acid-base balance, individual psycho-physiological constitution, lifestyle, the energetic subtleties of foods, and the seasons as they relate to one's individual constitution, as well as presenting a general process for how to individualize the diet. This approach is called— *Conscious Eating.*

Why are you interested in changing your diet toward becoming vegetarian?

■ *Something inside of me said it's time*

■ *Spiritual reasons*

■ *Desire better health*

■ *So as not to participate in the killing of animals*

■ *To protect the ecology of the planet*

■ *Desire to lose weight*

■ *All of the above*

VISION

BLACKBOARD SELF-REFLECTIONS

Preview of Chapter 1
Perspectives on Individualizing One's Diet

To create a healthy diet, one needs to understand more than simply about food; one needs to also understand one's physical, psychological, and spiritual self. It is important to have a template of conscious living which establishes food choices in their proper perspective in the context of Divine communion with prayer/meditation, love, wisdom, right companionship, and love and respect for oneself, others, Mother nature, and all of God's creation. For many, this means not living to eat or eating to live, but eating to enhance one's communion with the Divine. This chapter gives much "food for thought" and challenges the reader to look at his or her dietary motivations. What is it you really want out of life?

I. How to individualize one's diet
   A. Perspectives of diet
   B. Mental relationship with food
   C. Eating to enhance our communion with the Divine

II. Artful intelligence plus trial and error applied to individualizing diet
   A. Stabilizing time, emotional space, how much, and what we eat
   B. General purposes around which to organize a diet

III. Psychology of eating patterns
   A. Distinguishing between healthy intuition and unconscious habitual eating patterns
   B. Ways to become aware of nonfunctional eating patterns
   C. Resistence patterns and excuses people use to avoid changing

IV. Power of Divine Communion to change dysfunctional eating patterns

Chapter 1

Perspectives of Individualizing One's Diet

Because each one of us is a unique individual possessing his or her own distinct biochemical variations and functional capacities in the world, there is no set, rigid diet that applies to everyone. In order to develop an appropriate diet that gives maximum support to every aspect of our lives, we need to individualize it so that it is totally functional on all levels. **A healthy diet is one that does not barter that which is eternal for that which dieth in an hour.**

Although one usually thinks of diet in terms of the body, in the context of this book and of the cumulative contributions of ancient wisdom, the fullest understanding of diet is one which is intimately linked with spiritual life. Spiritual life is not something that occurs once a week on Saturday or Sunday, on special holy days, or just when one meditates or prays. The all-encompassing way of life represented by the Essene Tree of Life grows **all the time,** not just on weekends. The Tree of Life is a metaphor of balance and harmony of how we can live as true human beings on this planet. The roots of the Tree of Life are the universal laws of nature; its branches are the universal spiritual laws which reach to the heavens.

Diet, if looked upon from the perspective of spiritual nutrition, is not a religion or an obsessive, misdirected form of searching for God. It is simply part of a balanced, harmonious life. Developing such a functional diet for oneself is not a search for a perfect diet, because the only thing which is perfect is that which is beyond the body-mind complex, which is God, the ultimate Truth of the Self.

The most effective diet is one that is eaten in the context of the principles that sustain the Tree of Life itself. This template for the conscious living of a spiritual life includes: meditation and/or prayer; cultivation of wisdom; good fellowship of other conscious people; right livelihood; respect for the earth and its inhabitants; love of the family and of all humanity; respect for all peoples and cultures; respect for the forces of Mother Nature; respect and love of our own bodies and mind; and love for the overall totality of who we are.

The difficulty in developing a totally appropriate diet is not the food itself, but our mental relationship to food. Food is more basic than sex. Most people can survive without sex, but very few on this earth can say they do not need food to survive. Our relationship to food is a primary means of physical survival which enables us to relate to others and learn the lessons we need to learn while on this earth.

It is God's natural program that our first liquid food comes from the breast of our biological, earthly mother, herself a product of Mother Nature. Very few would argue that there is anything superior to mother's milk for the infant.

3

However, after solid food takes the place of human milk, the arguments start as regards what "should" be eaten. What one believes is "right" to eat is what one learned from parents and culture, for beliefs about diet are rooted in one's cultural and religious heritage. These beliefs are often very strong.

What we eat is both the cause and effect of our awareness. It reflects the totality of our ongoing harmony with ourselves, the world, the universal laws, and all of creation. Because the way, and what, one eats is often a source of security, people do not readily like to change their diets unless there is some significant reason to change, such as pain or disease associated with their present, particular eating pattern. This is why it is sometimes true that "there are no such things as incurable diseases, only incurable patients." This famous adage is based on the fact that many folks are simply unwilling to make needed dietary and lifestyle changes, even when their life depends on it.

For many people, eating may be a mechanism for suppressing a variety of feelings, avoiding sexual tensions, and/or avoiding certain painful aspects of their lives. Some people eat in an attempt to make themselves feel good. Others may eat in order to deaden themselves to their feelings or their lives in general. Some overeat in a conscious effort to self-destruct. For others, eating becomes an addictive way of handling life. Some are so afraid of their inner life that when God calls, they would rather reach for another plate of ice cream than heed this call.

Overeating is a way of numbing oneself to life. Nutrition in the context of the Tree of Life is eating when one is already glowing with life and joy, rather than as an attempt to gain this joy through the food. **Individualizing one's diet at the most refined level is eating to further enhance communion with the Divine. The art of conscious eating lies in creating an individualized diet that reflects and supports one's realization of the highest state of awareness and that is appropriate for the functions in the world of one's everyday life.**

Eating food appropriate to one's individual needs is a means of extracting energy from our environment in a harmonious way. In today's world of fast foods and food irradiation, the relationship to food has become confused and degenerate. Many of us are disconnected and perceive as foreign the natural foods that Mother Nature offers us. The natural way to eat somehow seems "old fashioned or strange." The diseases that unnatural diet causes are so rampant that they are thought to be an inevitable part of life. This is not the case. Western medicine approaches this problem in convoluted ways and continues to spend billions of dollars developing sophisticated technologies to treat headaches while continuing to bang its (and our) head against the proverbial wall. The one who chooses to stop banging his or her head against the wall by giving up destructive food habits is often ridiculed. Our culture has become so upside down that one who chooses to heal and maintain good health with a diet which brings him or her into harmony with nature is often considered the idealist and extremist, rather than practical and appropriate. If this seems far-fetched, consider all the people who have repeated triple by-pass surgeries for clogged arteries without eliminating the proven cause of the problem, which is to adopt a diet which does not clog the arteries.

To make the shift into harmony is a matter of making a conscious decision to make lifestyle changes. To do this, and to depart from the disease-generating practices of our culture, is considered heretical and seditious to our current, fast food lifestyle. Though it is difficult to change one's old habits and belief systems, this must be done if one values living a healthy spiritual life. When ambivalent to making these needed changes, some use the excuse that social forces are too powerful.

Nevertheless, in order to develop a totally functional diet for one's own particular life, one needs to be willing to examine these patterns and be willing to abandon what is no longer appropriate. Eventually, one begins to make food choices on the basis of what will maintain and enhance the blissful communion with God, as well as the feeling of well-being in mind and body.

As a meat-eating football player from the Midwest, I grew up without meeting a vegetarian until I was 28. Once I realized the spiritual, mental, and physical appropriateness of a vegetarian diet, it still took several years to finally complete the full transition. To make stable and lasting changes in one's diet, it is best to make step by step changes that can be incorporated into one's life in a way that is in sync with the overall context of one's life. One needs a solid support system if one is to make a successful, sustained, permanent change in the direction of high-level, physical, mental, and spiritual health. Making idealistic yet drastic changes often creates imbalances which often reverse themselves in short order.

Creating our own individualized diet is positively aided by a dose of artful intelligence as well as a trial-and-error approach. Gandhi, in his efforts to develop the appropriate diet for himself, would make one shift every four months. Often a change in diet or lifestyle may feel good the first week but may not be so good for us after several months. For example, I have observed many people who, in the first few weeks, felt much better when they were put on a high-protein diet for the treatment of hypoglycemia. After four to six months, however, they often found that though their hypoglycemia was in better control, they felt worse. This is usually because it takes a month or two to experience the toxic load that comes from the high-protein diet. Switching hypoglycemics to a low-protein, high, complex carbohydrate diet maintains a stable blood sugar and slowly removes the toxic load caused by the high-protein diet. This is the long-term solution that makes people feel better and is the more healthy solution to the problem.

The process of individualizing the diet is realistic and basic rather than idealistic. Idealistic or purist diets may even sidetrack us from our spiritual unfoldment. There is an interesting story of Buddha which makes this point quite nicely. In his ascetic stage Buddha was said to have spent several years eating just roots and tubers and standing on one leg in a river doing yogic austerities. He continued to get thinner and weaker until eventually he collapsed and was washed to shore. A little shepherd girl found him. She saw his emaciated condition and decided to feed him some raw milk and rice. In accepting this food, he let go of his ascetic concept of what was the "spiritually correct diet." Although he only was eating one meal of this food a day, he began to get stronger and sat himself under the bodhi tree; in short time, it is said that Buddha became enlightened. His diet was obviously not the cause of his enlightenment, but it was a functionally appropriate diet for him at that moment in time which helped to give him the strength to carry on his spiritual evolution. Diet is not the key, but it is a significant aid to enhancing all aspects of our lives, including the spiritual.

The art of conscious eating is learning how to eat just the right amount of food to maximize every aspect of our lives. It is not a deprivation or minimal eating diet. It is a pattern of eating that adds to our wholeness. It is a diet that requires some sensitive attention to the details of our daily activities. It is to let our hunger for the Divine be the overwhelming appetite and guide to our choice of diet.

Creating a Diet

In developing a diet, clarity of purpose is needed. Just as an architect does not design a building without knowing the purpose of the building, one is able to develop a more appropriate diet for oneself when there is a clear perspective in mind of what the purpose of one's life is and what must be done to support that purpose. Although this is an individual matter, I am taking the liberty to suggest four general purposes which may help the reader in designing a totally functional eating pattern:

1. To develop a diet which is an aid to spiritual unfolding; one that maintains, purifies, and honors the body as the physical aspect of the spirit and as the temple for the spirit in a way that keeps the mind clear, balanced, alert, and elevated. Such a diet helps our bodies to physically cope with the demands of everyday life.

2. To increase the ability to assimilate, store, conduct, and transmit the spiritual energies now being generated on our planet and also the energy released by one's own spiritual development. To develop a diet which supports these energies to either activate and increase one's energy potential for the awakening of one's spiritual energy or which further supports the awakened spiritual energy. When the spiritual energy in a person is birthed, it acts as

a neo-catalyst that works on all levels of body, mind, and spirit to enable the individual to better attract, hold, conduct, and be sensitive to, the energy and love of God's grace.

3. To develop a diet that balances all our subtle energy centers on a daily basis. This is the organizing effect of the "rainbow diet."

4. To develop a diet that brings us into harmony with the principle of noncruelty to animals, the universal laws of nature, and food-related, ecological issues, and that enhances peace on our planet.

There are many factors which play a role in how one goes about individualizing a diet, such as: one's biochemical individuality; associated lifestyle patterns; how well one digests proteins, carbohydrates, and lipids; the degree of one's physical activity; how much one meditates or prays each day; the functional status of the enzyme system; and one's present level of health, vitality, and detoxification. External factors, such as one's present diet in relation to the changing of the seasons and general climate, and the political and social context in which one lives, are also significant factors. Because of all these variables, one can see why following a fad diet that is recommended for everyone, or a computer recommended diet, has a limited value.

There is one computer program, however, which is superior. This is the magnificent, human biocomputer. The program of this biocomputer is built on both one's own inner sensitivity and one's observations of the results of one's choices. It is the one that helps us know how much, and what, to eat. To learn how to work this biocomputer one has to pay attention to inner messages and how one feels after eating food. **The process of individualizing one's diet requires trusting what is unfolding, cultivating artful intelligence, and trial and error experimentation.** To be effective at the art of observation one becomes both the scientist and the experiment. The general framework of this book can serve as a starting point for taking responsibility; the rest of the work of individualizing the diet is one's own.

If one is to experiment with food to determine specific effects of eating in a certain way, one must control variables such as when one eats, what one eats, how much one eats, the eating environment itself, and one's mental state in relationship to the food.

The timing of when one eats during the day, and the consistency with which one follows this schedule, needs to be stabilized. The regularity helps the body adjust its physiology. If one eats a food late at night when the digestive powers are diminished, most likely the food will have a different effect than if one eats the same food between 7-9 am or 10 am-2 pm, which are the times the digestive forces are the strongest.

Between 10 am and 2 pm is the optimal time to eat the biggest meal of the day according to the Ayurvedic system, and between 7 am and 9 am in the Chinese. One's own experimentation will uncover which is the best time. When one eats depends on one's constitution and daily schedule. For people who want to lose weight, not eating in the evening can be helpful because this is the time of weakest digestion. The key to timing, however, is to know when one is actually hungry and thirsty so one learns to eat only when one is hungry and drink only when one is thirsty. Finding the length of time between meals it generally takes to become hungry gives one a rather direct clue to how frequently to eat. A kapha constitution person may need to wait six hours while a vata needs to eat every 2-3 hours and a pitta every 3-4 hours. You'll learn about these constitutional types later.

The obvious but critical corollary is knowing **not** to eat and drink when one is **not** hungry and **not** thirsty. This may sound easy but it takes a high degree of discipline.

A stable emotional and mental environment helps to get clarity on how what one eats is affecting one. If one is centered and calm before eating, eats in a peaceful environment, and pays full attention to the food, the digestive process will be different than if one is emotionally upset, depressed, or angry and tries to eat during the stress of an important business luncheon, or while reading the newspaper or watching the news. Eating in a calm, uplifting environment and in a peaceful, inner state is beneficial to digestion.

How much one eats can dramatically affect how well one functions with a particular food. If one eats too much of any food, no matter how healthy it is, one will not get accurate information about that food. It is useful to allow time after meals for complete digestion. This also allows one to observe the digestive process. How good a food is for one goes beyond its immediate taste. It needs to be good in the context of the whole cycle of food preparation, digestion, assimilation, energization, and elimination. The effects of a food must be positive for the full cycle of the day and not just an hour after eating. It may take four months to understand the full impact of a particular food on one's system. As I pointed out before, some people initially feel well on the high-protein, flesh-centered diet traditionally recommended for hypoglycemia. Initially, this type of diet may make them feel good because it helps to balance the blood sugar. Also, the excess protein can reverse the flow of an uncomfortable detoxification process. There is also a stimulating effect in the meat from the adrenaline released by the dying animal. The high concentration of uric acid, which is close to caffeine in chemical structure, also may have a stimulatory effect. Initially these effects may seem beneficial. After several months on a high-protein, anti-hypoglycemia diet some people begin to feel toxic and arthritic and call me for advice on a different dietary approach to hypoglycemia.

Present Eating Habits I Want to Change

Daily Weekly

■	■	*Overeating*
■	■	*Red meat: hamburger, steak, ribs, roasts*
■	■	*Pork: chops, ham, bacon, sausage*
■	■	*Poultry: turkey, chicken*
■	■	*Fish: fresh, frozen, canned*
■	■	*Fried/fatty foods: potatoes, flesh foods*
■	■	*Junk foods: potato chips, candy, soda*
■	■	*Fast foods: McDonalds, Wendy's, Kentucky Fried Chicken*
■	■	*Dairy products: cheese, milk, yogurt*

VISION

BLACKBOARD SELF-REFLECTIONS

Once one has a clear feeling for how much food to eat, when to eat the food, and where to eat it, the next step is to look at what one eats. A good place to start is with one's current dietary intake. Begin to observe the response to the different foods in one's diet. One way to do this is to rotate one's food every three or four days so that the difference in how one feels with a particular food can be felt.

Feedback comes on several levels. On the physical level one may experience a full stomach, gas, and bloating from fermentation and putrification; increased mucous production; a sluggish mind and body; allergic response; and a feeling of low self-worth. If one is willing to pay attention, this data clearly gives indications that what one is eating is the probable cause of these very real symptoms.

Conversely, if the food one eats enhances, or at least doesn't interfere with, one's communion with the Divine and the flow of the cosmic energy in the body, the food one is eating is appropriate. If after eating, one feels heavy and slow because so much energy is needed for digestion that attention is drawn to the stomach, then one is eating the wrong food. If one's energy feels drained, or the communion with the Divine is blocked before, during, or after the meal, it is an indication that some factor in the process of eating needs to be changed. If one's ability to sustain meditation is enhanced and one experiences greater harmony with the forces of nature, this is strong evidence that what one is eating is appropriate. Eventually the diet pattern one develops will be totally adequate for every aspect of one's life.

Psychology of Eating Patterns

As we evolve in body, mind, and spirit, the dietary needs of our body also change. The diet not only changes with the seasons, but also with the maturation of our emotional, mental, and spiritual state. Remaining sensitive to our mind-body-spirit responses to our food plays an important role in helping us make the appropriate adjustments in dietary intake. These shifts are guided by intuition and aided by the awareness of changes in our tastes for different textures, foods, colors, and smells. As we become healthy, there is often a need for less food because the body is better able to assimilate the physical aspects of the food and the more subtle energies from which the food is condensed.

To successfully make the appropriate dietary adjustments requires that we be free enough psychologically to distinguish between healthy intuition (these subtle, internal feedback systems of when, where, how much, and what), and the responses from the unconscious drives of our habitual eating patterns, peer pressure, unconscious psychological needs, food transferences, and cultural and personal life patterns of how we use food. The key to this approach lies in identifying nonfunctional food patterns and being able to let them go if they are detracting from our love communion with the Divine or from our physical, emotional, and mental well-being. In this process, we need to ask questions of ourselves, such as:

Am I really hungry now?
Am I eating too rapidly and overriding the sensation of fullness?
Am I responding to other needs?
What am I trying to say by this food choice?
Are there alternative foods for filling this present desire to eat?
Are there alternative activities for filling this present desire to eat?

Some of these patterns are relatively easy to identify and dissolve. For example, I always considered my mother's cherry pie a love offering to me. I left for college with a very positive food transference to cherry pie. Over the years, I would always eat cherry pie with great joy. As my diet began to evolve, the way I felt after eating cherry pie began to change and I didn't feel the same afterwards. Even eating organic cherry pie did not reverse this trend. Because of the negative feedback from my post-eating experience and my awareness of my food transference, I was able to let go of my nonfunctional food desire for cherry pie.

If the process of letting go of certain food habits was always this easy, our culture would not have such a high percentage of the population eating such poor diets and living in such poor health. For many people, overcoming their food transferences and food issues can require intense and difficult work that takes them to the very core of their psychological beings. In the U.S. it is staggering how many people are overweight and obese (twenty pounds or more overweight).

In America there is such an abundance of food that people are literally eating themselves to death. Because of the abundance of food in our society, many ego defenses have developed around food. According to Dr. Cott, in his book, *The Ultimate Diet,* approximately eighty million people in the U.S. are overweight and forty-five million of these are obese. Forty percent of women between the ages of thirty to forty are obese.

Some of the more common negative beliefs and fears associated with being overweight have to do with the consequences people fear if they, in fact, lost weight and returned to normal weight and body shape. Many people fear that the opposite sex will be more interested in them sexually if they lost their fatty protection. Losing this protection brings up fears around sexuality, molestation, and intimate relationships in general. Some people even fear being rejected by jealous peers if they are too attractive. Others fear receiving too much attention and the demand for intimacy this would bring up. Fat can become a wall of protection against intimacy.

For others, food means love and attention. It is a way of feeling loved. Many have been programmed that eating is a way to get parental approval. Most people have been trained to please their parents by eating everything on their plate.

For some, overeating is a general, all-purpose way to stuff feelings of sadness, anger, rejection, fear, anxiety, and loneliness or to numb themselves to feelings and life in general. Not eating at all, or overeating, are ways to oppose a parent or spouse who wants you to do the opposite. For some, what they eat or do not eat may be one of the only activities in their lives that their parents or spouses cannot control. Eating may bring up many family, reactive patterns that we developed at the dinner table over years of programming.

Overeating may also keep re-creating feelings of guilt and low self-esteem. It is a great way to punish or be angry with oneself. Some even use overeating as a form of slow suicide. People who have experienced actual starvation situations may find themselves eating excessively as a compensation for, and avoidance of, their fear of starving again.

As we start to look at these many different psychological patterns, it becomes apparent that it is not only the actual eating habits that keep people unhealthy and overweight, but it is the negative thoughts they have created in relationship to the food that is also a contributing source of the problem. These disharmonious thoughts maintain inappropriate eating patterns. To use an analogy, fat sticks to our bodies the way these negative thoughts stick in our minds. When these contracting thoughts are released, a lot of blocked energy is simultaneously released. This released energy sometimes seems to rebalance the system and somehow enables us to release fat. Symbolically, and often literally, heavy thoughts add heaviness, thickness, and darkness to the body. Thoughts filled with light and love add lightness and fluidity to us. It is said that "angels fly because they take themselves lightly." While eating it is important to be joyous and think positive thoughts. Negative thinking or taking in negative thoughts from those sharing the meal, or from the newspaper or television, adds a heaviness to the food we are assimilating.

Food is love. Life is love. Contracting, limiting, and negative thought patterns keep us mired in chronic hunger, unconscious gobbling, and a state of chronic dissatisfaction with food intake. These heavy thoughts block us from the experience of love in our lives. No matter how much we try to eat in this blocked state, we cannot fully be nourished. We will feel nourished by food when the negative thoughts, which determine who we think we are—or aren't, are dissolved. Thoughts about food determine how we relate to food and ultimately to other people. Chronic overeating patterns usually fade away when dysfunctional thoughts associated with food are dissolved.

Negativity is often stored in excess fat as blocked energy. When we let go of such forms of negativity as self-loathing, guilt, grief, depression, loneliness, helplessness, anger, hate, fear of others, fear of life, self-pity, blame, and unconscious death urges, this negative, stored energy often leaves the body.

Then we are able to release the bulwark of fat which is used for protection from the pain of life. Eating then becomes filled with love and joy and the body and mind become lighter and happier.

A vegetarian diet, and particularly a raw food diet, can be threatening to some people because it directly forces them to face their food issues, and indirectly, their life issues. Live foods have so much nourishment in them that considerably less food is needed to get the same amount of nutrition. Needing less food for optimal nutrition, however, forces us to observe whatever food compulsions we may have. If we compulsively need to eat more food and the body actually needs less food, it becomes increasingly harder to deny this contradiction. Many negative thoughts may arise when beginning to eat less, particularly on a raw food diet or when fasting. Because of the highly energetic qualities of raw food, it seems harder to suppress feelings when eating it compared to when overeating cooked and nonvegetarian types of foods to numb ourselves to life. On raw foods, repressed emotions and thoughts seem to be more easily released by the body-mind complex.

As mentioned in the Ayurvedic section on sweet foods, sweet foods may create the illusion of fullness and a false contentment or a good feeling. Often when people are feeling bad, empty, or depressed, they turn to junk food, especially sweets, in a misguided attempt to create a temporary feeling of fullness and happiness. Instead of the alcoholic's illusion of drinking troubles away, those who turn to junk food to make themselves feel better try to eat away their sadness and emptiness. It is a double-levelled illusion. Junk foods are "shadow" foods with little nutrient value and great negative consequences to health. Junk foods are an illusion of real food. The idea that we can eat away our troubles is an illusion compounded on illusion. Unfortunately, many become addicted to this double illusion. The transition to living foods brings us immediately into the awareness of this double illusion.

Overeating, especially of junk food, may also represent a sweet, but slow suicide for some who are depressed. Carol Meer, a client of mine who had taken the Zero Point Process, a workshop that I offer which deals with dissolving negative thoughts and belief systems (described on pages 14 & 15), is currently overcoming her food addictions. In her transition to a live food approach she shared the following eloquent statement of the multiple meanings of overeating junk food from her May 1990 journal entry:

> "I have recently understood why I have eaten junk food for so many years. There are dead spaces...spaces in me that want death. Instead of going into myself and feeling and healing my death, I have "simulated" death by going in there with a strange reversal and eating dead food instead. Dead food is food that has no real vitality, but gives the sense of vitality or life. It is like artificial vitality giving one the false feeling

of having power and energy. It is, in fact, deception woven into deception."

Without the accompanying emotional-mental work to release the stored negative thoughts and identities in those "dead places," as Carol would say, it is difficult to heal oneself with simply a live-food diet. A live-food, or even healthy, vegetarian diet is a powerful aid to the healing process. The level of health created by such a diet creates a whole new experience and lightness in the body. The vibration of the somato-nervous system becomes so high that it literally forces the lower vibration, negative thoughts out of the system. These negative thoughts become incompatible with a higher vibration of energy that begins to fill the system. Metaphorically speaking, a live-food diet brings so much lightness to the system that "the light is able to dispel the darkness." Paradoxically, this is one reason I recommend that people make a slow transition to vegetarianism and particularly to a raw food cuisine. I see this releasing of stored negativity as a healthy healing process if one creates the proper psychological space to process these thoughts. For example, during our spiritual fasting retreats, we have a daily group process to help participants release and heal from these long-time stored negativities that come up.

Food is essential to our survival. It is more primary to our survival than sex. Psychological imbalances associated with food are associated with the survival energy center and consciousness. Working through our food issues helps us become conscious of our survival issues. These issues link our subtle survival center to the consciousness of survival issues of the whole planet. As we are able to come into harmony with our own survival issues, we become more and more able to eat in a way that is healthy for the survival of the whole planet, as well as ourselves. It is no accident that starvation is one of the critical issues our planet is facing today.

Once food compulsions and transferences are resolved and we overcome chronic overeating and lose weight, then the next subtle energy center and awareness issues often come to the surface. These are issues of sexuality and creativity. Throwing away the fatty protection frequently forces us to face our sexual power. In some cases, sexual obsessions that were buried underneath the food defense system begin to emerge.

Food difficulties are related to a whole complex of issues. Although a person may begin to lose weight after one session, time is needed to process and dissolve the thoughts that arise after the first layer has been dissolved.

Because of my background as a psychiatrist, I include psychologically working with people who are experiencing eating problems as part of my holistic approach. In order to speed the process and keep people independent, I teach a self-healing course on how to identify these limiting, negative thoughts that we have created in our own minds. This course, called the Zero Point Process, teaches people how to go prior to the onset of their thoughts about food and even prior to the formation of basic identities about food and the personality in general. This is the so-called "zero point." When we are able to do this, we can first witness these thoughts and then dissolve them. Once these thoughts are identified and dissolved, they no longer have any power over us. The techniques are powerful and simple Sometimes these issues can be cleared up in one hour. This depends, however, on one condition being present: it is whether the person is ready to let go of his or her dysfunctional thought patterns.

To successfully give up a thought pattern, people need to get in touch with both their desire and resistance to lose or gain weight. Some level of desire to change can usually be found. The process helps them get in touch with resistances so they do not deny them with affirmations and other avoidance patterns. Some of the resistant thoughts of which people become aware are: interpersonal manipulations around food; fears of change; self-mythologies; limiting self-concepts; negative self-images; unwillingness to give up family and cultural images; and unconscious secondary gain for being overweight.

Resistance Patterns and Excuses People Use:

1. I like to use my weight problem to punish myself; to show the world I am no good. I hold on to my guilt because guilt is the way I've always lived; it is what I am used to. I do not know what I would do if I were okay.

2. I like to complain and feel self-pity. It gives me sympathy and attention from my parents and from friends. I'd lose this if I lose weight.

3. Being overweight is a good and safe excuse for not succeeding. Success and power are a threat. I would have to give up being "not okay." If I am successful, people would become jealous and reject me.

4. Being overweight protects me from sexual intimacy and intimacy in relationships. It proves that no one wants me.

5. Food is safe sex. Food is sensual, accessible, and easy.

6. Food is my friend. It is my only friend and the only thing I can count on. It is someone to come home to.

7. Food makes me feel connected to life and the world.

8. Food is an addiction I cannot live without. It is an abusive lover.

9. Being overweight is a way to be loved and accepted by my parents. If I succeed and lose weight, it'll make my parents wrong because they said I was no good. My mother and father were both heavy and it would make me different from them. If I give up sweets, my mother would reject me. Sweets were the only form of love I got from my mother. I don't want to be rejected by my parents.

10. Being overweight proves life doesn't work. I enjoy being hateful. I can't let go of my resentments. If I felt good, I couldn't be as angry.

11. It is a sin to feel sexual and love my body.

12. If I got healthy, I would not have anything to talk or complain about. I am afraid to feel too good. I like to worry. I'm afraid to change my self-image.

13. Eating takes away my loneliness, grief, stress, and pain. Eating is a convenient way to stuff my feelings.

14. Overeating and being overweight is a way of numbing myself from the pain and responsibility of life. It allows me not to grow up.

15. I want to die. Life is just too much. I do not want to feel energetic and alive.

16. Lots of foods numb me to the peace and joy of my inner divinity and from my relationship with God. My inner light and God scare me. It is safer to eat some more ice cream.

Once the contracting and limiting thoughts are dissolved, one is free to become healthy. The idea is not to create anything new like a preconceived weight loss diet. Rigid diets can be a form of punishment in themselves. Rigid diets are potential traps for being wrong and guilty, because usually one goes off them eventually. Once the "food filter" or food transference blocks are removed, then one is spontaneously free to eat those foods and live in ways which bring health, love, harmony, and communion with the Divine. Overeating naturally fades when there is a reorientation toward eating to enhance health, joy, and communion. **The joy of Divine communion helps to decrease our physical appetite because we are already feeling satisfied from within.**

The body's desire for food has its roots in the soul's need for spiritual substance. When one is in touch with the Divine there is such a sense of contentment, joy, peace, and fullness that food has no power to throw one out of balance. The eternal craving for divine happiness is fulfilled on the deepest level.

If one surrenders to the divine unfolding, slowly and gently, harmony with the diet and body also happens. One spontaneously moves to a positive self-image. For example, one client who was ninety pounds overweight had tried many different approaches to lose weight. This person spontaneously went on a fast several days after a session using the Zero Point Process. What happened was that through the Zero Point methods she was able to dissolve her intense rejection and anger of her mother, who was a sleekly figured "health nut." As part of her rebellion against her mother, she had subconsciously created the opposing body shape in relation to her mother's. Unfortunately her rebellion made her an unhealthy, ninety pounds overweight. After this one hour zero point process, the client reported that it was the first time in forty years that she wasn't feeling constantly hungry. She was amazed how full and good she felt while fasting.

This subtle approach to trusting the unfolding, rather than trying to fit oneself into a rigid picture, does require some surrender to the mystery of our own unfolding. One time in the middle of winter, I was in Maine giving a Zero Point Process seminar. In order to create more heat to compensate for the sudden change from warm California to the winter cold of Maine, I found myself spontaneously increasing my food intake by about three times above the regular amount I usually eat. I did this with much gusto. My hosts, who had gone to a nutrition seminar where I talked about the dangers of overeating, were wondering what was going on with me. I shared with them that I had to trust my sudden increase in appetite. I explained that during the Zero Point Seminar I usually lost four pounds and perhaps my body was trying to compensate for that, as well as the cold. At the end of the seminar, although I ate three times as much, I lost my usual four pounds anyway. As soon as I left the cold of Maine my appetite immediately decreased to normal. In retrospect, I can look back and see that my body was eating more food to compensate for the shock of travelling from warm California to a very cold Maine. Attempting to be in control with a rigid diet creates the illusion that one is in control. It confuses the issue, because on the cosmic level one is never in control.

The gradual process of refining one's diet requires trusting one's observations and one's intuition. After a long period of time of eating soaked nuts and seeds with fruit in the morning, I noticed that I began to feel full after the usual six hours between breakfast and lunch. I also observed that my 24 hour urine indican, a toxin given off by pathogenic bacteria growing on partially digested food in the colon, and a sign of bowel toxins, had suddenly become positive. By eliminating the nuts and seeds in the morning and only having fruit, my bowel indican went back to normal and I was not feeling so full in the morning. This total picture was a sign to me that my body had just gone through another step toward optimal health. I now needed less food to support my lifestyle.

When the habituating thoughts that distort our eating patterns are dissolved, the balancing process can be quite delightful. One feels free to eat or not to eat. One begins to be spontaneously attracted to certain foods that one intuitively knows are appropriate. Food intake spontaneously drops and the joy of eating spontaneously increases. One actually pays attention to the food one is eating. The energies of the foods, their tastes, textures, and aromas are more sensuously experienced. Everything eaten in this way tends to be completely nourishing because a context has been created to receive, in an optimal way, the gifts of love given us.

Mind Over Matter Doesn't Matter

The mind plays an important role in the eating process on other levels too. Our attitudes and beliefs about what we are eating is at least as important as what we are eating. It is possible to overcome the natural laws by thinking so positively that even eating junk foods may become nourishing. I do not particularly recommend this practice, however, because it has us spending energy trying to overcome the natural laws rather than being in harmony with them. Although mind is stronger than matter, it requires extra energy and focus to convert junk food into something nutritious for the body. For most people this doesn't work too well anyway and can become a way of avoiding the healing process.

In the long run it is more healthy and harmonious to eat in a way that aligns us with the natural laws and ecology of our body and the planet. Author and religious leader Terry Cole Whittiker, who teaches people the power of mind over matter in everyday life, once taught that it did not matter what one ate because it can be transmuted by the mind. Although this is ultimately true, it has its price. The question can be asked, "Is this a worthwhile way to spend one's valuable mental energy, by using it to overcome the effects of junk food intake?" Once Terry Cole Whittiker experienced the power and higher vibration of a raw food diet, true to her dedication to her own evolution, she adopted more of a live-food diet. She is now recommending it to her students. Since being on such a high-powered diet she has lost fifty pounds and feels at least that many years younger in vitality.

When God, through Mother Nature, has given us the natural nutritional kingdom, why try to fruitlessly transform the worthless dust of junk food into the precious gold of whole, raw, organic food? Though blessing one's food can transform any food into a higher vibration food, why not seek and eat the highest vibrational food to begin with?

Become Your Own Scientist

The foods we eat are major factors in affecting our body, emotions, and mental and spiritual states.

Try observing how you feel after eating certain foods or eating too much. If your handwriting or vision are affected or your pulse increases by 20 beats after 30-60 minutes, then you might be allergic.

Experiment I.
Eat the same food at the same time for 4 days.

	What I Ate	How I Felt 1 Hour	How I Felt 2-3 Hours	How I Felt Rest of Day
B R E A K F A S T				
L U N C H				
D I N N I R				

Preview of Chapter 2
Assimilation of Mother Nature's Energies

The reader is introduced to the meaning of the idea that food is a love note from God. If we take time to read this note, the process of eating becomes a special time of enhanced spiritual awareness. It is a way to feel the Divine presence. This chapter also exposes the reader to the idea that assimilation is a dynamic interaction between the energetic forces of the food and the one who is eating. We are introduced to many meanings of assimilation. We are left with the questions—just what am I doing when I eat? Could I be more aware and what would it feel like? I invite you to explore this for yourself.

I. What is the process of assimilation
  A. Food as a love note from God
  B. Dynamic interaction between human and plant forces
  C. The many levels of assimilation
  D. Eating as a way to open one's heart to God

II. How we are prepared to receive the food is as important as how the food is prepared

III. Use it or lose it principle
  A. With assimilation
  B. Transition to a vegetarian or live food diet
  C. With synthetic vitamins

IV. Paradoxical assimilation

V. Colors of food as a coded message from God

Chapter 2

Assimilation of Mother Nature's Energies

A basic, ongoing, and primary way we all consciously or unconsciously relate to nature is through our food. Eating is an intimate way to extract life-sustaining energy from Mother Nature. In the process of digestive assimilation, the food, as part of Mother Nature, gives up its identity and takes on the identity of the one who has ingested it. We are actually assimilating the forces of nature, stored in our food, whenever we eat. Each bite we take brings us the experience of our loving connection with Mother Nature.

Food is a love note from God. Its letters are written by the rays of the sun. It says I love you and I shall take care of you and sustain you with the offerings of my earth. If we take time to read the love letter, by chewing carefully and feeling the messages that are stored in it from the sun, earth, wind, water, and even by those who have grown, harvested, and prepared the food, the assimilation of food takes on a whole new meaning. It is a specific way of receiving God's grace, a holy sacrament to be experienced slowly, carefully, and consciously.

Assimilation is the dynamic interaction of the forces of the food with the forces of our human organism. An old Arab saying highlights this point: "By eating we become sick, and by digesting we become healthy." **In assimilation, the physical and energetic forces of food interact with us on physical, emotional, mental, and spiritual levels.**

The idea that each food, as a particular energy, effects us on an emotional, mental, and spiritual level is a new idea for many people in our industrial civilization. But for thousands of years Ayurvedic physicians, Chinese acupuncturists, ancient healer priests and priestesses, and western herbalists have utilized this awareness in their work. According to *The Spiritual Properties of Herbs,* by Gurudas, "An herb as a natural substance provides healing, but it also provides a spiritual message."

One of the most significant developments in the awareness that plants, herbs, trees, and bushes can have their affect on emotional, mental, and spiritual levels was the pioneering work done by the extraordinary English physician, Dr. Edward Bach. In the 1930s, Bach gave up his job as a successful Harly Street physician and moved to the country where he communed with nature and developed the 38 Bach flower remedies. These remedies were prepared by an energy infusion process using the sun's energy. Each Bach flower prepared in this special way was found to have a specific emotional, mental, or spiritual energy that helped heal the person by bringing them back into harmony. Since 1972, I've been aware of the Bach flower remedies and the Bach Flower Society and have been very impressed with the thousands of reported healings which first take place on subtle energetic levels and then work themselves down to the physical.

I want to remind the reader that in the strict scientific sense, assimilation from nonmaterial sources has not been scientifically proven, nor has it been disproven. I ask the reader, in considering these and other untraditional ideas, to rely on his or her intuitive understanding in addition to the materialistic-mechanistic, left-brained ways of processing the world that is limited exclusively to the five senses. By including our intuition, we increase our ability to explore the concept that everything in nature is made of energy and that we are affected on multiple levels of body, mind, and spirit by the subtle energies and nutrients of our food. If we find this a useful concept to enhance the quality and clarity of our daily life and diet, then I heartily encourage all to use it.

Food, particularly plant food, is a condensation of the sun's energy, as well as more subtle energy from the stars and other sources in the universe. Though the magnitude of the influences of these celestial bodies is indeed subtle, scientists have discovered that the surface of the earth is constantly bombarded by radiation from different celestial bodies, including the moon, star systems and other sources of radiation in the universe. Plants take these radiations into their energetic systems and ultimately transfer them to humans when they are eaten by humans. From a spiritual perspective, these energies are simply just various condensations of the Divine cosmic energy. In the process of eating food the cosmic, solar, stellar, lunar, and other universal energies stored in the food are released so they can be absorbed directly into the human organism. We can experience the whole universe in each bite of our food.

Having now introduced and understood these ideas, we are ready to consider the many levels of assimilation. The basic question is "What goes on when one assimilates food?" The answer: On a basic level, energy that is locked up in the food is released.

Subtle Assimilation

From this point of view, what matters is not the quantity of solid or liquid food that we take in, but whether the food is assimilated totally and properly. To do this, we need to hold the food in the mouth long enough for this process to take place. The secret of digestion is to transform each element into a more subtle form. The idea is to chew the food so that it begins to release the stored subtle energy locked inside. Then subtle receptor centers in our palate and throughout the length of the digestive tract receive the essence of the food. Certain foods may release their essences at different times and locations in the gastrointestinal tract as the body's assimilative and alchemical forces work on integrating the food so that it becomes part of the body's substance. The essence released from the food may gravitate to different organs, glands, and subtle energy centers in the body. This is done by thoroughly masticating the food until the solid food is transformed into a liquid state, which then begins the process of the release of energy from the solid food.

For many years I have been reminded, in word and in print, about the importance of chewing each bite 40-100 times. This practice of thorough chewing is called "fletcherizing," named after Dr. Fletcher who popularized this practice. As for myself, I never could quite get myself to consistently and fully chew my food in this way, even though I understood intellectually that thorough chewing helped enzymes work more efficiently and thus improved assimilation.

It is true that masticating food meticulously breaks open the cells of the foods in order to release the naturally occurring food enzymes within the plant. One of these enzymes is cellulase, which humans do not have in their own system. This cellulase released from the plant by chewing dissolves a significant amount of the thin film of cellulose which covers all plant surfaces and hinders assimilation until the cellulose is more completely digested.

Despite all this information, it was only when I began to think in terms of a subtly experienced energy release that the whole process of chewing became intriguing to me. The whole alchemical process of releasing the subtle energies stored in the food seems to take place without any special effort on our part, except of course, the act of chewing our food sufficiently. The process of chewing becomes less a mechanical chore and more spontaneously interesting when we focus on the subtle release of energy with mastication. Cultivating this subtle awareness brings us into greater harmony with this delicate interchange of ourselves with nature.

Developing this subtle awareness is easier when we do not talk much at meals or do distracting things while we eat. Reading the newspaper, watching T.V., business meetings, and engaging in a lot of verbal interaction distracts our attention away from the assimilation process. If we focus on absorbing the energy from the food we will derive greater good from our food. There is usually plenty of time left over for socialization with others after the chewing and subtle assimilation part of the meal is completed. For many, this approach to assimilation requires a change in eating styles. I personally found it a challenge to let go of glancing through the newspaper while eating breakfast.

This concentrated focus on the Divine gift of food can be a powerful spiritual practice. Not everyone makes time to pray, study the scriptures, or think about God each day, but most everyone makes time to eat. **If our heart and mind are focused on experiencing food as a love note from God, eating becomes not only a way to nourish and love ourselves, but each meal becomes a time for enhanced spiritual awareness and gratitude to God. It becomes a way to directly experience a meaning of "give us this day our daily bread."** It provides a regular opportunity for the conscious eater to take the time to receive and read God's love note, rather than toss it unconsciously into the garbage can of the stomach. **Eating consciously is a way of opening one's heart to God. It is a way to feel the Divine presence.**

To intimately interact with nature through the medium of food requires that one maintain some degree of awareness and thoughtfulness. In this state one can sense a subtle fullness in the mouth and palate when the energy is released and therefore one does not have to clutter the mind counting chews. Food is also transformed from its solid form to a liquid state, then to a gaseous state, and from a gaseous state to a more subtle or etheric state. This not only involves chewing well, but also breathing in a way which enhances the liberation of this subtle energy from the food. Taking a pause and a deep breath four or five times with meals is an important aid to this assimilation process. This may be one reason the Essene Jesus, in *The Essene Gospel of Peace Book I (p. 39)* said:

"And when you eat, have above you the angel of air, and below you that angel of water. Breathe long and deeply at all your meals, that the angel of air may bless your repasts. And chew well your food with your teeth, that it becomes water, and that the angel of water turns it into blood in your body. And eat slowly, as if it were a prayer you make to the Lord." For I tell you truly, the power of God enters into you if you eat after this manner at his table...."

Preparing Ourselves to Eat

How consciously prepared one is to eat food becomes as important as how one has prepared the food. There is a wonderful story about the Greek sage Epicurus (342- 270 B.C.). The word Epicurean, which means "one with sensitive discriminatory taste in food," is derived from his name. News of how wonderful it was to dine with Epicurus had travelled far and wide. One day a king who had heard of his reputation arrived to feast with Epicurus. He was shocked to see Epicurus sitting in a simple setting with just a piece of bread and some salt. The king, possessing some wisdom in his own right, kept his mind open enough to observe the fine level of consciousness and joy with which Epicurus, and eventually he himself also, ate the bread and salt. As the king grew more ecstatic with each bite, he decided to offer Epicurus anything he wanted, up to half his kingdom. He was shocked again to hear Epicurus turn down his request with the comment, "it is enough to be, nothing more is needed." The king pressed his request again and in order to please the king, Epicurus made a request for one pound of butter. His lesson to the king was that a good meal depends on the consciousness of the eater and how he/she celebrates it. It is not how elaborate the food, dining hall, or material lifestyle of the eater is. It is the state of consciousness that counts in extracting joy from our interaction with nature.

The practice of being conscious of the experience of energy being released from food seems also to be conducive to bringing about a shift in how the food is prepared. It is much easier to experience the unique energy of one specific food when that one type of food is all that is in one's mouth. Because of this, I find myself preparing food in larger, bite-sized, and identifiable pieces. For example, I might have just three or four items in my salads, which are cut in big enough pieces so that I can easily identify their tastes as I eat them. In this way I can experience the play of the different tastes and energies.

The interplay of a single spice, or combination of spices, with the food is another way of experiencing the delicious mix of energies. Spices tend to bring out and accentuate the different tastes of the individual foods. Each spice has its own unique herbal energy and taste that balances and harmonizes one's own constitutional psychophysiology. This balancing and healing effect adds an additional dimension to the assimilation process. How spices affect specific constitutional psychophysiological types will be discussed later in the book and the recipe section. In the food preparation section we have designed recipes that include this new approach to preparing food. It also turns out that when we prepare and eat just a few varieties of food in our meal, it is easier to assimilate and digest. As Jesus says, in the *Essene Gospel of Peace Book One (p. 37)*:

> "And when you eat at her table, eat all things even as they are found on the table of the Earthly Mother. Cook not, neither mix all things with another, lest your bowels become as steaming bogs."

Art of Relating to Food

Another aspect in the art of consciously eating food is how one regards the food itself. If one sees nature as a servant existing only for personal needs, then one fails to fully appreciate the food and other gifts of nature. If one sees humanity as one strand in the web of life rather than egocentrically as the whole web, a much broader awareness of the nature of our union and harmony with nature develops. To experience oneself as interwoven with nature leads to receiving our food with more love and gratefulness. If food is eaten with a prayer of gratitude and respect for the life force it bestows and the sacrifice it is making for the survival of the human body, the food will carry the love of this prayer inside. The power and sacredness of the eating process is enhanced by the awareness that each particular fruit or vegetable is giving up its own individual existence as part of the evolutionary process so that it may be assimilated into the greater existence of the human body. In this larger context, eating becomes a sacred act in which food is an offering to the digestive fire to honor and appease the spirit of one's human form. In addition to making an offering to oneself, in some traditions an offering to nature or God is also made. In some of the American Indian traditions, such as with the Cherokee Indians, a food offering is made to the four directions and to some aspect of nature, such as a plant or a tree. In the Hindu tradition an offering before eating is made to God. Food may also be given to a sacred fire, an animal, or another human being as a way of allowing one to experience the joy of providing food, as well as the joy of receiving it. I witnessed this offering in almost every home I visited in India. This offering before eating, of feeding some of nature's children, is a way of thanking Mother Nature for her food offering. It is another reminder that one's food is connected to all God's children.

Thoughts Affect Foods

In addition to the physical nutrients and the plant's energy, one also inadvertently assimilates the state of mind of the people who grew, harvested, and prepared the food. If the food is grown and harvested by an organic farmer who is very much committed to caretaking the land and its produce, it is likely that this will produce a different energy than that of food grown by an agribusiness corporation. Personally caring for the land in a natural way creates a different effect than using synthetic fertilizers which deplete and imbalance the soil, or using pesticides and herbicides that are toxic for those who eat the food and for those who are harvesting the food. Food harvested by a worker who feels exploited by the working conditions has a different energy than food harvested by one who is connected with his or her garden and who harvests with gratefulness, love, and joy. If food is prepared with love as an offering to God and with the consciousness of the essential oneness of the person preparing the food and the person eating the food, the food itself will be absorbed and elevated by that consciousness.

Marcel Vogel, who had been a research scientist at IBM for 29 years, has been able to experimentally show that when water is infused with the thoughtform of love, its structure changes and the taste is sweeter. He did this by having people project loving thoughts into water and then he tested it in two ways. One was a subjective taste test in which people were asked to taste the two different waters. They all found that the water infused with love tasted sweeter. He also tested the water with nuclear magnetic resonance equipment and found that the bond angle of the oxygen and hydrogen water infused with love was actually changed. In other cultures, the food preparers are encouraged to chant the name of God while preparing the food for this same reason.

An interesting story of a monk living in the forest in India helps to illustrate this point. He was living in a simple setting, meditating regularly, and eating pure food that he gathered from the land. In this region it was customary that the kings and wealthy people invite the monks to stay with them during the monsoon season. It was considered a blessing for the king to invite this monk to stay with him. The king, being of a greedy nature, also had a greedy cook. During the time of the monsoon, the monk had to eat the food prepared by the greedy cook of the greedy king. Over time the pure mind of the monk began to have greedy thoughts as a result of eating the food that had taken on the greedy thoughts of the cook. One day, near the end of the monsoon, the monk impulsively stole the necklace of the queen. The palace was in an uproar about this and, of course, no one suspected the monk. After a short time, the monk announced he was leaving. He returned to the forest with the necklace. After a few weeks of eating his own food, his mind began to clear. One day he looked at this necklace and could not figure out what he was doing with this useless piece of jewelry. When it became clear to him what had happened, he returned to the king with the necklace. The king, of course, wanted to know why he had done it. The monk explained that the food he had been eating while he was in the king's castle had been permeated by the greedy consciousness of the cook and had temporarily infected him with that greed. When he began to eat his own pure food prepared with love, his mind cleared and the greed left.

For similar reasons, I regularly prepare my own food. I go to my garden and pick the vegetables to which I am most drawn. I thank the individual plant for feeding me and try to pick it with love in an awareness that the food is an offering. While eating, I try to maintain the imagery of where I picked the food. This helps me maintain an intimate interface with nature. It also keeps the food from being anonymous.

Imagery of Foods

The way food is served in most restaurants, supermarkets, and in fast food restaurants has little imagery or energy of its connection to its origin. Some people who have never lived in the country may think that food grows on a grocery shelf, but most understand that food is grown in the context of Mother Nature's energies of the sun, wind, earth, and rain. The active awareness that what one eats comes from Nature's bountiful earth rather than from a grocery shelf or fast food bag, honors Mother Nature. The Ten Commandments say to honor our mother and father. To me, this includes Mother Nature, who I refer to as the Earthly Mother, and God as the Heavenly Father. I have observed an added joy in eating and an appreciation for food in myself and others who re-create the poetic images of the source of their food, such as visualizing an apple tree when eating apples, or imaging beets in the ground when eating beets. I also think about all the forces of nature that have helped create the plants. I see the sun shining on the beet, the rain nourishing it, the wind caressing it, and the earth giving it nutrients and acting as its home. With each bite, I am taking in, and being energized by, all these forces of nature. It's a delight! When these multiple insights are included in the eating process, it helps in our taking into ourselves the full nurturing qualities of nature, which are love.

Energy Needed to Assimilate

In the process of eating we are penetrated by the forces of the food. If these forces are too strong for us, and we are not able to muster enough assimilative energy to match the forces of the food, we can become sick. A classic example of this is overeating in a foreign country and getting "tourista." We get tourista because included in the new foods we eat in foreign countries are new types of bacteria that we are not accustomed to taking into our bodies. When we eat just a little of this food, the hydrochloric acid in our digestive system is able to neutralize and digest the bacteria. But if we overeat, we are sometimes not able to secrete enough digestive enzymes to destroy the bacteria. Consequently, the bacteria start to digest us in the sense that the bacteria create a pathological condition in our bodies. The practical side of this is not to overeat while travelling and to take some extra digestive enzymes, such as betaine hydrochloride, with each meal. By following this simple rule, my own family did not have digestive or parasite problems in about eighteen months in India as well as on several trips to Mexico. Other people who have followed this basic advice have also done quite well.

Food Stimulates Inner Forces

Digestion involves overcoming and assimilating the energetic forces in our foods by stimulating our inner forces to respond. This constant stimulation of our digestive forces by our food is actually very healthy. There is a general principle in the functioning of the human body which is called "use it or lose it." For example, in walking, the muscle and skeletal system is strengthened by constantly overcoming the forces of gravity. When gravity is absent, as in the case of the astronauts who live for periods of time in a gravity-free environment, it was found that they began to lose bone and muscle mass unless they did specific exercises.

The concept of our inner forces meeting the outer forces of food will be explored more in depth later in the book in the sections on transitioning to vegetarianism and raw foods. Those who eat primarily cooked foods, which have lost some of their energy through the cooking, stop exercising their full digestive energies and may lose some digestive power over time or even generations.

When live foods are introduced too quickly, I have observed that people sometimes have trouble digesting them. If one doesn't understand this principle and doesn't give oneself time to develop the digestive power by making such a transition slowly, it is very easy to become discouraged in the transition process. A classic case of this is my observation of the people visiting the United States from India. In India, most of the food needs to be cooked for hygienic purposes. When people from India start to eat raw salads, they may develop some discomfort. On a more subtle level, in the transition to vegetarianism from meat-eating, some people may have some difficulty responding to the forces of stored sunlight that is released by the plants. Plants store light through the process of photosynthesis. During the process of assimilation, this light is released from the plant into our own systems. According to Rudolf Steiner, if one is prepared, an equal and opposite inner light is activated to match this. By this process, one increases the strength of the inner spiritual light which is the original sustaining energy which keeps us alive. Heavy meat eaters become deprived of this light stimulation, because the plant light has been released into the animal and is not transferred to the human. Some people who have come from generations of meat eaters need time to build up this light. To use a physical analogy, if one were doing push-ups, one does not immediately start with 100 push-ups, and then when one fails, make the pronouncement that because one wasn't able to do it, that doing push-ups are too difficult for nonpush-up people. If one wants to succeed, one starts with 5, 10, or 20 push-ups and works up from there. One usually isn't discouraged if one can't start with 100 push-ups, and so in the same way one should try not to be discouraged if one is slow in making the transition to vegetarianism or raw foods.

Supplements Affect Powers of Assimilation

Understanding the dynamics between the body's energies and the external energy of foods gives us an understanding of how the body might be affected by vitamin and mineral supplements, specifically the chronic use of high-potency, synthetic vitamins, minerals, free amino acids, and other supplements. For example, for vitamin Bs, a high-potency, synthetic nutrient is anything over 5 to 10 milligrams. B vitamins less than these potency levels are usually from natural food sources and are not synthetically made. I believe that it is a credible hypothesis that the use of high-potency B vitamins makes it too easy for the body to take in these nutrients in that the body doesn't have to work to extract and absorb them from the food. It is comparable to a person getting a car and no longer walking regularly. Without the vital exercise of walking, they lose their stamina and strength. It is possible that this same principle of "use it or lose it" is operating when one excessively uses synthetic, high-potency supplements.

Stating this possibility does not mean that I am against the use of supplements. I find that often at the beginning of the process of healing and rejuvenation, clients may need a good deal of nutrients to get the body going in the direction of a healthier state. As their bodies progressively begin to heal and get to a higher level of health, their ability to assimilate improves and they make the transition to food concentrates along with, perhaps, a minimal amount of supplements.

29

Assimilation Aspects of Withdrawal

I am suggesting that synthetic supplements should be used with the aware-ness that assimilation involves a dynamic interaction between our bodies and the forces in the food. Because of this, we should be cautious concerning the idea that all we have to do to get our nutrients is to mechanically load the system with high-potency, synthetic nutrients. Although there is not hard data to prove it, the indiscriminate, excessive use of high-potency, synthetic nutrients may act more as a stimulant and may cause some energetic imbalances. In addition, the body may become less able to assimilate nutrients from food when, and if, the synthetic vitamins and minerals are withdrawn for some unexpected reason.

In some of my clients, I have discovered that during withdrawal from fast foods, sugars, and drugs that these people first sometimes feel weaker before they become stronger. In addition, paradoxically, if they backslide and eat the old energetically disruptive junk food of their old diet, they will curiously get sort of a false sense of feeling stronger. Let me explain. Most people test weak to white sugar. During withdrawal from white sugar, some people test stronger with it in the beginning, although later they will test weaker. This can occasionally be true for junk foods. This doesn't mean one goes out and resumes eating junk foods; it means that, knowing this, one should try harder to resist the craving. The actual process may be that the physiology and cell memory, a metaphor for the body's subtle ability to remember substances to which it's addicted or allergic, goes through a temporary adjustment period in which it switches from unhealthy metabolism to a healthier metabolism. An analogy to this is what we see in some people going through withdrawal symptoms from alcohol. A drink of alcohol will decrease the hangover effects or the symptoms and for a short time make the person feel stronger and better. This paradoxical effect is sometimes seen with allergies when we crave the very things to which we are allergic. After this period has passed, people usually test weaker with the particular junk food or drug from which they have withdrawn and become worse when they are exposed to it.

Another energetic quality of food involves the actual colors that Nature bestows on our food. These colors can be viewed as different frequencies of condensed sunlight which aid our balanced development on a variety of body, mind, and spiritual levels. Each specific color frequency stimulates and nurtures specific subtle energy centers, different nervous system plexuses, our autonomic nervous system, and the various glands and organs. This principle, which I call the "rainbow diet" is described in detail in my book *Spiritual Nutrition and The Rainbow Diet* and will be clarified later in this book.

It is fascinating to me how understanding the process of assimilation on a deeper level brings us into such an intimate interrelationship with Nature. The very process of assimilation is a way to experience the manifestation of the Divine through nature in our everyday life, no matter where or how we live.

TUNING IN TO THE LOVE NOTE OF GOD'S FOOD

1. *Close your eyes and take a deep breath.*

2. *Hold the food in your hand and feel texture, weight, smell, shape, color and any subtle message.*

3. *With eyes still closed, imagine the food in its natural setting.*

4. *Thank God for the food and take one bite.*

5. *Chew slowly and experience juices, texture, and tastes.*

6. *Feel any energy release into the soft palate.*

VISION

BLACKBOARD EXERCISE

Preview of Chapter 3
Personalizing Your Diet to
Your Body-Mind Constitution

This chapter gives specific information on how to organize your food intake to enhance your personal body-mind (psychophysiological) constitution and health. It explains the best foods and lifestyles to emphasize for the three major psychophysiological constitutions as well as how to shift your diet to adjust to the seasons and even the time of day. These constitutions are best thought of as tendencies rather than absolutes. In this chapter you are going to learn several new words from an ancient culture such as dosha, pitta, kapha, and vata. These words come from the Ayurvedic system of healing which is a comprehensive system of medicine developed more than 5000 years ago. The term Ayurveda means "science of daily living." As you read this chapter you will begin to recognize your predominant psychophysiological or body-mind type as well as those of your family and friends. It is fun to be validated for who you are. There is also a questionnaire that can help you identify your primary and secondary constitutional tendencies. As you understand these types, you will begin to appreciate the unique needs of each individual and why there is no one general diet that is correct for everyone. Once you understand this, you become free from the tyranny of trying to fit into the newest fad diet that comes along. You become your own researcher and begin to trust your own knowledge of what are the best food choices for you. Are you ready to be empowered in this way? Are you ready to become more independent in taking responsibility for your own health?

I. The Ayrvedic Tridosha System and discovering your personal body-mind constitution
   A. Vata: Air/Ether, kinetic energy movement of intestines, muscles, and nerve impulse
   B. Kapha: Water/Earth potential energy, body fluids and mucous
   C. Pitta: Fire and metabolism, balances potential and kinetic energies
II. Finding your dosha type
   A. Characteristics – physical and psychological
   B. Images
   C. Food tastes
   D. Spiritual task
   E. How to recognize imbalances
III. Cycles
   A. Life Cycle
   B. Day cycles and timing of meals
   C. Seasons' effect on diet
IV. Dual Constitutions
V. Chapter Summary

Chapter 3

Personalizing Your Diet to Your Body-Mind Constitution

In order to artfully and intelligently develop an individualized diet, it is useful to be aware that different foods have specific effects on our body-mind complex. These effects go beyond simply feeling recharged from eating a particular food. Ayurvedic and Chinese healing systems, which have been successfully used for thousands of years, both recognize the importance of the specific energies of foods and herbs in rebalancing and healing the body. Western herbalists also share a similar awareness about the use of herbs. The Ayurvedic and Chinese also are cognizant that our foods help to balance the relationship of our body energies with the changing seasons of the environment. In the Ayurvedic system, the individual body-mind or psychophysiological constitution is called one's dosha. The tridosha system, which is part of the Ayurvedic system, offers a simple, yet relatively complete way to understand how the foods we eat directly affect our health and well-being. Tridosha means three doshas or constitutions, which are called vata, pitta, and kapha. Please remember that all the suggestions that are made in this food and dosha section are only tendencies. Your personal exploration with these tendencies in mind will reveal what works best for you.

Ayurvedic Tridosha System

The tridosha system of the science of Ayurveda is particularly useful in helping maintain the awareness of nutrition as the interaction between the forces of food and one's own dynamic forces. In the tridosha system, the five basic elements of creation, which are earth, water, fire, air, and ether, manifest in the human psychosomatic complex as a balance of three dosha essences named vata, kapha, and pitta. Vata is associated with the energy of air and ether, kapha is associated with the energy of water and earth, and pitta is associated with the energy of fire and water. Often they are thought of as vata/air, kapha/water, and pitta/fire.

One is born with a permanent constitutional complex combination of all three doshas. In other words, the dosha combination for each person is genetically determined. These dosha types influence all our biological and psychological tendencies. A person's constitutional type predetermines which doshas tend to become imbalanced more easily than others. When the doshas are in balance, it means there is a healthy psychophysiological state. If the doshas are temporarily unbalanced, one may feel a subtle disharmony in the body-mind complex. If the doshas are chronically imbalanced, the result may be disease.

33

A rough translation of the word dosha given by Dr. Robert Svoboda in his excellent book, *Prakruti*, is "things which can go out of whack." The vata energy goes out of balance most easily for everyone. The next most frequent dosha to go out of balance is pitta. Kapha is the least likely to go out of balance. The three dosha energies work together in the body to maintain health. All three doshas are needed to maintain the life of every cell and organ. All three doshas must be balanced to maintain optimal health. For a body organ to remain alive, vata energy is needed for movement of nutrients and oxygen to the organ and for the removal of wastes. The pitta energy is needed for the organ to metabolize the nutrients to make energy for the cell to live. The energy of kapha is needed to maintain the structure of the organ so assimilation, metabolism, and elimination of wastes can take place. In disease, one or all three elements may be off. For example, to conceptualize a knee problem using the understanding of the dosha energies, one might say if kapha energy is decreased in the knee joint there is not enough lubrication; if there is excess dryness and pain on movement, there is a painful vata imbalance. In addition, if there is redness and heat in this joint, a pitta imbalance is also indicated. If all three types of symptoms are happening, then there is a pitta, kapha, and vata imbalance.

Energy Characteristics of the Three Doshas

The doshas may be understood as three forms of energies operating simultaneously in the organism. Vata is kinetic energy operating in the body. Vata may also be understood as catabolic, or the energy involved with the breakdown of the tissues and aging. Vata is the force which tends to predominate in the senior years. It regulates all physical and psychological movement including the flow of thoughts in the mind, the movement of breath, the movement of nerve impulses in the nervous system, and the function of the muscles. In terms of digestion, vata supplies the energy for chewing, swallowing, assimilating food, and expelling wastes. At the cellular level, vata is responsible for the movement of cellular nutrients into the cell and the removal of wastes out of cells. On the level of mind, vata influences the rapidity of the thought process. It influences the flow of impulses in the nervous system. All movement in the body from peristalsis (muscle movement) of the stomach, small intestine, and large intestine, and the entire muscle system, is influenced by vata.

Kapha can be thought of as stored or potential energy. It governs biological strength, vigor and natural tissue resistance. Kapha lubricates the joints, moisturizes the skin, gives support to the heart and lungs, and helps to heal wounds. The anabolic or growth forces in the body are activated by the kapha energy. Kapha is the energy that tends to predominate in children up to puberty. This is the time of active growth. It is also the time that children tend to have illnesses arising out of excess mucous conditions such as colds, flus, and earaches.

Kapha controls body lubrication, form and stability. It affects the tissues and wastes of the body that vata moves around. Kapha should not be thought of as simply mucous. It is the force in the body which causes the mucous to accumulate or dissipate. The secretions which lubricate and protect the digestive organs and all the joints are energized by kapha. It affects the structure of the body cells. Kapha gives stability to the mind and power to long-term memory. It helps the mind focus on particular thoughts and chosen topics of concentration. A kapha dominated personality is stable. Kapha represents the tendency to accumulate energy and form. It is stored potential energy. For example, a person whose predominate dosha is kapha more easily puts on weight than a person whose predominate energy is vata. The tendency of a predominantly vata person is to readily expel energy. Because of this, vata dominated people tend to be thin and active, and kapha people tend to be heavy and more inert.

Pitta is the energy that balances the vata kinetic energy and the kapha potential energy in the organism. Metabolism is the main influence of pitta. It primarily affects cellular metabolism and the endocrine or glandular system. Pitta directs digestive nutrients to provide energy for cellular function. The metabolic heat and fire in the body is ruled by pitta. On the mind level, pitta is the energy that processes new data.

These dosha forces have certain qualities and properties which characterize their energetic effects on the body, which helps us better understand their effects on us. Vata and kapha seem to be almost completely opposite in qualities. Vata as kinetic energy promotes change and movement; kapha as stored energy promotes lubrication and stasis. One of the functions of pitta is to balance the opposing forces of kapha and vata. Pitta people seem to be naturally gifted managers of the flow of all sorts of energies. It is fascinating how a person's dosha constitution determines the mental and physical pattern of energy utilization in everyday activities. The dosha type affects how one works with such basics as: exercise, sex, money, and way of organizing one's business and daily schedule. Even one's sleep and dream pattern is influenced by the balance of the doshas.

The body regularly discharges these dosha forces as part of its efforts to maintain health. Kapha is expelled primarily as mucous; pitta is excreted via acid and bile; and vata is eliminated as gas and muscle or nervous energy. For example, if the system has an excess of kapha energy, one will be discharging more mucous. If there is excess vata it may be noted as flatulence or muscle twitching.

In each person there is a constitutional balance of these forces which informs us of the tendencies by which doshas are most easily imbalanced. The dosha type, as distinct from dosha energy essences, is a descriptive pattern of our psychophysiological makeup with which we are born and which does not change during our life. Each dosha personality I'll be describing, however, is more of a pattern of tendencies for how the mind will respond to different life situations rather than one's specific individual personality. The dosha can be thought of as a genetic precondition for acting in a certain general psychological or physical way to the environment. For example, as a kapha it is easier for me to stay peacefully at home than be out socializing at parties, whereas a vata dosha person may be out socializing. Our constitutional dosha balance influences how the body and mind will tend to react when experiencing a particular stimulus, such as food, weather, or emotions. It also influences our lifestyle, form of expression, interaction in the world, and even marital compatibility. As we develop in body, mind, and spirit toward more health in our lives, the doshas do not imbalance as easily.

Finding Your Constitutional Dosha Type

There are ten possible constitutional types: vata, kapha, pitta, vata-pitta, pitta-vata, vata-kapha, kapha-vata, pitta-kapha, kapha-pitta, and vatta-pitta-kapha. A particular dosha constitution indicates a heightened tendency to manifest imbalance or disease in a particular way as characterized by the dosha. For example, those with a vata imbalance will imbalance in typical vata ways such as with large intestine difficulties and gas or nerve or muscle problems. Usually people have a combination of doshas such as pitta-kapha or vata-pitta. The dosha mentioned first is the primary dosha to most easily go out of balance. The dosha mentioned second, such as the vata in a kapha-vata, will go out of balance next most frequently. Those who have a vata-pitta-kapha dosha combination either have the most difficulty with their health or are the healthiest. Those who have the most trouble with their health are those for whom all their doshas equally become easily imbalanced. Those with the best health do not have any dosha that readily becomes imbalanced. These are the people who seem to have good health no matter what they do to their bodies. The majority of people make up the other nine possible constitutional types.

See pages 38-40 for a self-interview to help you gain some clarity on your dosha constitution. Mark each answer to each question from 0-3. Three means it describes you most of the time and zero means it doesn't describe you at all. Add up each column. The column with the highest score is your primary dosha. The combination of this questionnaire and this chapter should give you a good feeling for your dosha constitution.

Usually people are not purely kapha, pitta, or vata, but predominantly one and secondarily the other. If one dosha scores much higher than the other two, one is considered a single dosha type. The single dosha can have a score which is as much as twice as high as the next one, but it can be less. In a double dosha type, the dosha that represents the greatest percentage of one's qualities is your predominate constitution type of the pair. The second dosha may be almost equal or considerably less. Occasionally, two doshas are equal, and the third dosha is higher than both. The third is the dominant dosha; most likely one of the two that are tied on the self-interview will emerge as the secondary dosha as you further study and understand your characteristics.

By understanding one's constitutional dosha tendencies it is possible to more intelligently select the most appropriate lifestyle, environment, and dietary pattern for conscious eating. One's dosha type serves as a guideline for selecting the types of foods to eat according to the seasons, time of day, and many other factors, all of which, if wisely chosen and carried out, will contribute to the balancing of one's doshas. The more balanced the doshas are maintained, the healthier one is.

Images of Vata People

The animal archetypal images of people with predominant vata constitutions are: goat, rabbit, camel, or crow. Vata possesses the qualities we commonly associate with air and wind. Vata energy dries, cools, and roughens like a desert wind. It has the irregular, inconsistent quality of wind coming and going. Like the wind, vata energy is light with little form and much movement. Changeable like the wind is a central vata theme. Their mental and physical energy comes in bursts of wind. The images of vata are somewhat like a cross between a hyperactive child and the brilliant, but ungrounded futurist or theorist who has difficulty manifesting his or her vision. The vata person can be a great visionary who exhausts easily from the stresses of life. Vata people have a tendency to use up their energy quickly.

Physical Characteristics of Vata People

People with a vata constitution are generally thin, flat-chested, have noticeable veins and muscle tendons, and have difficulty gaining weight. The quality of dryness of the vata energy leads to a tendency to have dry, cracked skin and a thinness of the body. They tend to be more dark-skinned as compared to others of the same racial background and tan easily. The skin of a vata person chaps easily and is prone to eczema and psoriasis. Oiling the skin is both balancing and healing for a vata, especially if regularly done. Rubbing oil on the skin, especially sesame oil, seems to balance the vata tendency for roughness, dryness, irritability, and lightness. This also seems to be emotionally soothing for those with a vata constitution.

The hair of vata people tends to be dark, coarse, and curly. Because of the quality of variability, head hair may be oily or dry in different places. The nails of a vata person are usually rough, irregular, and show marked ridges or depressions. The color of the finger just below the nails may look slightly bluish

Dosha Constitutional Types

Instructions: Mark each column from 0-3. Three means *most often describes you* and zero means *doesn't describe you at all*. Put your score in the column on the right side of each Dosha category. Add up the total of each column and put total on the bottom for each column.

Characteristic	Kapha		Pitta		Vata	
Gait, Pace	Slow graceful		Brisk		Fast, irregular	
Body Type	Heavy bone structure, wide shoulders/hips		Proportional, balanced		Tall, thin, small, thick irregular prominent joints poorly proportioned, imbalanced	
Structural Abnormalities	Rare		Rare		Sclerosis, nasal sepal defects, bow legs	
Fingers & Toes	Short & square		Medium		Long, thin, tapered	
Joints	Well-lubricated		Average		Crack easily	
Body Weight /Dynamic	Tends to gain weight easily/lose weight with difficulty		Maintains a steady weight, gain slowly or lose easily		Variable, irregular, often hard to gain weight	
Location of Weight Accumulation	Below waist		Weight deposited evenly		Accumulates around waist	
Endurance	High stamina		Medium stamina		Irregular, low stamina	
Physical Activity	Avoids exercise, but better from it.		Likes regular exercise, vigorous okay		Active, irregular	
Sex Drive	Low & steady		Moderate		High, erratic	
Fertility	High		Medium		Low	
Menses	Painless		Moderate cramping		Irregular, misses period	
Menses Flow	Light		Bleed heavily, bright red		Scanty, clots, dark	
Appetite & Thirst	Moderate, eats slowly		Excessive, sharp hunger, does not miss meals		Irregular, extreme, eats quickly	
Taste Preferences	Warm, bitter, spicy, sweet		Cooling, sweet, bitter		Warm, sweet, sour, salty	
Taste in Mouth in Morning	Sweetish		Sour, metallic		Astringent, bitter	
Digestive Power	Mild, slow		Strong, fast		Irregular, problem with gas	
Food Tastes Which Create Imbalance	Sweet, sour, salty, dairy		Salt, pungent, sour, hot		Bitter, astringent, pungent	
Food Tastes Which Create Balance	Pungent, bitter, astringent		Sweet, bitter, astringent		Sweet, sour, salty	
Food Qualities Which Create Balance	Warm, dry, light		Cold, heavy, dry		Heavy, oily, warm	
Food Qualities Which Create Imbalance	Oils, cold, heavy		Oily, hot, light		Cold, dry, light	
Best Climate	Warm, mild		Cool		Warm, hot weather	
Worse Climate	Cold, damp		Hot		Cold, windy	
Stool	Well-formed		Yellowish, well-formed		Hard, dark colored	
Bowel Functions	Regular, once a day, slow		Regular, two times daily		Variable, diarrhea, constipation	
Face	Strong jaw, broad, muscular		Well-proportioned		Narrow, dry, irregular, unbalanced	
Teeth	Strong/white		Medium-sized		Protruded, big, crooked, uneven, buck	
Teeth Sensitivity	No problems		Prone to cavities Soft, easily bleeds, canker		Brittle, sensitive to cold & sweet	
Subtotal Chart 1						

Constitutional Types			
Characteristic	**Kapha**	**Pitta**	**Vata**
Gums	Decay resistant	Soft, easily bleeds, canker sores	Emaciated
Eye Type	Large with large pupils, white sclera, long dense eyelashes	Proportional, light sensitive, yellowish sclera, short eyelashes	Small, dull, dry & close or far apart
Eye Color	Blue, milk chocolate	Green, light blue, red	Black, grey, slate blue, dark chocolate
Hair Quality	Smooth, oily, thick, straight	Wavy, fine	Dry, curly
Hair Color	Light-dark brown, medium blonde	Light brown, red, light blonde	Dark brown, black
Skin Characteristics	Thick, no skin problems	Delicate, irritable, rashes, pimples	Patchy, variable, chaps easily, bottom of feet tend to crack, eczema, psoriasis
Skin Color	White	Red, yellowish, coppery	Dark complexion
Skin With Age	Smooth, few wrinkles	Freckles, moles, pigmentation	Dry, flaky, cracked
Skin Response to Sun	Tans evenly	Burns easily	Tans easily
Nails	Strong, large, symetrical	Soft, strong, well-formed, pink	Hard, brittle, irregular
Pulse Quality	Slow, broad, cool	Firm, jumpy	Shallow
Pulse Rate	60-70 / minute	70-80 / minute	80-100 / minute
Perspiration	Moderate	Profuse	Scanty even in warm weather
Strength	Strong, sturdy	Moderate	Variable to weak
Voice	Low-pitched, resonant, drone	Intense, enthusiastic	High-pitched, wavering, weak
Vocal Habit	Silent, speaks slowly	Vocal, good public speaker	Very talkative, but variable
Pain Tolerance	Would rather avoid pain	Moderate, faces pain	Low, sensitive to pain
Worse From	Lack of exercise	Acid food & acid system	Wind, overexertion of any sort of emotional or physical extremes
Travel	Likes to stay home	Adventurer with a purpose, explorer	War...
Natural Immunity	Moderate	High	Weak
Tendency for Disease	Mucous accumulates, colds, flus	Inflammations, heart, skin	Body pain–frequent, nervous system, muscle & joint problems
Communication Pattern	Slow, cautious communicator, quiet	Concise, clear	Loves to talk alot, gets off subject
Personality Trait	Serious, patient, regular	Strong, forceful	Chaotic, spacy, flexible
Personality Imbalance	Inertia, complacent, greedy, stubborn	Domineering, angry	Ungrounded, poor life or task focus
Emotions Which Create Imbalance	Complacence	Anger, jealousy, grief	Fear, anxiety
Mental State	Calm, steady	Intelligent, aggressive	Alert, restless, quick
Humor	Serious, quiet humor, slow to laugh	Intense laugh, sharp, sarcastic, biting	Quick wit, joyful, punster
Friendships	Few, steady, loyal	Utilitarian	Changes, brief, many
Subtotal Chart 2			

39

Constitutional Types			
Characteristic	**Kapha**	**Pitta**	**Vata**
Competitiveness	Not aggressive	Very aggressive	Variable
Forgiveness	Slow to forgive, forgets with difficulty	May hold grudge with eventual forgiveness	Forgives & forgets easily
Decision-making Style	Slow, deliberate	Comprehensive, clear	Impulsive, short-sighted
Ability to Grasp Information	Slow, comprehensive, but works logically with material once comprehends	Insightful, takes in information easily	Quick, makes theoretical connections
Mode of Receiving Information	Sensate, feeling, intuitive	Visual intake of information	Receive information auditorily, through intellect; auditory senses acute; noise level is painful
Follow-through	Completes everything, strong perseverance, detail oriented	Completes work quickly	Inconsistent, incomplete
Typical Role in Organizations	Bureaucrat	Executive leader, good organizer	Doesn't do well in organizations, inspirational, visionary
Concentration Ability	Steady, strong	Moderate	Erratic, variable
Speech	Harmonious, slow	Sharp, cutting	Fast
Voice Tone	Low-pitched	Medium-pitched	High-pitched, dissonant, cracks easily, hoarse
Emotional	Calm, greedy	Irritable, aggressive	Fearful, insecure, anxious
Temperament	Attached	Jealous, fiery	Impatient, fragile
Stress Response	Insensitive, withdrawal, complacent	Anger, jealousy, hatefulness	Fear, anxiety, panic
Mental Stability	Calm, tolerant, complacent	Irritable	Easily knocked off center
Mental Style	Stable, logical	Judging, artistic	Inspired, theoretical
Memory	Good long-term	Good short-, moderate-, long-term	Good short-term, weak long-term
Faith–commitment	Steady, loyal	Fanatical	Fickle, changeable
Financial Style	Wealthy, frugal	Saves, buys luxuries when appropriate	Poor, spends quickly
Dreams	Water, romantic	Fire, violence, war	Fearful, flying, running
Sleep	Easy, long, deep, excessive	Short, sound	Insomnia, scanty, irregular, grinds teeth
Stress Tolerance	High	Medium	Low
Typical Livelihood	Professional	Executive, engineer, builder, professional	Artist, theoretician, visionary
Type of Appreciation	Grateful	Demonstrably appreciative	Fickle
Life Style	Home-oriented, accumulates money	Well-organized, pragmatic life	Exciting, irregular life style on every level
Subtotal Chart 3			
Subtotal Chart 2			
Subtotal Chart 1			
Totals			

or gray in color. Nail-biters are often vatas. Irregularity also shows up in the teeth. A vata's teeth may be bucked, crooked, and uneven. Teeth tend to be brittle and overly sensitive to hot and cold. The jaw is often out of alignment with the rest of the mouth. Gums may recede early in life and there may be an astringent or bitter taste in vata mouths.

Because of the vata quality of coldness they crave the sun. Their circulation is usually poor and so their skin is cool to touch. Their innate coldness leads to scanty sweating. They love external heat sources such as the sun, saunas, and hot springs. Vata people love warm climates and more easily go out of balance in the windy cold time of the year, such as in the fall and the winter. A smart vata will dress warmly and may put cayenne powder in his or her socks and shirts during cold weather.

Vatas may be tall or short with narrow shoulders and/or hips. They tend to have long fingers and toes. The vata quality of irregularity leads to unbalanced body proportions and structural abnormalities, such as deviated septums, scoliosis, or bowed legs. The irregularity of a vata may also manifest as fluctuations in weight. These are also the people who seem to be able to eat almost anything without gaining weight.

Typical eye colors of vatas are grey or slate blue. They may also be dark brown or black. Vatas are erratic eaters. They often are in a hurry to eat but may take more food than they can eat. They also may eat too much and have trouble digesting it all. Their appetites are variable from day to day and they often need to have snacks between meals. If breakfast is missed they usually function poorly because of the vata tendency toward hypoglycemia. The vata tendency to irregularity does not easily hold blood sugar levels stable. Unless they eat a heavy breakfast they will usually want to eat an early lunch. Those with a vata constitution have a harder time fasting unless they get juices every few hours.

Vata people tend to have irregular bowel function. Sometimes they have constipation and sometimes diarrhea. Their tendency to be irregular and to become dry gives some vata women irregular menstrual periods. Sometimes vata women miss their periods or they have scanty flow. Cramping with their periods is sometimes accentuated, as muscle spasms and cramping is a vata tendency.

Food Needs of Vata People

Vata people can eat a raw food diet if they eat heavier, oily foods, such as avocado and soaked nuts and seeds, both of which have water to balance their dryness and oil to balance their lightness. Heating herbs help vatas by giving their raw food the warmth it needs. Since vatas have a tendency to be cold and to get cold, warming up food to 118°F in the sun or the stove is an especially good practice for a vata who likes raw foods. Vatas are imbalanced by the dryness of dried fruit, but can eat some if they add back the water element by first soaking the fruit in water. Vatas should eat at regular intervals and not go too long without eating. Blending raw vegetables into a liquid soup form is good for vatas in that it supplies the water element in an easily digestible way while still preserving the enzymes. This blending process and soaking of nuts and seeds helps to minimize the gas that vata people tend to have because of the inherent air quality of their basic constitution. In general, vata people are best maintained in balance with soupy, oily, salty, and warm foods. This is particularly true for those vatas who have been successful on a raw food diet.

Psychophysiology of Vata People

The vata psychophysiological type tends to be active and restless but often has low endurance. They have fluctuations in their energy and have a tendency to expend energy quickly–they love to burn it up as soon as they get it. The tendency is to overextend themselves and burn themselves out like a match which flames brightly and then exhausts itself. Exercise often tires them out. Like their energy, their pulses tend to be fast, thin, and irregular. Their sexual activity tends to mirror this as well. They may have intense interest in sex which peaks when it is expended in lovemaking. They have a tendency for sexual overindulgence which often leads to exhaustion.

Creativity comes easily for a vata person. They have alert, active, and restless minds which verbalize rapidly. Sometimes they can become mentally fatigued easily. They are quick to understand things intellectually. Vata people often are the visionaries, artists, and people who theorize. They love excitement and variation in lifestyle. When in balance, a vata person is vivacious, energetic, talkative, gregarious, and enthusiastic.

Their sensitivity to subtle energies, desire for harmony, and open-mindedness make it easy for them to pursue a spiritual life. Sometimes their will power is weak and needs to be exercised to increase it through balanced, harmonious discipline. They tend to have quick memories and forget easily. Often they are very sensitive to environmental activity and are affected by noise and pain. Loud music may actually be painful to them. They think predominantly in words. I often think of vatas as people whose nervous systems have less insulation. They are knocked off their "center" the most easily compared to the other dosha types. Balancing vata in general can miraculously clear up many nervous system imbalances.

This thinner insulation makes them sensitive to changes in the environment. Vatas also have a tendency to insomnia. They either have difficulty falling asleep or they awaken early. They dream frequently and often have flying dreams or dreams which are intense and active. Because of the sensitivity of their nervous system they tend to be nervous, anxious, and fearful. Vatas may be irritable and anger easily, but it is an anger that fades easily. Vatas' active minds require continual stimulation. They make friends easily, but often the relationships are not sustained. Often these people appear to be "space cases." Vatas are receptive and open to spiritual development. It even comes easily for them, but they have a tendency to have poor follow-through. They may move from one stylish social group, or experimental activity or group, to another.

Spiritual Challenge for Vata People

One of the most important spiritual challenges people with vata constitutions have to learn is how to regulate their energy and balance their lifestyle so they do not fall into the imbalancing syndrome of overextension of their energies and chronic exhaustion. As a medical doctor I have instructed my vata clients in mastering and developing a balanced, regular, harmonious lifestyle. They become quite pleased with the improved quality of their health and spiritual life. Balance is one of the hardest achievements for a vata. It is, however, this stability that allows them to manifest their vision.

How to Recognize an Imbalance in the Vata Dosha

I can often recognize an imbalance of vata on the psychological level as nervousness, fear, anxiety, insomnia, pain, tremors, and spasms. This vata imbalance may also reveal itself in its drying tendencies as rough skin, arthritis, emaciation, stiffness, constipation, general dryness, thirst, insomnia, excessive sensitivity, and excitability. Vatas have a tendency to large intestine disorders and to suffer from excessive gas. A vata disorder may also manifest in the muscle system with low back pain or in the nervous system with sciatica, paralysis, and various types of neuralgias. Almost any sort of psychosomatic symptom can be connected to a vata imbalance.

These vata imbalances more often manifest during weather conditions such as cold, windy, stormy weather. I once was able to solve the problem of insomnia of one of my vata patients by suggesting that this person turn off his fan at night. The wind from the fan was causing a vata imbalance and the consequent insomnia.

It seems that with vata people, anything which is excessive, such as strenuous exercise, mental work, extreme diet changes, grief, anger, suppression of natural urges, severe weather conditions, or any activities taken to the limit, will cause an imbalance. A calm, stable environment will usually bring a vata person back into balance.

Several of my predominantly vata clients have found that to successfully live in the world they need to pay constant attention to keeping their lifestyle and diet balanced. I have found that high-functioning vatas approach their vata constitution as a spiritual challenge. When they don't, pure vata types have difficulties adjusting to society. To illustrate with a case example, when one of my patients first came to me she was a typical, thin, high strung, anxious vata who was in constant turmoil with her husband. She was unable to commit herself to the role of mother and frequently spoke about "skipping out" as she had done in the past. She was using marijuana and other stimulating drugs. She was on a heavy flesh food diet and she ate at irregular intervals. She often tackled projects in the work world that would overwhelm her. She was depressed and angry with herself and her work. After eighteen months of nutritional and dietary work, homeopathy, family therapy, and meditation training, her life was transformed into a model of balance and harmony that she could hardly believe. Her marriage became a happy one, she began to enjoy her motherhood, she meditated on a regular basis, she changed to a balanced, vegetarian, 80% raw food diet, and got off drugs. She stopped taking on those stressful extra projects and focused on making her home her own Garden of Eden. A key component in her success was increased self-understanding, which included an understanding of her vata constitution, and committing herself to not creating stressful situations on any level in her life. By seeing her vata constitution as a spiritual challenge, rather than a limitation, she has turned her chaotic, unhappy life into one experienced by her as blessed.

Another vata constitution patient that came to see me was already on a spiritual path and quite aware of her vata constitution. One major balancing factor for her was her sticking to an 80-90% raw food, vegetarian diet. She was extremely sensitive and when she wandered from it, her mind and body would go out of balance. One typical characteristic of vatas is what I call time disease. They tend to overextend, stress out, and go into crises. A major improvement in this person's vata balancing effort was when she became strong enough to refuse to let herself be overworked by the demands of the spiritual group she belonged to. Healthy vatas usually have learned to "say no" and have become experts in their own time and stress management strategies.

My constitutional type is kapha-vata. One way my vata manifests is in the muscular skeletal system. By doing stretching and breathing exercises regularly, I have found a way to keep my vata balanced. Travelling is a vata stress for me so it is a time when I pay particular attention to hatha yoga and other vata balancing factors. Because travel is potential stress for my constitutional type, I have found that the day after I arrive at my destination I eat lightly and only do light yoga and exercise. When I travel, I keep myself warm and avoid cold breezes that are imbalancing to vata. These might seem like little things, but to me they have meant the difference between feeling great and full of energy or suffering with a stiff neck or some pulled muscle.

Your physical, emotional, mental, and spiritual needs are relatively unique.

A "Conscious Eating" approach is best developed from sensitivity to your own uniqueness.

VISION

BLACKBOARD FOOD FOR THOUGHT

Summary of Ways to Imbalance Vata

1. Avoid calm, soothing environments.
2. Be excessively physically and mentally active with travel, overscheduling, overworking, excessive fasting, or extended periods of any extreme.
3. Live chaotically without any regular schedule or rhythm connected with the natural earth cycles, such as working a graveyard shift, eating irregularly, and being on the run.
4. Don't get enough sleep, rest, or meditation.
5. Live in a windy, cold environment.
6. Use of cocaine, speed, and other drugs.
7. Overly act out or suppress feelings.
8. Eat dry, frozen leftovers; cooling, light, bitter, astringent, & pungent foods.
9. Engage in worry, fear, and excess mental activity.

Summary of Ways to Balance Vata People

1. Live in a warm, moist, tranquil environment with a minimum of wind. Keep warm.
2. Live moderately and in a balanced regular way in harmony with earth cycles. Always be gentle to oneself. Avoid all physical, emotional, and mental excesses.
3. Eat warm and moist foods which have some oil content and which do not stimulate gas (such as beans). Avoid drinks and foods which have been chilled, frozen, or have ice cubes.
4. Eat foods which have sweet, salty, and sour tastes and are not light and dry (such as dried or dehydrated food).
5. Get adequate sleep.
6. Meditate regularly to maintain a calm mind.
7. Try to make the environment as secure and safe as possible.

Images of Kapha Dosha People

Kapha characteristics are almost opposite the characteristics of vatas. The symbolic animal is the elephant, bull, horse, sea turtle, or lion. They have the physical characteristics similar to that of most football lineman. Kaphas are the quiet, heroic work horses of the world who do their work without complaining. Kapha men and women are the quiet, family oriented, homebody and homebuilder type people who are comfortable with the status quo. They tend to store and steward their energy in every aspect of their lives whether it be body or money energy. They have pack rat tendencies in that they collect and hold onto everything, including possessions, money, the past, people, energy, words, and their weight. Kapha possesses many of the qualities of earth and water combined, such as we experience with mucous or mud. Kapha is inert, thick, heavy, sluggish, stable, viscous, sticky, cold, and slow-moving. A couch potato is an image that fits a kapha who is in a kapha imbalance.

Physical Characteristics of Kapha People

Weight is one place kaphas regularly tend to store energy. Kapha females and males have a difficult time losing weight. Females have a tendency to gain weight, especially in the lower part of their bodies, such as the hips and buttocks. Kapha women tend toward water retention, especially premenstrually. The menstrual periods of kapha women are usually regular without excessive blood flow, and generally not too difficult.

Kaphas have heavy bone structures with wide shoulders and hips. Fingers and toes are usually short and squarish in relation to the rest of the body. The tendency to store energy is reflected in kapha's thickness and tendency to be heavy, to gain weight easily, and to store it most obviously in the hips and downward in the body. They are well-proportioned in terms of the relative sizes of body parts and their joints are well-lubricated.

The skin of a kapha person is well-oiled, tans easily in the sun, and is smooth and thick. They may have a few freckles and an occasional mole. Their skin may be cool, but not cold, because they usually have good circulation. Kaphas usually perspire moderately. Typical kapha hair is oily, slightly wavy, thick, and brown or dark brown. Their nails are strong, large, and symmetrical as are their teeth. The tongue of kaphas is rarely coated. A sweetish taste may be present in their mouths when they become imbalanced. Kapha eyes are often large and liquid, blue but also milk chocolate in color.

Exercise is very beneficial for kapha people. They tend to do poorly if they do not get sufficient or regular exercise. Paradoxically, they are not motivated to exercise until they actually begin to experience the sense of well-being regular exercise gives them. They often have good muscle tone and coordination and are best able to endure vigorous exercise of the different dosha types.

In the realm of sexual activity they tend to have a lower sex drive compared to the other doshas since they inherently like to conserve their energies; but, as with exercise, when they actually reap sexual satisfaction this encourages them to engage in sex more often because the experience was positive. Kaphas, as part of their homebuilding energy, are also very fertile. Like their physical attributes, a typical kapha pulse is slow, full, rhythmic, and strong.

The sleep of a kapha person is usually deep and long. They are the longest sleepers of the three doshas. They characteristically awake refreshed and alert. However, if they take naps during the day, they usually awake groggy and slow. Rarely do they have insomnia. Their dreams are usually calm and peaceful.

47

Food Needs of Kapha People

The digestion in a kapha is slow and regular. Digestion is especially slowed if oily or fatty foods are ingested. Kaphas have a tendency to move their bowels one time per day. Their appetites are moderate and they are the least thirsty of the three dosha types. Excess water may throw them into imbalance. My experience is that these people do better on less than the commonly recommended eight glasses of water per day. In my laboratory I'm able to test for optimal hydration. Often those with a kapha constitution who drink 6-8 glasses of water per day test as overhydrated. Because I eat primarily fruit and vegetables, if I, as a kapha-vata, drink more than four glasses of water per day I test as overhydrated. Excess fluid may precipitate a kapha imbalance, especially if it is a time of day when the kapha forces are strongest, such as 6 am to 10 am and 6 pm to 10 pm.

Kaphas are balanced by a diet that is light, warm, and dry. Oily, fatty, fried, salty, sweet, cold, and heavy foods create a kapha imbalance. The all-American diet of high fat and sugar content plus excess salt is the worst for kaphas. Fast foods are a disaster for them. Most dairy products are also imbalancing for a kapha constitution. Raw foods with an abundance of bitter and astringent greens with some heating and pungent herbs is the best type of diet because of kapha's tendency to gain weight and have slow digestion,. The lighter kaphas eat at each meal, the easier their digestion and the better their health will be.

Psychophysiology of Kapha People

The typical kapha personality is calm, quiet, steady, relaxed, and serious. They are the easy going types who are the most unlikely to become upset by stress. Intellectually, they may at first be slow to comprehend, but once they grasp a concept they are able to work with it and hold on to it. In concert with their mental activity, they tend to speak slowly and carefully. They may be temperamentally disinclined to talk in that they do not initiate conversations easily unless they feel they have something of use to say. The voices of kapha people are often low and sonorous. There is a certain sweetness about kaphas in tone, voice, and manner.

Tolerance, calmness, forgiveness, and love are predominate kapha characteristics as are righteousness, generosity, patience, humility, steadiness in relationships, and stability of mind. There is a tendency to avoid confrontations. Kapha people often withdraw when confronted. There is a turtle quality about the social interaction of a kapha. Sweetness in their human interactions will lure them out of their shell.

Sometimes kaphas tend toward complacency and avoidance of change. They have a tendency toward inertia, as is typical of a tendency to store energy rather than expend it. But once the ball is rolling they can have strong emotions. They tend to procrastinate if they feel under pressure. Kaphas take a long time to make up their minds, but once committed to an action or a friendship, they are very loyal to the commitment. An imbalance of the kapha personality may manifest as passivity, inertia, oversensitivity, possessiveness, or greed. Overattachment and greed are the two most common kapha imbalances.

Kapha types tend to experience their world, and express themselves, through their senses and emotions. They are linked to the material world. They tend to accumulate possessions. Their tendency to familiarity, long-term commitments, and the material world makes them be home- and family-centered in their desires and skills. A kapha mind retains information well, but they are not particularly the theorizers of the world. They are good at running things and settling down once they are built rather than explorers who discover the land. Kaphas think in terms of stabilizing systems rather than creating systems. They are conciliators. This makes them good managers and bureaucrats. The tendency to resist change makes them sometimes inflexible. Kaphas are the solid citizens of the world who enjoy their lives and do not make too many waves unless they are pushed too far.

Spiritual Challenge of Kapha People

A main spiritual task for a kapha is overcoming the tendency for inertia and complacency in a way that brings them into an active personal interaction established in the moment with people and the Divine. Kaphas may become stuck in the orthodoxy of a particular form of spiritual ritual or routine and lose the meaning and passion for the Divine in the process. The key task is how to use their groundedness and their tendency for form to support and sustain an active, dynamic, expanding spiritual life that will transcend the form in order to keep them in communion with the Divine.

How to Recognize an Imbalance in the Kapha Dosha Person

Symptoms of a kapha derangement are a sense of heaviness, drowsiness, constipation, itching, skin disease, dullness, inertia, depression, edema, swelling of joints with fluid, and excess mucous production in the eye, ear, nose, throat, and lungs. Kaphas have a tendency toward upper respiratory infections, colds, and flus. A kapha person can be thrown out of balance by eating too much sweet, cold, damp food, such as ice cream. Their imbalance is worsened by cold, damp weather. They are put in balance by warm, dry weather and warm, dry food. They are made better by plenty of exercise, heat, such as a sauna, a mucousless diet, plenty of raw food, periodic fasting, and a warm, dry, climate. Avoidance of sweets is important for kaphas because of their tendency toward a "sweet" complacency, inertia, and a "stuck in a rut" lifestyle which sweets amplify. Natural, raw, unprocessed, nonfiltered honey is a notable exception to the sweet danger, for a little bit of honey helps to heat, nourish, and rebalance kaphas.

Those who tend to imbalance toward kapha are sensitive to cool and damp weather. In India, where the change of seasons is distinct, many people with asthma get worse in the rainy season, which is a cool and damp time of year. Because of my own kapha tendencies, I do not eat watermelon in the morning or after the sun goes down. These are the times kaphas are most easily imbalanced. In fact, if I have too much of any fluid or watery fruit in the morning I may get a slight accumulation of fluid in the nose which will go away if I sit in the sun for a few minutes. When I have eaten watermelon at these kapha-vulnerable times, even in the summer, I feel an immediate mucous buildup within a half hour. It took me a long time before I figured out that a raw diet alone was not enough to balance the tendencies for kaphas to produce mucous. By getting into the sun or heat, such as a sauna, and using a little cayenne in the morning, this tendency to have too much fluid and mucous has faded away.

The above case is instructive in that the timing of foods is important. The same watermelon taken during the pitta time of day, which is 10 am–2 pm, feels quite balancing, especially if I have been out in the summer sun. Because of this, the only time I even consider having watermelon is during the hot summer. This is one example of how one balances food, environment, and dosha.

Summary of Ways to Imbalance Kapha People

1. Become a couch potato by overeating fatty, oily, fried foods, getting no exercise, and napping after meals.
2. Eat at least one sweet, oily dessert and lots of ice cream and other dairy products each day while watching T.V.
3. Overeat and concentrate on sweet, oily, salty, and cooling, frozen, chilled, and watery foods. Eat an excess of wheat bread and pastries.
4. Avoid all exercise.
5. Suppress all creativity and do one's best to become inert mentally and physically. Create no waves in your life or job and do a lot of repetitive work.
6. Use tranquilizers to excess and hypnotics.
7. Avoid all emotional expression and all conflict.
8. Live in a wet, humid, cold climate.

9. Be a collector.
10. Become deeply involved in ritual and orthodoxy.

Summary of Ways That Balance Kapha People

1. Lead an active, creative, and stimulating physical, emotional, and mental life. Have daily exercise and stimulating friends and work environment. Minimize T.V. viewing.
2. Eat foods which are warm, dry, pungent, bitter, and astringent. Minimize sweet, salty, oily, heavy, and sour foods.
3. Eat an 80% raw food diet.
4. Eat the minimum to feel satisfied.
5. Minimize fluid intake to 3 or 4 cups per day.
6. Express your feelings in the moment.
7. Throw away the turtle shell you wear and try to interact with the world.
8. Maintain only those spiritual practices which keep you in contact with God's divine nature and purpose for you.

Images of Pitta Dosha People

The archetypical animal of the pitta dosha is the tiger, cat, or monkey. A football quarterback who is balanced and well-coordinated, a warrior and the stereotyped image of a corporate leader are all archetypal examples that portray the pitta person. For females, the proverbial "Amazon woman" comes close to representing this archetype. The "hot-blooded" teenager is another image. The elemental image is fire. Fire is hot, intense, fluid, and light. It burns you if you get too close, but is inspiring at the right distance. Pittas are hot in every aspect of their lives. The key word-image for pitta is intense.

Physical Characteristics of Pitta People

A pitta person usually has a medium-framed, well-balanced physical body of average weight. Pitta people tend to deposit weight evenly over the body and can gain or lose weight easily. A pitta type person is physically graceful and strong, and their physical structure reflects this. The skin of a pitta person is usually light or coppery and sensitive to the sun. They have many freckles and usually become sunburned before they tan. Skin problems are interrelated to a pitta person. The pitta person's skin can become irritated easily and is prone to rashes, inflammations, and pimples. These tendencies can become much worse in the summer.

51

The heat of the pitta makes them warm-bodied and warm to the touch. Their tendency to perspire, even in cold weather, makes them sometimes have sweaty palms. Their heat is reflected in red hair or light-colored brown or blonde hair. Early baldness or the hair changing to white or gray at an early age is an indication of pitta. Nails are strong and rubbery with a pink hue because of their warm blood under the skin. Pitta eyes may be hazel, green, red, or light blue. They may have a charismatic fire in their eyes that radiates out in all directions. They have medium-size mouths with teeth that are prone to cavities and gums that tend to bleed. Pitta tongues and mouths are prone to canker sores. Body heat may manifest so strongly that their tongues may be deep pink to red or even bleed at various times. A sour or metallic taste may occur in their mouths early in the morning if there is an imbalance.

Pitta people have strong digestive fires and good appetites. They are the least affected by poor food combining because they digest so well. A good appetite is common. They may become irritable if they do not eat when they are hungry. Eating usually calms them down. Pittas usually like cold drinks. Their bowel function is regular and frequent, but may feel hot on excretion. Stools may be yellow or orange. If this stool color is too intensely yellow or orange, it suggests a pitta imbalance. Because of their innate heat, pitta women bleed more heavily and for a longer time during menses. The menses blood is usually bright red. During menses, pitta women may have moderate cramps and loose stools.

Until they overheat, pitta people enjoy vigorous exercise. Pittas do not need exercise as much as kaphas. Pittas can fatigue more easily. After a good workout they will usually be hungry and thirsty as compared to a kapha who may not be hungry. The pulse of a pitta is regular, full, and strong with a medium speed of about 70.

The sleep habits of pittas are generally regular and problem-free. They do not have insomnia unless there is particularly excessive stress or too much work worry. They sleep lightly and wake up alert. They do not need as much sleep as a kapha person. Pitta dreams are active, intense, often in color, and are often vividly remembered upon awakening. Their dreams may involve being chased or chasing someone as well as involve themes where there is much heat or light.

Food Needs of Pitta People

The best diet for a pitta is bland raw food. They are the most sensitive of the three doshas to toxins in the food, air, and water. It is most important for them to eat organic food and have only filtered water. Other polluters, such as alcohol, coffee, marijuana, and cigarettes, et cetera, also throw them out of balance. Sweet-, bitter-, and astringent-tasting foods, which are cool and heavy, are the most balancing. Spicy, oily, salty, and sour foods tend to imbalance them. Overeating is another major hazard for pittas since one of their major tendencies is acid indigestion. Pittas do best on a low-protein diet since protein, especially from flesh foods, creates a metabolic stimulation and heat of about 30%.

Psychophysiological Characteristics of Pitta People

The pitta personality is ambitious, intense, and competitive. There is much fire in their makeup which is reflected as a tendency to anger easily. The mind of a pitta usually has good comprehension and intelligence. At work, they know how to pace themselves. They tend to live by their watch and do not like having people waste their time. They are good managers and executives and exhibit great leadership qualities. They naturally tend to take command of situations. Whereas vatas may be the ungrounded theoreticians, the pittas are the engineers that manifest the plan or ideas on the physical plane. Unlike the kaphas, they have minimal interest in the day-to-day running of a business. They are not the sustainers the kaphas are. The essence of the pitta mind works visually and there is usually no difficulty visualizing or remembering a visual scene. The pitta memory is good. Like the kaphas, they do not easily forget a slight.

These people are strong leaders that may tend to dominate those around them. They are outgoing and make friends easily. Pittas believe in fair play and have a warrior's courage. When in balance, they are happy, confident, and friendly. If angered, they tend to be hurtful or vengeful. They are also easily imbalanced by the toxic emotions of others such as hostility, hatred, and jealousy. It is characteristic of them to become angry and hostile under stress. They tend to be impatient with those who do not catch on as fast as they. This tendency can lead to arrogance. The pitta fire is sometimes revealed in sharp sarcasm and in an undertone of impatience. They are often dedicated to self-growth and may rise to leadership roles in tightly knit, intolerant organizations, whether they be spiritual, cultural, athletic, or business settings. They work well with energy and often spontaneously create a well-organized and balanced lifestyle. Their money is spent appropriately and not impulsively and excessively as do vatas.

How to Recognize an Imbalance in the Pitta Dosha

When pittas are out of balance, their psychological symptoms tend toward vanity, intolerance, pride, aggressiveness, stubbornness, hatefulness, jealousy, and excessive anger. Chronically angry individuals are highly suggestive of a pitta imbalance. They may experience acid indigestion and sourness or burning in their mouths, eyes, skin, small intestines, and stomachs. Other signs of pitta imbalance may be fainting, excessive perspiration, restlessness, increased thirst, desire for cold drinks, and even delirium. Excessive environmental heat may cause all of these symptoms. Heat stroke occurs more frequently in pittas than the other doshas. Other causes for a pitta derangement may be strong anger, grief, excess physical exertion, fear, and too much salty, pungent, acid, dry, or heating foods. Pittas are rebalanced by cool weather, nighttime, sweet foods, cold baths, and clarified butter (ghee). Although in the Ayurvedic system ghee is recommended for balancing aggravated pitta, I do not necessarily recommend it for general use because it is a dairy product and a cooked oil.

An example of a predominantly pitta constitution is my son, Rafael. When we were in India on vacation he was in fine health until the hot season arrived. As the temperatures went above 95° F he began to develop heat rashes on his body, canker sores on his tongue, and generalized exhaustion. He also began to get colds. When the cooler monsoon season came, his health immediately returned to its prior excellent condition. In the same heat another women was so pitta that she literally became disoriented. In her delirium she felt that she was going to die. She required a variety of cooling foods and homeopathic remedies to return her to normal functioning.

Spiritual Challenge for Pitta People

The central spiritual challenge for a pitta is how to transform the tendency for anger and irritability into a feeling of calm and love. This does not mean the suppression of feelings as much as learning how to express emotions in an unharmful way without judgment. To develop the awareness and expression of unconditional love is the culmination of this spiritual challenge.

Summary of Ways that Imbalance Pitta People

1. Live in a hot, dry climate, exercise in hottest time of the day, and wear tight clothing.
2. Avoid cool and peaceful places, relationships, and lifestyles.
3. Act out all aggressive, angry feelings and thoughts. Be a bully.
4. Work in a high-stress, competitive job.
5. Keep life as frustrating, warlike, argumentative, and agitating as possible. Associate with people who share and encourage these toxic behaviors.
6. Do not meditate.
7. Drink alcohol in excess and use marijuana, speed, and cocaine.
8. Eat large amounts of spicy, hot, oily, sour, acid-producing, and salty foods. Indulge in large amounts of red meat, tomatoes, hot peppers, garlic, onions, sour foods, yogurt, and caffeine.

Summary of Ways to Balance Pitta People

1. Live in a cool and calming personal, social, and work environment.
2. Avoid excess heat, humidity, and steam in the environment, such as hot tubs and excess sun, as well as in all relationships and activities.
3. Meditate regularly and strive for peace with self, friends, and humanity.
4. Learn to express feelings and thoughts in constructive and supportive ways to those around you.
5. Focus on being in a state of universal, unconditional love.
6. Eat cooling, sweet, bitter, and astringent foods with an emphasis on fruits and vegetables.
7. Eat a bland, 80% raw-food diet.

The Effect of the Time Cycles on the Dosha Energies

Not only can individuals be described as being a particular dosha, but times of the day, the seasons and periods in the life cycle (teenage, middle age, old age, etc.) also possess the dosha qualities.

The seasons, the time of day, and one's age have an intimate effect on the energy and manifested qualities of the doshas.

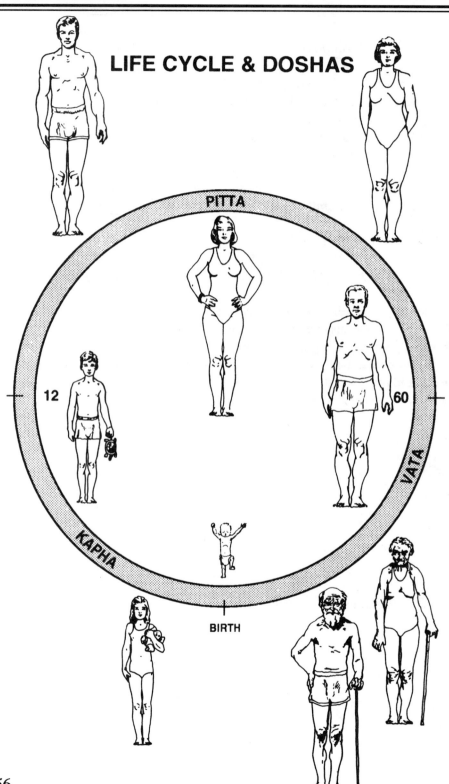

LIFE CYCLE & DOSHAS

PITTA

12

60

VATA

KAPHA

BIRTH

Dosha Energies of the Life Cycles

In addition to one's given dosha constitutional type, from birth to the teen years the kapha dosha is the predominate force since kapha governs growth. Because kapha is predominant, no matter what one's constitution, kapha will tend to go out of balance the most easily during these years. This is why one sees a tendency for so many colds, flus, runny noises, and earaches in young children. These mucous conditions are typical of imbalanced kapha energy. This is often made worse by the excess consumption of dairy products in our culture. It is also true that many in our western culture are outright genetically predisposed to be intolerant of dairy. During these years it is best to slant the diet toward those foods which balance kapha. That means minimal ice cream, cake, cookies, candy, and dairy.

From puberty to the sixties, pitta predominates. It is most obvious in the teenage years when the fire of life begins to express itself in such well-known forms as high sexual energy, pimples, heightened emotions, and rock and roll music. During the teenage years, more emphasis should be put on avoiding pitta-imbalancing foods, such as hot, spicy pizzas and Mexican foods. Alcohol, marijuana, and other drugs should be avoided, especially after the teen years and early twenties. Young adults need less focus on the pitta-imbalancing foods and more attention on avoiding foods and habits which imbalance their particular dosha.

After ages sixty or seventy, the vata force tends to predominate. Of course, if one doesn't take care of oneself, pitta will "burn out" more quickly and the vata phase will arrive sooner. The vata phase shows itself with the tendencies toward arthritis, emaciation, nervous system disorders, sensitivity to cold weather, and a decrease in the power of both digestion and memory. These vata imbalancing tendencies are balanced in the same way that one balances vata as outlined in the vata section.

Dosha Energy Cycles of the Day

The day cycle begins with the movement of vata from 2 am to 6 am. The vata force creates movement and lightness and is the upward awakening force. Kapha predominates from 6 am to 10 am. It is the time that those with a predominant kapha constitution are most easily thrown out of balance. Kapha people do well not to eat or drink too much for breakfast, especially if the food is still cold from being in the refrigerator. People with the constitution of a kapha may even want to take a little ginger or cayenne to bring heat to the system and clear the mucous at this time.

24 HOUR DOSHA CYCLE

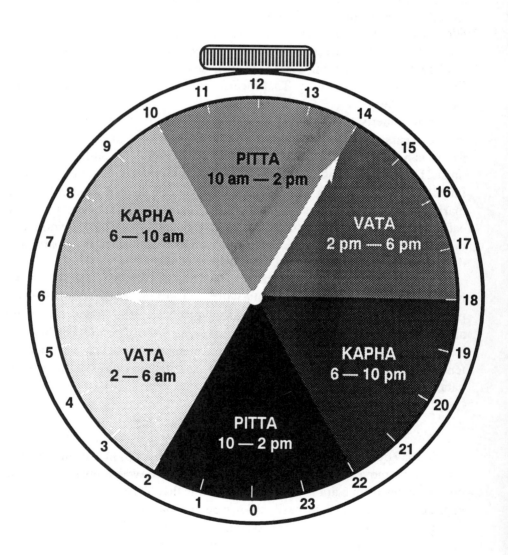

From 10 am to 2 pm pitta predominates. This is the time of best digestion for most everyone. Because of this it is the optimal time to eat the largest meal of the day in the Ayurvedic system if all other factors are in balance. Whereas a kapha or vata person may enjoy some sun and do exercise to warm up, the pitta person will do well to avoid the sun and other heating activities during this time of day.

From 2 pm to 6 pm the vata dosha predominates. This is the time of day that many people may experience bloating and fatigue. Kapha then begins to predominate from 6 pm to 10 pm; therefore, it is better to eat early in the evening because kapha has a slowing force on digestion. It is particularly advisable for kaphas to eat lightly and earlier in the evening. Pitta begins to predominate from 10 pm to 2 am. Pittas may find that their appetites are stimulated during this time. Although generally it is not recommended to eat late at night, pittas can get away with it if they eat lightly.

The Changing Dosha Forces of the Seasons

The seasons and the change of seasons have a powerful effect on the balance of the dosha. By maintaining an awareness of the predominate dosha imbalancing force with each season, one is able to shift diets, clothing, and lifestyle to maintain the doshas in a balanced state.

The healthy practice of eating with the seasons is well-known in Chinese medicine also. In the Ayurvedic system, the change of seasons are times of significant dosha imbalance. The peak energy change times are the equinoxes on March 21 or 22 and September 21 or 22, and the solstices on June 21 or 22 and December 21 or 22. During these transition times when the natural energies are in the extremes, it is beneficial to eat lightly and be particularly careful to follow a balanced, harmonious lifestyle.

Fall is usually a time of cooling temperatures and of increased wind. These two forces aggravate the vata dosha. For vata people in particular, it is important to dress warmly in order to minimize exposure to the cold and wind. It is a time to eat more warming foods and to increase the intake of foods which have a more sweet, salty, and sour taste. These are foods which balance vata. Moderate amounts of pungent and warm foods may have a healing effect at this time. In the Chinese system, fall is a time when the air element (vata) and lungs and large intestine meridians tend to become most easily imbalanced. Fall is an important time to make sure one's bowels are moving regularly and to eat high-fiber foods, such as fruits and vegetables, to aid the elimination process. It is also a time to work on the assimilation of vitamin O, oxygen, with a focus on breathing exercises to build lung function. Ginger root is a good tonic for the whole system and especially the lungs and sinuses during this time. Other good lung teas to have during this time are burdock and comfrey. Coltsfoot is another good general

EATING WITH DOSHAS
OF THE SEASONS

SUMMER

SPRING

Eat more sweet, cool,
bitter, astringent, raw, and high
water content foods: fruits, melons,
vegetables, greens, sprouts

Eat similar to
winter but increase raw
food, greens, sprouts,
vegetables, fruits and low
fat foods and
decrease grains

Eat more sweet,
naturally salty, sour,
warming, heavy and high
fiber foods: ginger, grains,
vegetables, soaked nuts
and seeds

Eat more pungent, bitter,
astringent, warm, dry and light
foods: ginger, cayenne, vegetables,
grains, greens and sprouts

WINTER

lung herb to have occasionally. Licorice root is good for the adrenals and a mild laxative to support the bowels. Grief is the emotion in the Chinese system which is associated with the lungs and large intestine. Repressed grief can inhibit the function of these organs so the fall is a significant time to get in touch with one's grief and express it and release it.

Winter is a time of dampness and coldness. Damp and cold imbalances kapha and kapha-vata most strongly. Disorders of excess mucous such as bronchitis, colds, flus, and pneumonia happen more frequently during the winter. Heating activities, such as physical exercise, saunas, certain breathing exercises, consuming warming herbs, and eating foods that are dry, pungent, hot, bitter, and astringent, will help to balance kapha. The winter is a time for kaphas to minimize fatty, oily, sweet, sour, salty, and dairy foods. It is distinctly not a time to eat ice cream. Raw, unpasteurized honey in small amounts, although a sweet, is a warming kapha balancer. In the Chinese system, it is a time for the water element to become most vulnerable to imbalance. This often correlates with the tendency for the mucous imbalance of the kapha during this time. The kidneys and bladder meridians are most easily imbalanced at this time. This is a time to take in herbs which support the kidneys, such as juniper berry, flaxseed, marshmallow root, nettles, fenugreek seeds, cornsilk, and parsley teas. Ginger and cayenne are particularly good for this season as well. Aerobic exercises that heat the body and stimulate circulation, and hatha yoga to keep the muscles loose, are also good for maintaining balance during this season. According to the ancient Chinese system, the kidneys are said to hold fear. Winter is a good time to make yourself feel safe and secure and even to work on your fears. Meditation and prayer is both soothing to the mind and helps to eliminate fear.

Spring, with the melting of the snow and the arrival of wind and rain, is another time of kapha and kapha-vata imbalance. In addition to the balancing activities recommended for winter mentioned above, it is also a good time to fast to clear out the excess kapha buildup from winter. It is a time to eat more lightly and eat more raw fruits, vegetables, and raw, soaked nuts and seeds, and cut down on grains. Spring is the time for green foods, sprouts and salads; they should be eaten abundantly. In the ancient Chinese system, it is the time the element, wood, which involves the liver and gallbladder, is most easily imbalanced. So these need the most support during the spring. Sour foods are particularly balancing for the wood energy as well as for vata. Lemon is a great cleanser for the liver. Foods which imbalance kapha, such as alcohol, fatty, fried, oily foods, dairy, and excess of grains, also stress the liver. These should be avoided, as well as junk foods and processed foods. By avoiding these foods it gives the liver a chance to do its spring cleaning. A short fast during this time is also beneficial for this cleansing process. Herbs that are supportive of this process are dandelion, chaparral, milk thistle, barberry, and chelidonium. In the Chinese system, the liver is where anger is stored. During this spring season it is beneficial to the liver and the whole organism to begin to express these feelings in ways that are not harmful to others.

In late spring and summer the pitta energy of the sun predominates. Those who are predominantly pitta will do best to avoid the noontime sun, excessive physical exertion, and oily, hot, salty, and sour foods. Balancing agents are cool baths, and sweet, cool, and high-water-content foods, such as watermelon and cucumbers. Food with sweet, astringent, and bitter tastes are also good for balancing pitta. Late spring and summer is a time to maximize raw foods, sprouts, salads, greens, fruits and vegetables in the diet. It is a time to minimize grain and dairy. Stimulants such as coffee and tobacco are best avoided. It's a time for less heating grains and beans. In the Chinese system it corresponds to the fire element. The heart and small intestine meridian are the most easily imbalanced. Hawthorn berry is a good herb to take occasionally to support the heart, as well as peppermint, tansy, and sorrel. Although ginger is good for the heart, it is also heating and is best taken in the fall. The emotions associated with the heart and small intestine are joy and sorrow. If there is some sorrow, try and let it be released so the joy of the summer can be expressed without any holding back.

Dual Dosha Constitutions

Rarely do people just have one dosha. Most people have a constitution which is a mixture of two doshas. One is usually the primary constitutional energy and the other is the secondary constitutional energy. The combination dosha constitutions are vata-kapha, kapha-vata, pitta-kapha, kapha-pitta, vata-pitta, pitta-vata, and vata-pitta-kapha. In denoting a combination dosha, the predominant dosha is indicated by it appearing first in the abbreviation. A vata-kapha, for instance, would be more vata energy than kapha. A kapha-vata would have more kapha than vata.

Under certain conditions either one or the other dosha may be in imbalance at a particular time. Although a two-dosha constitution can be thought of as a dual constitution, it still is one constitution with more tendencies of which to be aware. Sometimes these tendencies cancel each other out and other times they may reinforce each other. Often the symptoms of only one dosha aspect will appear at a time if one is living in a way that is imbalancing that particular dosha.

An example of how one learns to work with this is my experience with my constitution which is kapha-vata. The vata and kapha tendencies amplify each other in their coldness. Yet the kapha gives some protection against the cold that a regular vata does not have. Kapha-vata types tend to have a low digestive fire, are sometimes constipated, and produce much mucous. My raw food diet minimizes the mucous production and stimulates bowel function by its high fiber. After several years on raw foods, my body heat has increased as my circulation and overall health has improved. Because most of the energetic and nutritional value remains in fresh live foods, I am able to eat less and get the same, or more, nutritional value than if I ate more cooked food. Less food means less strain on my kapha-vata low digestive fire. The digestive fire and general health of a kapha-vata is made better by pungent, salty, and sour foods.

As the seasons change, one dosha may tend to predominate. Warm weather is best for me since vata and kapha both do better in warmth, but being aware of vata imbalances in the fall, and kapha tendencies to imbalance in the winter and spring, allows me to be more in tune with the appropriate foods and balancing activities.

The vata creative, theoretical, explorer, and spiritual tendencies balance my kapha tendencies to be too grounded and routine. The kapha grounding tempers my vata spiritual, inspirational life. My homebody kapha aspects are what allows me to be grounded enough to write books, be happily married since 1967, and to raise and support my two college student offspring. My dosha tendencies express themselves in different ways. If I fast too much, I tend to lose my kapha buffer and fall into vata imbalances. However, my kapha dosha makes it easier for me to regain lost weight after fasting.

Food selection of a dual dosha requires some awareness and trial and error. For example, oily foods such as an avocado, which are not the best for a pure kapha, turn out to be balancing for me, particularly during the summer when it is easy to get too dry. By understanding one's dosha characteristics, one learns to use the tendencies of the different doshas to best advantage.

Each combination has its own unique limitations and strengths to work out. Vata-pitta people need warmth, but their pitta dosha limits their tolerance of heat. They like to eat, but their vata tendencies limits how much they can eat without getting indigestion. An imbalanced vata-pitta may not be able to control their fiery emotional constitution and will alternate between pitta anger and vata fear. A vata-pitta has the pitta leadership drive and some of the lack of confidence of a vata. This can blend to make a humble and good leader, or result in the possibility of becoming a domineering, insecure leader. A balanced vata-pitta combines the vata capacity for original thought with the pitta ability to manifest the theory. Vata-pitta types have a tendency to amplify instability if they get imbalanced. Since vata and pitta are balanced by the moderate intake of sweets, vata-pitta people are balanced by a moderate use of sweets, such as sweet fruits and grains. Sweets that are helpful do not include white sugar, which imbalances everyone.

Pitta-kapha types combine the pitta leadership, ability to balance energy, and adaptability with kapha's stability. Pitta's strong metabolism balances a kapha's tendency to a slow digestion, and adds to the kapha's strong physical body to bring robust health. The mental stability, calmness, and patience of a kapha helps to modify the anger, impatience, and irritability of the pitta. The pitta-kapha can do well in any climate. Pitta-kaphas tend to imbalance with an excess of oil. Pitta's overconfidence combined with the kapha's lack of openness to change, may result in poor response to feedback. The pitta-kapha combination amplifies the lack of spiritual discipline, drive, and insight of the kapha. Pitta-kaphas tend to be the great business leaders, school principles, warriors, and athletes, but not the great saints.

Marriages may often serve to balance a mate's dosha. My wife is vata-pitta and this adds fire to my kapha-vata. My kapha adds stability to her vata-pitta. We chose to live in Northern California because it is neither too warm for her pitta nor too cold for my kapha-vata doshas. A marriage of the doshas doesn't always work out so comfortably. The marriage of a predominate vata and pitta type might amplify instability, anger, and fear. The polarity between the pitta need for coolness and the vata need for warmth is ground for a continual struggle between opening the windows to bring in the cool breeze and closing the window and turning on the heat. The vata will choose sweet, sour, and salty food whereas the pitta does better with sweet, bitter and astringent foods. It takes some insight and tolerance to work this out in marriage and have the balancing foods for each dosha at a shared meal. Knowing one's constitution can be of help in finding an appropriate mate as well as an appropriate diet.

Dietary Patterns for Dual Constitutions

When a person has a dual constitution there are two guidelines to follow. Eat to balance the dosha by the seasons or any other imbalancing force at that time, and that of trial and error. The trial and error element is created by the merging of the two doshas. For example, I find that avocado, which is aggravating for a kapha but balancing for a vata, works well for my kapha-vata constitution in all seasons. Generally, those with kapha-vata constitution may get the best results by eating foods which decrease vata in the summer and fall and decrease kapha in the winter and spring. This means more pungent, bitter, and astringent foods in the winter and spring, and more sweet, sour, and salty foods in the summer and fall.

Pitta-kapha constitutional types do best following a pitta-decreasing diet in the late spring through the fall. Bitter and astringent tastes help to decrease both pitta and kapha. In the summer there can be more sweets and cooling foods and in the winter and spring, more mild, pungent, and heating foods. Salt and sour tend to aggravate both pitta and kapha so they should be minimized.

Vata-pitta constitutional types do well if they follow a vata-decreasing diet in the fall and winter and a pitta-decreasing diet in the spring and summer. Sweets help to decrease both vata and pitta, and pungent, spicy foods may aggravate both vata and pitta. In the summer there can be more bitter, astringent, and cooling foods, such as raw salads. In the winter there can be more sour and salty foods to balance the vata.

Summary

Small imbalances in the dosha system create the seeds for the growth of future disease. Maintaining the doshas in balance helps to bring us toward an optimal level of health. Although our focus is on food, everything we eat, think, say, feel, or act on affects the overall state of harmony and balance in our lives and therefore requires some attention.

The awareness of our dosha constitution increases the knowledge of how to change food and other lifestyle habits to prevent disease and create optimal health. Knowing one's mind-body type makes disease prevention and treatment considerably more specific and individual. The dosha constitution helps us understand how nature specifically intended us to live. Simply eating the foods which balance our doshas can exert an astonishing balancing influence on every aspect of our lives. Eating what is specifically best for ourselves, and not trying to fit into any external, generalized dietary concepts, is a major step in developing an individualized diet.

Did you find your constitutional type?

- *Vata*
- *Pitta*
- *Kapha*
- *Vatta-pitta*
- *Pitta-vata*
- *Vata-kapha*
- *Kapha-vata*
- *Pitta-kapha*
- *Kapha-pitta*
- *Vata-pitta-kapha*

In order to find the best dietary intake for your body, mind and spirit it is important to discover your constitutional type.

VISION

BLACKBOARD SELF-REFLECTIONS

Preview of Chapter 4
Foods Which Can Balance or
Unbalance Your Constitution

Some foods work better with some types of people and do not do well with other types. In this chapter you will get a detailed discussion of what food and food categories work best with the different constitutional types. Understanding this information is part of the process of conscious eating. This does not mean you necessarily cut out all the other types of foods that are not optimal for you, but that you begin to explore what works best for you and minimize those foods that tend to unbalance your constitution. Are you ready to take the time to understand what foods are best for your psychophysiological constitution? Are you ready to make the changes necessary to take advantage of this understanding?

I. Vata food guidelines
  A. Food varieties
  B. Blended and pre-blended foods
  C. Oils, vegetables and salads
  D. Soups
  E. Fruits
  F. Nuts & seeds
  G. Grains
  H. Legumes
  I. Dairy
  J. Spices and herbs
  K. Drinks
  L. Sweets
II. Kapha food guidelines
III. Pitta food guidelines
IV. Guideline chart

Chapter 4

Foods Which Can Balance or Unbalance Your Constitution

Guidelines and Perspective for Vata Food Intake for Vata People

Vata people are most balanced when they eat regular and small meals three times a day plus snacks. Excesses in eating, both in timing and amount of food at one time, may lead to vata imbalance. Anorexia nervousa and bulimia are examples of this type of imbalance.

For vata, meals are best if they are limited to a small number of food varieties at one meal. This is because of the tendency for vatas to get imbalanced when there is too much variable input. According to some Ayurvedic thinking, several foods made into a soup is easier for vatas to assimilate than if these foods were eaten at the same meal separately. The fire and water used in cooking serve as alchemical agents to transform the separate ingredients into a unified whole that is easier for vatas to handle.

This same thinking seems to be found in some western, natural, herbal healing traditions, as well as in Chinese food preparation. In the Chinese system, there is a definite awareness of the synergistic effects of combining their herbal medicines. In other words, the energies of each individual element combine together in a way which enhances their separate qualities, as well as create a new whole that is more effective than the herbs or foods taken separately. In this way they form a third, more complete energy with the qualities of both merged in a way that makes its effect stronger than the qualities of the two taken separately. In my own food experiments with live, unheated soups and blended foods, the same principle of synergistic improvement of foods for vatas is created. This has been the experience of others as well. The change agent in this case is the blender's ability to breakdown the individual identities of the foods into one identity and to break open the cells so that the enzymes further the digestive process. These foods are easier to digest and often are given to people who are recovering from illnesses or who have digestive disorders. Those with vata constitutions and others whose digestions are compromised due to ill health have been able to successfully digest blended foods that, in their separate, preblended state, would not be the best food combinations. For example, people are able to assimilate, without digestive difficulties, blended combinations, such as bananas or figs with grains, tahini and fruit, and fruit and vegetable juices. Each of these becomes its own synergistic food. In addition, the liquidity of these blends counters the vata dryness.

The traditional Ayurvedic teachings discourage vatas from eating a lot of raw foods, but in my clinical research I have found that many vata constitutional types such as vata, vata-kapha and vata-pitta, do quite well with live foods if they follow certain principles. Vata-pittas do particularly well with raw food because they have the additional fire of the pitta energy to give heat to the system. One approach is the use of soaked nuts and seeds, particularly in the seed sauce form. There are many raw foods which are high in oil content, such as avocado, nuts, and seeds, which I have found to be balancing for vatas. Sprouted or soaked grains can be blended with water or juices, which balances the dryness of the sprouted or soaked grains. Warming the blended grains, raw soups, and blended vegetables adds the heat to compensate for the vata coolness. A warmed, blended, soaked, raw grain cereal in the morning is very soothing for vatas (please see recipe section). Warm-to-the-finger-touch temperature, approximately 118° F, does not destroy enzymes, and supplies the needed warmth for a vata. Some people have even benefited by placing their food in an oven for a minute or two to bring the food up to body temperature.

Using herbs to balance vata by improving digestion, adding heat and water to the system, and decreasing the vata tendency for gas are general strategies for a healthy vata eating style. Vatas have less vata imbalance from gastric stress if they eat simple meals because the dryness and the instability of the vata digestive system doesn't handle a lot of different food types at one time. Blended foods and soups help with this. Food-combining practices and mono meals have the most relevance for vatas. Using these practices, I've witnessed a growing number of vatas doing extremely well on live foods. Some even find themselves getting imbalanced if they go off the raw-food diet. Some of my vata clients who are primarily eating live foods have even begun to change the traditional attitudes of their Ayurvedic teachers. There are also some modern Ayurvedic practitioners who are beginning to acknowledge that this raw food approach for vatas does work to produce the best health for their vata clients.

The key taste for a vata is sweet because it satisfies and calms the system and makes it feel secure. Salty tastes add some heat and sour tasting foods increase acidity. Bitter-, pungent-, and astringent-tasting foods tend to create emotional instability by "drying out" the nervous system. Heavy, oily, and hot foods balance vatas. Cold, dry, light foods tend to imbalance the vatas. **Vata people are benefited by a warm, oily, sweet, salty, watery, soupy cuisine.** Pungent spices are okay unless used in excess. Actually, any taste in excess may eventually imbalance vata, and any food in excess aggravates vata. Cold foods, gassy or carbonated drinks, and ice water aggravate vata. A little warm water with ginger at the beginning or end of a meal is soothing. Ginger is the best spice for vatas. It is most important for those with vata constitutions to eat in a warm, comfortable, calm setting and perhaps meditate before eating.

Vatas may have the full range of **vegetables and salads**, particularly if they are combined with high-oil-content foods, such as avocado or soaked nuts and seeds. These high-oil-content foods can be made into salad dressings or blended with vegetables in the form of raw soups. Although I do not generally recommend extensive use of extracted oils even if they are cold pressed, a person with a predominate vata constitution may find that a little of these extracted oils provides a balance in the transition to eating only foods that have naturally occurring oil in them. Combining the watery vegetables, such as cucumber and squash, with the dryer, bitter, and astringent ones, such as the leafy greens, can balance the drying effects of these bitters. The dryer greens are still best taken as a minor, rather than a major, part of the diet. The vegetables which help to balance vata are asparagus, beets, carrots, celery, cucumber, garlic, green beans, okra, parsnips, radishes, turnips, sweet potatoes, zucchini, and onions (if cooked). The cabbage (bras-si-cae) family, which tends to produce air (gas), and the nightshades, from which allergies may produce joint pains, should be taken in moderation and with an experimental attitude to see if one is affected by these foods. Vegetables which cause gas, such as the cabbage family, and vegetables with a lot of ruffage, should be minimized or blended into raw soups for the vata raw-food person. The blending creates more water in the food and releases the cellulase enzymes stored in the vegetables for digesting the cellulose film on the vegetables which is so hard for vatas to digest. Warmed vegetables are easiest for the vata constitution to consume, but raw vegetables, leafy greens, and sprouts that are balanced by oily dressings and warming spices are neutral to balancing for vatas. Often just warming the vegetables to 118° F, which doesn't destroy the enzymes, supplies enough heat to balance the vata person.

In summary, although traditionally prepared raw vegetables can be unbalancing to vatas, blending the vegetables into soups, juicing them, warming them to 118° F, adding spices that are warming or adding digestive stimulants, and using oily or creamy dressings, make it possible to eat most raw vegetables without aggravating the vata dosha.

Many **fruits**, especially sweet fruits, are balancing for vatas, except for astringent, unripe, drying, and dried fruits, which are aggravating for vata. Unripe fruits like unripe bananas, are astringent and therefore mildly aggravating for vata. Ripe bananas, however, are balancing. Dried fruits, unless reconstituted in water, may accentuate the dryness and thus also cause imbalance. Astringent fruits, such as unripe persimmons, cranberries and pomegranates, are best taken in moderation, if at all. Apples and pears may have a slight drying effect but can be neutral in their effect on vata if they are taken with some warming spices like ginger or cinnamon. Melons in excess can unbalance vata. Mangos and green grapes are particularly good for vata. The fruits which seem to be the most balancing for vatas include: apricots, avocados, bananas, berries, cherries, coconuts, dates, figs, citrus, melons, nectarines, papayas, pineapples, and plums. Some fruits are good for all three doshas. They are called tridoshic, which means balances all three doshas. They are: mangos, raisins, sweet grapes, sweet cherries, sweet apricots, fresh sweet berries, and pineapple.

Nuts and seeds which have a high oil content may be balancing for vata if eaten in small amounts. Almonds are the best nut, and sesame seed is the best seed, as it is heating and oily. One reason for avoiding nuts and seeds in excess is because they are concentrated foods. They are not easy to digest and may cause gas, especially since vata digestive energy is usually not very strong. Soaking overnight alleviates some of this difficulty. Overnight soaking washes away inhibitory digestive enzymes and starts a predigestive process for proteins and fats that makes assimilation easier. Seeds and nuts are well-absorbed by a vata person when made into seed sauces and seed milks. In this form they are predigested. Liquid has also been added which makes them less concentrated and less dry. Seed and nut butters are also a more assimilable form.

Grains are generally good for vata. Wheat and rice are the most balancing and soothing. A warm oat cereal in the morning is also quite nourishing. Amaranth and barley are balancing in moderate use. Millet, buckwheat, corn, and rye, although listed as aggravating, can be eaten in moderation if cooked in plenty of water and a little oil is added to them to make them less drying. Yeasted breads are not as balancing as nonyeasted grain preparations because yeasted bread has the gas of fermentation.

Legumes are not easy for vatas. Legumes tend to be gas-producing. Mung beans, garbanzo beans, tofu, and black and red lentils are also acceptable (if cooked well, and if certain spices are used, such as asafoetida, cumin, ginger, and garlic). These are the safest beans that a vata should even attempt to eat. In general, I have observed that the legumes, whether sprouted or cooked, tend to produce gas in many people who are not even predominantly vata. Even frequent use of tofu for a vata person may cause a vata imbalance. If eaten in small amounts, however, an aggravation in vata can be avoided. Garbanzo beans, if made into a spiced humus (see recipe section), are acceptable. Sprouted legumes tend to be aggravating for everyone, especially vata, and should be minimized.

Oils are generally good for vata. Sesame seed oil is particularly good. Safflower oil is the least balancing. Although I generally do not recommend free-flowing oils, limited amounts may be balancing for vata constitutions at different stages of their health evolution. The oils should be cold pressed and fresh so that some enzymes are preserved. I do not suggest cooked oils because the fatty acids become transformed from a cis to the trans configuration. A cis structure for fats is the same number of atoms as a trans structure, but its shape is curved rather than a straight line like trans structure. The cis structure is biologically active because of the electromagnetic field of the curve, whereas the trans straight line structure is not biologically active. The cooked fatty acids become incorporated into the cell membrane and because they are not biologically active, they consequently have the effect of weakening cell membrane structures in the body.

All **dairy** products are good in moderation. The oily and watery qualities of dairy products may be balancing for a vata person if they are consumed in a raw

VATA FOOD GUIDELINES

BALANCING FOODS

FRUITS
Sweet Fruits
Apricots
Avocados
Bananas
Berries
Cherries
Coconuts
Dates
Figs (fresh)
Grapefruit
Grapes
Lemons
Mango
Melons (sweet)
Oranges
Papaya

FRUITS (CONT.)
Peaches
Pineapples
Plums
Raisins

VEGETABLES
Asparagus
Beets
Carrots
Cucumbers
Dulse
Garlic
Ginger (fresh)
Hijiki
Horseradish
Jicama
Kelp
Kombu

VEGETABLES (CONT.)
Green Beans
Leafy Greens*
Lettuce*
Okra (cooked)
Okra
Onion (cooked)
Olives
Parsley*
Potato (sweet)
Radishes
Spinach*
Sprouts*
Squash
Zucchini

GRAINS
Amaranth*
Barley*

GRAINS (CONT.)
Oats (cooked)
Rice (all types)
Rice Cakes*
Wheat

LEGUMES
Aduki[A]
Alfalfa Sprouts*
Clover Sprouts*
Garbanzos, sprouted,*
(in spicey hummus)
Black & Red lentils*
Mung*
Tofu

NUTS
All nuts are acceptable in
small amounts

SEEDS
All seeds, soaked
All seeds, dry*
Psyllium*

SWEETENERS
All sweeteners are acceptable except white sugar

CONDIMENTS
All spices are good

DAIRY
All dairy products are
acceptable (in moderation)

OILS
All oils are good

* Okay if eaten in small amounts

UNBALANCING OR AGGRAVATING FOODS

FRUITS
Dried Fruit
Apples
Cranberries
Pears
Persimmons
Pomegranates
Watermelon
Prunes

VEGETABLES
Broccoli
Brussels Sprouts
Cabbage
Cauliflower
Celery
Eggplant
Ginger (dry)
Mushrooms

VEGETABLES (CONT.)
Onions (raw)
Peas
Peppers
Potatoes (white)
Tomatoes

SWEETENERS
White Sugar

GRAINS
Buckwheat
Corn
Millet
Oats (dry)
Quinoa
Rye

LEGUMES
Black beans
Black-eyed peas
Kidney beans
Navy beans
Pinto beans
Split peas
Soy beans
White beans

form and if the person is not allergic to dairy products. The only exception to the balancing effects of dairy is use of hard cheeses, which are drying for vatas.

Sweets, such as grains, sweet fruits, vegetables, and honey, are all acceptable, except for white sugar and any foods containing white sugar, such as baked goods and candy.

Spices and herbs are generally balancing for vata. Ginger is the most balancing herb. The ones which are the best are those which aid the digestive process, minimize gas, and bring warmth to the system. The sweet spices, such as cinnamon, fennel, and cardamom, are also good. Asafoetida is particularly good for those with gas problems. Garlic is another excellent vata-balancing herb. Cumin is also beneficial. The one danger for vata is to use too many hot spices which may eventually aggravate vata. Coriander, saffron, parsley, and fenugreek are neutral to unbalancing for vata. Cayenne in small amounts is good for its heating quality, but in excess may sometimes be too activating and drying.

Drinks that aggravate vata: contain caffeine; are carbonated, ice cold, or cooling; or are astringent and bitter. Cathartic drinks, such as prune juice, also aggravate. Most teas are acceptable unless they are bitter, astringent, diuretic, or drying teas. Blackberry, cornsilk, dandelion, and yarrow teas are best avoided because they have these vata-aggravating qualities.

Guidelines and Perspective for Kapha Food Intake for Kapha People

Those with a predominant kapha constitution: kapha, kapha-vata, or kapha-pitta, generally do well on live foods. Kapha-pitta people have the easiest time being on raw foods because the pitta energy gives additional gastric fire for the winter. Raw food can tone up the digestive power of kapha and kapha-vata people so that they may do quite well all year. Because kaphas tend to have excess mucous, the living foods help them feel better because raw foods are less mucous-producing than the same foods in cooked form. Kaphas do best if they avoid fried, fatty, oily, heavy, and cold foods. These foods further slow and strain the already slow digestion and increase the tendency to gain weight. Because of their slow digestion and tendency to gain weight, kaphas generally do well on just two main meals a day which are separated by at least six hours. It is best for their system if they avoid snacking between meals and train themselves to not overeat.

Sweet, sour, and salty foods imbalance kaphas. Pungent, bitter, and astringent foods tend to balance them. Watery foods eaten during seasons or day cycles in which kapha tends to be imbalanced should be eaten with great care, if at all (the times of day for kaphas to be particularly vigilant are between the hours of 6 am and 10 am, and 6 pm and 10 pm during the winter and spring seasons and when it is raining).

Vegetables are a particularly balancing food for kaphas. Leafy green vegetables, because of their dry, astringent qualities, are probably the most healing for a kapha person. Vegetables and warmed, raw foods, in combination with pungent spices, make an excellent diet for kapha. By eating some astringent and bitter foods at the beginning of the meal, kaphas create a stimulant to digestion that helps their whole process of digestion. Having a salad first or some fresh, raw ginger in a little warm water or in the salad dressing are examples of this. Raw vegetables also supply fiber to stimulate the bowel function.

The sweet, sour, and watery vegetables may be neutral to aggravating unless taken during a season and time of day when kapha is less likely to be aggravated. Cucumbers are neutral because they are watery, yet bitter and astringent. Tomatoes are the least aggravating for kapha. Black and green olives, which are oily and salty, aggravate kapha. Sweet potatoes, because of their sweetness, also aggravate. Warmed, raw, leafy greens and vegetables are excellent for kapha. Root vegetables are acceptable, but because they have more earth quality, they may reinforce the inertia of a kapha person who is already too earthy and fixed. Good vegetables for kaphas are pungent and bitter ones, such as asparagus, beets, broccoli, brussel sprouts, cabbage, carrots, cauliflower, celery, eggplant, leafy greens, lettuce, mushrooms, onions, parsley, peas, peppers, white potatoes, spinach, and all types of sprouts.

Fruits which are drying and astringent, such as pears, apples, and pomegranates, are the best fruits. Fruit juices can be taken if they are diluted by 33 to 50%. Sour juices, such as orange juice, are best taken in minimal amounts. Bananas, if spiced with herbs like dried ginger, are neutral for kapha. Sweet and sour fruits are neutral to aggravating for kapha unless eaten in the right season and time of day. For example, on our fasting retreats, when we served watermelon juice in the morning, several kapha people got congested because the morning is a time of kapha aggravation. When the watermelon juice was given at the pitta time of day (10 am- 2 pm), all the kapha people who had previously gotten congested, did well. Particularly good fruits for kaphas are apples, apricots, cranberries, mangos, peaches, pomegranates, dry figs, persimmons, prunes, raisins, berries, and cherries. Oily fruits, such as coconuts and avocados, should be eaten in moderation for the pure kapha, but can be eaten more liberally for the kapha-vata or pitta-vata types.

Nuts and seeds are heavy and oily and therefore are best eaten in minimal amounts. Nuts and seeds that are soaked or sprouted do well for a kapha type on a raw diet, however. The partially digested oils in sprouted and soaked seeds allow kaphas to comfortably have adequate amounts of the essential oils without suffering any ill effects. Although kaphas don't do well on large amounts of oil, there is a minimum amount of oil the body needs for its basic functioning. The best seeds are sunflower, pumpkin, and flax seed.

Grains are not the best food for kapha because they are heavy and mucous-producing and kaphas already have a tendency to produce excess mucous. Millet,

KAPHA FOOD GUIDELINES

BALANCING FOODS

FRUITS
Apples
Apricots
Berries
Cherries
Cranberries
Figs (dry)
Mango
Peaches
Pears
Persimmon
Pomegranate
Prunes
Raisins

VEGETABLES
Pungent & bitter vegetables
Asparagus
Beets
Broccoli
Brussels Sprouts
Cabbage
Carrots
Cauliflower
Celery
Dulse* (rinsed)
Eggplant
Ginger (fresh or dry)
Hijiki* (rinsed)
Horseradish
Jicama
Kelp* (rinsed)
Kombu* (rinsed)
Leafy Greens
Lettuce
Mushrooms
Okra
Onions
Parsley
Peas
Peppers
Potato (white)
Radishes
Spinach
Sprouts

GRAINS
Amaranth
Barley
Buckwheat
Corn
Millet
Oats (dry)
Quinoa
Rice,* basmati
Rice Cakes
Rye

NUTS
Almonds,* soaked

LEGUMES
All legumes & tofu
(warm) are good except
kidney beans,
soy beans, black beans,
mung beans

SEEDS
Chia
Flax*
Pumpkin
Sesame*
Sunflower
Sprouted and soaked
seeds are okay

SWEETENERS
No sweeteners
except raw honey
and fruit juice
concentrates

CONDIMENTS
All spices are good
except salt

DAIRY
No dairy except ghee
& goatmilk

OILS
No oils except
almond, corn,
flaxseed or sunflower
in small amounts

*Okay if eaten in small amounts

UNBALANCING OR AGGRAVATING FOODS

FRUITS
Sweet & Sour
Fruits
Avocado
Bananas
Coconuts
Dates
Figs (fresh)
Grapefruit
Grapes
Lemons
Melons
Oranges
Papaya
Pineapple
Plums

VEGETABLES
Sweet & Juicy
Vegetables
Cucumber
Olives
Potatoes (sweet)
Squash
Tomatoes
Zucchini

GRAINS
Oats (cooked)
Rice (brown)
Rice (white)
Wheat

SEEDS
Psyllium

SWEETENERS
Barley malt syrup
Brown rice syrup
Fructose
Molasses
Sucanat
White sugar

LEGUMES
Tofu (cold)

NUTS
Black walnuts
Brazil nuts
Cashews
Coconut

buckwheat, corn, and rye, which are heating and drying, are the best grains for a kapha. Wheat, which is cold, oily, and heavy is the worst grain for a kapha. Rice and oats are moderate aggravators. All raw, sprouted, and soaked grains are acceptable.

Legumes are a heavy food that is not needed for the kapha constitution because legumes are concentrated foods and body builders. Since kapha bodies almost effortlessly build and add weight to the point of excess, they don't need this extra push. Black beans, mung beans, garbanzo beans, pinto beans, and red lentils are safe legumes for kaphas. The heaviest legumes, such as black lentils, kidney beans, and soy beans, are best taken in minimal amounts. A little tofu, although a soybean product and high in fat, can be eaten by kaphas.

Oils in the extracted form are specifically aggravating. In minimal amounts, almond, sunflower, and corn oil can be tolerated.

Dairy is heavy, oily, cooling, and sweet. With the exception of ghee and raw goat's milk they are very aggravating for a kapha constitution.

Sweets aggravate kaphas into the heaviness of mental inertia and physical weight gain. Raw honey, which is heating, specifically balances kapha; taken at one tablespoon or less per day, honey is acceptable.

Spices in general are beneficial to kapha. Garlic and ginger are two of the most healing herbs for kapha. With the exception of salt, which is specifically aggravating for kapha, the same spices and herbs which benefit vatas are also an aid to kaphas. Kaphas are significantly aggravated by salt; this includes canned soups and juices with salt already added, most processed and junk food because of their added salt, and salted potato and corn chips. A minimal amount of miso soup is neutral, but in excess will aggravate kapha. Tamarind is another spice that aggravates kapha. Sea vegetables are fine if they are soaked and rinsed with fresh water.

Drinks that are warm and pungent are balancing to kapha. Sour, salty, and carbonated drinks are aggravating. This includes miso in excess. Cold soy milk is also aggravating.

Guidelines and Perspective for Pitta Food Intake

A bland vegetarian diet which is predominantly raw is best for the pitta, pitta-vata, and pitta-kapha individuals. Flesh food, eggs, alcohol, salt, caffeine, coffee, tobacco, mustard, garlic, onions, ginger and other stimulants aggravate the emotional and physical heat and natural aggressiveness of pitta. Fruits, vegetables, and sprouts with some grains are the bulk of the diet. Foods which are sour, such as citrus, yogurt, sour cream, vinegar, and dill pickles, also aggravate pitta. Lemon, although sour, can be tolerated in small amounts because of its overall alkalinizing and liver-purifying effect. It is best for a pitta to avoid pungent foods and herbs, such as cayenne, mustard, catsup, barbecue sauce, and salsa. The cold tastes, which are bitter and astringent, such as the leafy green vegetables, are balancing. Foods which are sweet tasting are also balancing, except honey and molasses, which are heating. High-protein foods increase the metabolic heat by 30% and should be kept to a moderate intake. Foods which stress the liver are usually aggravating, such as coffee and alcohol. Such foods as carrots and beets, which purify and cleanse the liver, are balancing or neutral to pitta, even though they are considered slightly heating. Balancing herbs for the pitta are coriander, cardamom, fennel, and tumeric. Fruits and vegetables are the most balancing for pitta. Pittas do best when they avoid salty, pungent, and sour tastes, as well as hot, light, and dry foods. Pitta people have a speedy metabolism so they generally need to eat three main meals a day, separated by at least four hours. If necessary, light snacking two to three hours after a meal is acceptable.

Vegetables are very good for pitta. The exceptions are tomatoes, which are heating and pungent, and vegetables like radishes, raw onions, hot peppers, and raw garlic. White or yellow onions will become sweet on cooking and may be eaten in moderation. Although beets, carrots, and daikons are slightly heating, they can be eaten unless pitta is already aggravated. The vegetables which are most balancing for pitta are: the whole brassicae family, such as cabbage and brussel sprouts; asparagus, cilantro, cucumbers, celery, cress, leafy greens, green beans, lettuce, mushrooms, okra, peas, parsley, potatoes, and sprouts; and the squash family.

Sweet fruits, such as apples, figs, raisins, sweet grapes, sweet plums, prunes, sweet berries, and melons, are most balancing for the pittas. Sour fruits, such as citrus, sour cherries, and pomegranates, should be minimized. Well-ripened, sweet, citrus fruits are acceptable because for pittas the sweet taste is balancing. Other fruits that are balancing are mangos, avocados, persimmons, and apricots.

Nuts and seeds are best used sparingly because they are hot and oily. If they are soaked or sprouted, they can be used in moderation. Coconut, which is cooling, is very balancing for pitta. Sunflower and pumpkin seeds can be eaten, especially if soaked.

Grains that are heating, such as corn, millet, buckwheat, and rye, are best avoided or minimized. Barley, which is cooling and drying, is the best grain. It also helps to reduce stomach acid, which is a pitta tendency. Rice and wheat, which are sweet and heavy, are also good. Sourdough breads and other yeasted breads create a sourness which aggravates pitta.

Legumes should be taken in moderation because of their high protein content and tendency to produce gas if taken in excess. The least aggravating legumes are mung beans, garbanzo beans, tofu, and black lentils.

Oils are generally aggravating for pitta. Small amounts of coconut, almond, olive, soy, and sunflower oils are okay. Coconut, with its oil, is beneficial to pitta because it is cooling, but should be used in moderation because of the high

PITTA FOOD GUIDELINES

BALANCING FOODS

FRUITS
Sweet Fruits
Apples
Avocado
Dates
Figs
Grapes (dark)
Mango
Melons
Oranges (sweet)
Pears
Pineapple (sweet)
Plums (sweet)
Pomegranate
Prunes
Raisins

VEGETABLES
Sweet and Bitter Vegetables
Asparagus
Broccoli
Brussels Sprouts
Cabbage
Cauliflower
Celery
Dulse (rinsed)
Green Beans
Hijiki (rinsed)
Jicama
Kelp* (rinsed)
Kombu (rinsed)
Leafy Greens
Mushrooms
Okra
Peas
Parsley
Peppers (green)
Potatoes
Sprouts
Squash
Zucchini

GRAINS
Amaranth*
Barley
Oats
Rice, basmati
Rice,* brown
Rice, white
Rice Cakes
Wheat

LEGUMES
All legumes acceptable
except lentils
Tofu

NUTS
No nuts except coconuts

SEEDS
Flax*
Pumpkin
Psyllium*
Sesame*
Sunflower
Sprouted and soaked
seeds are acceptable

DAIRY
Butter (unsalted)
Cottage Cheese
Ghee
Milk

OILS
Coconut
Olive
Sunflower
Soy

SWEETENERS
All sweeteners are
acceptable except
molasses and cooked
honey
Raw honey*

CONDIMENTS
No spices except
coriander, cinnamon,
cardamom, fennel,
turmeric, and a little
black pepper

* Okay if eaten in small amounts

UNBALANCING OR AGGRAVATING FOODS

FRUITS
Sour Fruits
Apricots
Berries
Bananas
Cherries
Cranberries
Grapefruit
Grapes (green)

VEGETABLES
Pungent Vegetables
Lemons
Oranges (sour)
Papaya
Peaches
Pineapple (sour)
Persimmon
Plums (sour)
Beets
Carrots
Eggplant
Garlic
Horseradish
Onions
Olives
Peppers (hot)
Radishes

Spinach
Tomatoes

GRAINS
Buckwheat
Corn
Millet
Quinoa
Rye

DAIRY
Buttermilk
Cheese
Sour Cream
Yogurt

SEEDS
Chia

OILS
Almond
Corn
Safflower
Sesame

SWEETENERS
Molasses

percentage of saturated fats it contains. Sunflower and pumpkin seed oil are fine for pitta people.

Dairy products have variable effects. Sweet dairy is acceptable. Sour dairy products and hard cheese aggravate. Ghee, which is a clarified, raw, unsalted butter, is very balancing and calming for pitta.

Sweets are cooling to pitta. Even white sugar, which I do not recommend, can help to cool pitta. Honey is moderately heating, but can be used in minimal amounts. Molasses is heating and is best avoided.

Spices that are hot or pungent are aggravating to pitta. Cardamom, cinnamon, coriander, and fennel are balancing. Black pepper can be occasionally used and cumin, although somewhat heating, can be used in moderation.

Drinks that are cooling, sweet, bitter, and astringent are balancers. Pittas need a lot of water. Carbonated drinks and alcohol aggravate pitta. Salty drinks and an excess of hot teas are imbalancing to pitta. Sour drinks and citrus in excess, including orange juice, may also aggravate pitta.

DRINK GUIDELINES

VATTA	PITTA	KAPHA
BALANCING DRINKS		
Apple Juice*	Apple Juice	Apple Juice
Carrot Juice	Carrot Juice*	Caffeine*
Coconut Milk	Cold Drinks	Carrot Juice
Grape Juice	Coconut Milk	Coffee**
Grapefruit Juice	Grapefruit Juice*	Cranberry Juice
Mango Juice	Grape Juice	Grape Juice*
Miso Broth	Mango Juice	Grapefruit Juice*
Orange Juice	Miso Broth*	Mango Juice
Papaya Juice	Orange Juice*	Miso Broth*
Prune Juice*	Papaya Juice*	Orange Juice*
Soy Milk* (if warmed	Prune Juice	Papaya Juice*
and spiced)	Soy Milk	Pear Juice
		Prune Juice
		Soy Milk* (if warmed
		and spiced)

* Okay if taken in small amounts
** Okay for Kapha but not healthy for anyone

VATTA	PITTA	KAPHA
UNBALANCING OR AGGRAVATING DRINKS		
Alcohol	Alcohol	Alcohol
Caffeine Drinks	Caffeine Drinks	Carbonated Drinks
Carbonated Drinks	Carbonated Drinks	Cold Drinks
Coffee	Coffee	Coconut Milk
Cranberry Juice	Cranberry Juice	
Cold Drinks		
Pear Juice		

Preview of Chapter 5
Subtle Food Messages From Nature

In this chapter you will learn about some of the silent messages Mother Nature is continually giving to us about the qualities and energies of the food we eat. These communications come in terms of tastes, colors, and qualities. You will learn about the six tastes, six qualities, directions of action of foods, and the color code of foods as explained through the rainbow diet. The rainbow diet is like learning how to select a good wardrobe, it helps us to color coordinate our foods with the energies of our own bodies. As we select our foods and eat them, are we ready to listen to and act on these silent messages? Are we ready to read these love notes from God?

  I. Mother Nature's Clues

 II. Six Tastes

    A. Sweet

    B. Sour

    C. Salty

    D. Pungent

    E. Bitter

    F. Astringent

III. Six Food Qualities

    A. Heavy

    B. Light

    C. Oily

    D. Dry

    E. Cold

    F. Hot

IV. Direction of Action of Foods

 V. Rainbow Diet

Chapter 5

Subtle Food Messages From Nature

It is apparent to the reader by now that food is more than just carbohydrates, proteins, and fats. The spectrum of nutrition ranges from undifferentiated energy to various levels of differentiated energy, which energies play an important role in balancing, building, healing, activating, and cleansing the glands, organs, nervous system, tissues, and more subtle elements of the body, such as the dosha energies and subtle energy centers. Each food has a particular taste, quality, shape, and color that is part of Mother Nature's clues and efforts to communicate with us. Each food has its own "personality" that affects our psychophysiological and spiritual nature. For example, the golden colored mango and papaya have the shape and color radiance that matches the pineal and pituitary. I have developed the system of the rainbow diet, as explained in detail in *Spiritual Nutrition and the Rainbow Diet,* which correlates the colors of the foods with the subtle energy centers, organs, glands, and nervous system. The Chinese system has classified the yin and yang effect of the foods according to color. The more red a food is, the more yang it is; the more a food is toward the purple side of the rainbow, the more it is considered yin. In the Ayurvedic and Chinese system, the tastes and food qualities are very important clues to the energetic effect of the foods.

The Six Tastes

There are six tastes and food qualities that help to inform us as to how a food will tend to affect and interact with our doshas. Each taste is, in a way, nature's way of signalling us as to how the food will energetically act on our body and mind. The six tastes are: sweet, sour, salty, bitter, pungent, and astringent (see p. 84).

The **sweet taste** can be experienced by the varying degrees of sweetness that are in sweet fruit, sugar, milk, rice, and grains. Sweetness increases kapha and decreases pitta and vata. Sweetness has the qualities of being cooling, heavy, and oily. It relieves hunger and thirst and nourishes the body. Because it increases kapha, sweetness increases tissue mass. Sweet is the overwhelmingly predominant and favorite taste in America, creating a kapha imbalance which contributes to the obesity of millions of overweight people. Eating sweets gives satisfaction and a sense of fullness on the mental plane. For those who feel lacking in their lives, sweets can become addicting because it supplies the short-term illusion of mental and physical satiation. Sweets have a cooling effect on the pitta anger and a temporary calming affect on the vata fear. Too much sweets may contribute to complacency and greed, especially for kaphas, who have a propensity for manifesting that tendency anyway.

The **sour taste** (lemon and yogurt) imbalances kapha and pitta. The sour qualities are heavy, heating, and oily and therefore are balancing for vata. Sour-tasting foods usually improve digestion and appetite. Sour grapes is a term that relates to a certain feeling of being deprived or bitterness about lacking something in life. An overindulgence in sour foods may lead to envy or jealousy about what is lacking. This sourpuss tendency to envy and possess creates an imbalance in pittas. Not only does it amplify these tendencies, but these tendencies create anger. The greed tendency of kaphas may be amplified by sour foods. Sour is balancing for vatas by creating mental heat.

The **salty taste** is heavy and heating. These qualities help to balance vata and imbalance kapha and pitta. Salt increases digestive fire and helps to clean the body of wastes. Salt enhances all our appetites for life and physical indulgence in the senses. In excess, it can contribute to imbalancing the mental state of kapha. It reinforces the kapha tendency toward complacency and sense indulgence. The heat of pitta is also aggravated by salt, especially if the desires fired up by the salty food are not expressed. The vata mind, which is sometimes too ungrounded to indulge in the earthy senses, is brought more into balance by salt, in a way that draws awareness to the physical level.

Pungent foods (spicy foods such as ginger and cayenne) are heating, light, and dry. The heating and drying qualities of pungent foods help to balance kapha. Pungent foods aggravate pitta and vata. Pungent foods, such as cayenne, are good for reducing mucous and stimulating gastric fire in the kapha dosha. The anger and irritability of pitta is aggravated by pungent foods because fire brings out an extroverted energy and a desire for external stimulation. These qualities of pungent foods help kaphas come out of their complacency and inertia.

Foods of **bitter taste** (spinach and other leafy greens) are cooling, light, and dry. Foods of bitter taste balance kapha and pitta but may tend to aggravate vata. Bitter-tasting foods dry and purify secretions and increase appetite, which is perfect for kapha. Bitter foods tend to amplify dissatisfaction, criticism, and grief. Mild dissatisfaction may be a stimulus to change and thus is good for balancing the complacency aspects of kapha. These same qualities of bitterness bring out insecurity and fear in vata because it enhances the tendency to change and enhances the dry sadness of excessive dissatisfaction.

Astringent foods are those which make the mouth pucker. Examples are unripe persimmons, turmeric, and okra. Astringent foods are cooling, light, and dry. Because of this, they tend to aggravate vata and balance pitta and kapha. These foods purify and reduce secretions, as well as dry out the body, which is excellent for kapha. Their drying and shrivelling energy create introverted tendencies. If this withdrawal is excessive, it causes mental contraction that brings out fear and anxiety. This may imbalance the vata mind. This same contraction energy helps to balance the extroverted energies of the pitta personality.

In general, the bitter, pungent, and astringent tastes imbalance vata and decrease kapha. The tastes of bitter, pungent, and astringent have a "lightness" quality to them, and helps to free kaphas from their tendency to be complacently attached to the body and the desires of the material world. Sweet, sour, and salty tastes increase the attachment to the body and worldly desires. Because of this, sweet, sour, and salty tastes decrease vata, as vatas need to increase these attachments because of their lack of groundedness. Perhaps the food industry is aware of this because there is so much emphasis on sweetness and saltiness in most fast foods. Eating these processed, empty, foodless foods feeds the life of the senses.

Pittas are balanced by sweet, bitter, and astringent foods. Pungent, salty, and sour foods imbalance pitta. Vatas are aggravated by excessive amounts of any taste. My experience in eating in the homes of Ayurvedic physicians is that they would serve meals with all the tastes to create a general balance. The wisdom of eating in a way that maintains one's own dosha balance requires artful intelligence, intuition, and trial and error concerning what tastes of foods are balancing and when to eat these foods.

The Chinese medicine system has also systematized the meaning of the tastes of foods. They recognize five flavors (tastes): pungent, sweet, bitter, sour, and salty. According to the Chinese system, each taste affects specific organ systems.

Pungent foods act on the lungs and large intestine. They also induce perspiration.

Sweet-flavored foods act upon the stomach, spleen, and pancreas and neutralize toxins.

Bitter foods act upon the heart and small intestine. Bitter foods are also said to reduce fever and induce diarrhea.

Sour foods act upon the liver and gall bladder. They also stop diarrhea and perspiration.

Salty foods act upon the kidney and urinary bladder and also soften hard masses and tissues.

Food Qualities

The six major food qualities in Ayurveda are: **heavy** (cheese, yogurt, wheat); **light** (barley, corn, spinach, apples); **oily** (dairy, fatty foods, avocados); **dry** (barley, corn, potatoes, beans); **hot** food and drink (hot tea); and **cold** food and drink (iced tea). Generally, heavy, oily, and hot foods tend to balance vatas and imbalance kaphas. Hot, light, and dry foods tend to balance kaphas and imbalance pittas. Pittas are more balanced by heavy, oily, and cold foods.

The Six Tastes

SIX FOOD QUALITIES

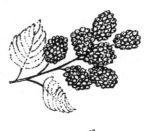

	VATTA	PITTA	KAPHA
HEAVY	YES	YES	NO
OILY	YES	YES	NO
HOT	YES	NO	YES
LIGHT	NO	NO	YES
DRY	NO	NO	YES
COLD	NO	YES	NO

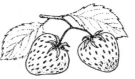

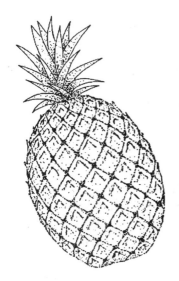

SIX TASTES GROUP

	VATTA	PITTA	KAPHA
SWEET	YES	YES	NO
SOUR	YES	NO	NO
SALTY	YES	NO	NO
PUNGENT	NO	NO	YES
BITTER	NO	YES	YES
ASTRINGENT	NO	YES	YES

In the Chinese system, foods are considered for their medicinal qualities by flavor, energetic quality, direction of action in the body, and specific affinity for different organs and glands. The energy of the different foods is broken into five energetic categories:

Cold energy (very yin), such as banana, grapefruit, kelp, lettuce, persimmon, sugar, water chestnut, and watermelon.

Cool energy (slightly yin), such as apples, barley, tofu, mushrooms, cucumbers, eggplant, oranges, mangos, spinach, strawberries, and tangerines.

Neutral energy (balanced), such as apricots, sesame seeds, soybeans, cabbage, carrots, celery, eggs, corn, apples, figs, honey, kidney beans, milk, olives, papaya, peanuts, pineapples, plums, potatoes, pumpkin, radishes, rice, sunflower seeds, and sweet potatoes.

Warm energy (slightly yang), such as asparagus and malt.

Hot energy (very yang), such as vinegar, cinnamon, cloves, cayenne, dates, garlic, ginger, green onion, nutmeg, raspberries, and black pepper.

Foods in the Chinese system are also seen to have a directional influence on the flow of energy in the body. The foods which have an **upward** movement are those which move energy from the lower parts of the body toward the chest and head. Their tastes may be neutral, pungent, sweet, and bitter. Some of these foods are: apricots, sesame, soybeans, cabbage, carrots, celery, sunflower seeds, apples, figs, grapes, honey, kidney beans, milk, peanuts, rice, and sweet potatoes. Some of these foods, by moving the direction of energetic flow upward, are said to alleviate diarrhea and prolapsed organs.

Outward-moving foods move toward, and affect, the surface of the body. Their tastes may be pungent or sweet. Some of them are good for inducing perspiration and reducing fever. Examples of outward-moving foods are: black pepper, ginger, cinnamon and red pepper.

Inward-moving foods tend to ease bowel movements and abdominal swelling. Examples of these foods are: hops, kelp, lettuce, salt, and seaweed. These foods have cold, bitter, or salty tastes.

Downward-moving foods are said to relieve nausea, vomiting, hiccupping, and asthma. Their tastes may be sweet or sour. Examples of downward-moving foods are apples, bananas, barley, tofu, cucumbers, eggplant, lettuce, mango, persimmons, spinach, wheat, and watermelon.

Foods may also be classified as to how they move nutrients. Honey is a "delivery system" which enhances the movement of nutrients. Olive oil is considered an obstructive food because it slows down the movement of nutrients.

It is significant that both these ancient medical systems of India and China, which have been used for thousands of years with impressive results, equally go to great lengths to delineate the energetic properties of foods and how these energies influence the flow and balance of the body's energies. Based on this understanding of the energetic qualities of foods, the Chinese, and also the Ayurvedic system, prescribed specific foods to rebalance the energy of a person. For example, if a person was suffering from a deep, inner cold, both systems would probably prescribe the heat-producing herbs cayenne, black pepper, and ginger. Though these two great healing systems might use different terms and concepts to describe the action of these foods, they would both share a basic understanding of what tastes and qualities of foods are needed to remedy the situation.

The Secrets of the Rainbow of Foods

The next step in this connection back to Mother Nature and health is the understanding of vegetarian foods and their multiple colors as condensations of sunlight. The color of foods is a secret, silent communication of Nature about the characteristics of Her gifts to us. This is discussed in great depth in *Spiritual Nutrition and the Rainbow Diet* .

Dr. Bircher-Benner and Rudolf Steiner, two great minds from the earlier part of this century, have said that raw foods contain the sunlight energies which are stored in their living tissues through the process of photosynthesis. I feel these sunlight energies are stored in photosynthesis-activated carbon-hydrogen bonds just waiting to be released into receptive, happy humans who appreciate the secret gifts of Mother Nature. Although it isn't completely understood how these energies are stored, particular energetic vibrations are stored as indicated by their colors. This forms the basis of what I call the Rainbow Diet. The Rainbow Diet says that the outer coverings of the plant is the key to understanding and recognizing the particular light and micronutrient energies that are stored in that particular vegetable, fruit, grain, or grass as they occur in nature. It is a way to tune in to the color-coded secrets of nature.

Each of the seven primary color foods associated with the seven primary colors of the rainbow relates to a specific subtle energy center in the body and its associated glands, organs, and nervous system plexuses. For example, the green-colored vegetables are high in magnesium and calcium, which is beneficial for heart function. The heart center is also associated with the green color. The basic survival center in the body is associated with red. Red fruits and vegetables, such as red peppers and rose hips, are very high in vitamin C. The adrenals, which are one of our primary survival glands, often nicknamed the "flight or fright gland," have the highest concentration of vitamin C. The vitamin C in the red fruits and vegetables also is important for the function and strength of connective and muscle tissue, which are another part of our survival system. As we get more sensitive to the colors of fruits and vegetables, we become drawn to the color we need to assimilate to balance, build, heal, and cleanse our system on any particular day.

The general principle of the Rainbow Diet in practice is to eat a full spectrum of colored foods throughout the day to cover the full spectrum of our physical and subtle biological systems. Generally, the red, orange, and yellow colors are taken at breakfast. This includes a wide variety of fruits, vegetables, nuts, seeds, and grains. At lunch the green color predominates, but yellows (which includes grains, nuts, and seeds) and blues are also included. Green salads, grains, nuts, and seeds, and blue-green sea vegetables are the mainstay. The evening meal is the top end of the rainbow with blue, indigo, and purple or gold. This is easier in the summer when the blue and purple fruits are in season. The gold includes grains, as well as golden fruits like papayas and mangoes. Reddish-purple beets and red and purple sea vegetables are also included.

The gradual incorporation of a rainbow awareness is a way to organize and be sensitive to our patterns of taking in food during the day. By bringing in this full spectrum of light to our systems, we are energized by the full spectrum of light from the sun. As we become more sensitive to these subtle clues of Mother Nature as to what is in the different foods, we find that we are spontaneously drawn to the different colors of the foods depending on our particular needs. Yes, Mother Nature feeds us with her benevolent light energy as well as her physical nutrients.

RAINBOW DIET SPECTRUM

Breakfast: Primary colors are red, orange, yellow (apples, oranges, bananas, etc.) — fruits, vegetables, nuts, seeds, grains, and all white foods.

Lunch: Primary colors are green, yellow and blue — green salads, grains, nuts, seeds and sea vegetables.

Dinner: Primary colors are gold, blue, indigo, and purple — includes grains, golden fruits, papayas, mangoes, redish-purple beets, red and purple sea vegetables, and all white foods.

"At the end of the rainbow, you'll find a pot of plenty."

BLACKBOARD FACTS

Preview of Chapter 6
Food Effects on Body, Mind, and Spirit

This chapter introduces you to the powerful affects our food choices can have not only on body, but also on the emotional moods, mind, and spirit. The effect of diet on spiritual receptivity, strength of moral character, clarity of mind, and the enhancement of the spiritualizing energies in the body is something well known in the Judaic-Christian traditions as well as other traditions around the world. Food choices may have either a dulling or enhancing effect on our ability to receive God's grace. Are you ready to consider how what you are eating may be affecting your mind and spiritual sensitivity?

   I.   Historical observations

  II.   Creating of three states of mind and lifestyle from diet

      A. Sattvic

      B. Rajasic

      C. Tamasic

  IV.   Fast foods and effect on American culture

   V.   Chinese approach to food and mind-body

      A. Yin

      B. Yang

      C. How to balance for a spiritual life

  VI. Enhancing spiritual energy and sensitivity with diet

 VII. Hypoglycemia and the mind

VIII. Effects of overeating or excess acid

  IX. Timing of eating and the mind

Chapter 6

Food Effects on Body, Mind, and Spirit

"Let Food Be Thy Medicine"

Hippocrates taught this message in 431 B.C., yet in the 1990s its meaning is just beginning to influence public and medical opinion. Food can be looked upon as possessing several levels of energy. **Particular energies exist within each food that affect our physical functioning, the nature of our thoughts, and even the expansion of our consciousness.** The color of the outer coating of a food, the five (Chinese) or six tastes (Ayurvedic), their aromas (which I haven't yet worked out), and the six qualities, are several systems with which one can tune into these more specific food energies. Foods can also be classified by their shapes, yin or yang energy (Chinese), and the three gunas (mental state characteristics in Ayurveda).

For thousands of years different cultures have been aware that the types of food we eat have subtle effects on the mind. Herodotus, the Greek historian, reported that grain-eating vegetarian cultures surpassed meat-eating cultures in art, science, and spiritual development. In his writings it was his view that meat-eating nations tended to be more warlike and more focused on expression of anger and sensual passions. It is said that the ancient, Egyptian priesthood ate specific foods to increase their spiritual sensitivity and awareness. In India today, the Brahmin priests still prepare their own food and eat separately from people of other social classes. They also keep themselves on a vegetarian diet that is aimed at enhancing the subtle spiritual qualities of the mind. The implication of this practice is that the dietary patterns of a social group affect the spiritual consciousness of that group. The logical extension of this is that the type of diet a whole nation follows may affect the mental state of that nation. Rudolf Steiner, the founder of biogenic gardening, the Waldorf School, and Anthroposophical medicine, felt that the spiritual progress of humanity as a whole would be enhanced by a progressive increase in a vegetarian eating pattern. Conversely, he felt that an overemphasis on a flesh-eating diet would exert a negative influence regarding an interest in spiritual life.

Ayurvedic physicians and yogis have been aware for thousands of years that a dietary pattern specifically affects the state of a person's mind. They divided the types of foods and the states of mind into three categories: sattvic, rajasic, and tamasic. A sattvic state of mind is clear, peaceful, harmonious, and interested in spiritual life. Sattvic foods help to create this state. This is typified by the mental states of spiritual monks of many religious traditions. A rajasic state of mind is active, restless, worldly, and aggressive. Rajasic food creates this mental state. It is the diet for warriors and the stereotypic image held of corporate executives.

A tamasic mental state is lethargic, impulsive, cruel, violent, and morally and physically degenerate. It is the state of the stereotypical drug addict or other types of criminals. Tamasic foods help to create this state of mind.

Consciously or unconsciously, **people tend to choose the diet that reinforces and reflects their own mental and spiritual state of awareness.** Spiritual aspirants have a tendency to gravitate to sattvic-centered diets. A sattvic diet is made of pure foods which keep the body-mind complex clear, balanced, harmonious, peaceful, and strong. Sattvic foods are easy to digest and result in a minimal accumulation of toxins in the system. In the Ayurvedic system of medicine these sattvic foods include: all fruits, vegetables, edible greens, grasses, beans, raw milk, honey, and small quantities of rice or bread preparations. It is basically a vegetarian diet. From the Western Essene tradition of the West and the spiritual nutrition perspective, a sattvic diet would be essentially a vegetarian diet with approximately 80% raw and 20% cooked foods. It is a diet with an abundance of different sprouts consisting of: legumes, grains, seeds, immature greens, and grasses; fresh fruits and vegetables; soaked nuts and seeds; grains, legumes, and honey; and occasionally raw milk and yogurt.

Rajasic foods are more stimulating to the nervous system. They include: coffee, green or black teas, tobacco, fresh meats, and large amounts of stimulating spices, such as garlic and peppers. These foods are sought as stimulants by people who consciously or unconsciously use them to help carry out worldly activities. The imbalanced stimulating effects on activity level may propel the eater of primarily rajasic foods into a state of agitation, restlessness, and eventual burnout as these foods push our mind and body beyond their natural limits. Coffee addiction and hypoglycemia are typical imbalances which may result from a rajasic diet. Rajasic foods include flesh foods and spicy, cooked foods with rich oily sauces. It is a diet which includes butter, cheese, eggs, sugar, and oily, fried foods. The taste stimulating effects of these foods tends to distract one from inner, somatic messages and propel one outward into stimulating physical, emotional, and mental activities, but often in an imbalanced way.

Tamasic foods are stale, decayed, decomposed, spoiled, overcooked, leftover, heavily processed, and fast foods. They basically include what one might call synthetic foods. These are foods which are chemically treated with preservatives, pesticides, fungicides, artificial and processed sweeteners, artificial colors, sulfites, and nitrites, etc. Alcohol, marijuana, cocaine and other drugs of today's addicted society fall into the category of tamasic foods. Cocaine and amphetamines are initially rajasic in their stimulating effect, but the end result of long-term use is often an exhausted tamasic mental and physical state. The addicted mind set that accompanies cocaine or amphetamine abuse, even during the stimulation phase, falls more into the degenerate tamasic category. Any flesh foods which have not been freshly killed are tamasic foods because within a short time they begin putrefying. This includes almost all meats found in the supermarket. These foods have almost no positive energetic life force left in them. These foods do, however supply us with the toxic chemical breakdown products that affect the functioning of our mind and irritate our nervous system. These foods accelerate more premature aging and chronic degenerative disease. They tend to bring out the worst psychological characteristics because of the irritable, negative, lethargic state they create in us. The tamasic state that I am referring to can be described as that "raunchy, yuck" state that some people experience when they overeat, particularly of tamasic foods. While in this imbalanced energy condition it is difficult to meditate or be in harmony with one's self or the environment.

In assessing the American fast food diet, which is eaten by hundreds of millions in this country, it becomes obvious that this is a strong tamasic diet that also has stimulating rajasic overtones. This type of diet, along with its accompanying drug use, contributes to the fact that **Americans rank 21st in life expectancy** and number one in murders among the industrialized nations. According to federal statistics, the U.S. has more than 20,000 murders per year, which is more deaths per year in peacetime than averaged in Vietnam during the war. The FBI estimates that the national homicide rate increased by 5% in 1989. The rate of homicides increased in some of the major cities by 10-20%. Experts are predicting continual increases in violence, as our society seems to have taken violence for granted and accepted it as part of our way of life.

Further evidence of the link between a tamasic type diet and social violence has been supported by consistent research findings on teenage offenders. When the teenager's diets were changed from their typical high white sugar, fast food, tamasic type diet, a marked decrease in the teen's acting out, violent behavior occurred. For example, Mrs. Barbara Reed, a probation officer at Cuyahoga Falls, Ohio, found that when she switched offenders from what was essentially a tamasic diet of fast foods, et cetera, to a diet higher in fruits and vegetables, every one of the 252 teenagers in her case load stayed out of court as long as they maintained themselves on the healthy diet. A two-year, scientifically precise study with 267 subjects by Steven Schoenthaler, Ph.d., published in the *Journal of Biosocial Research*, showed that while the average American eats approximately 125 pounds of white sugar per year, juvenile delinquents in custody averaged about 300 pounds per year. When this sugar intake was significantly reduced, junk food was reduced, and fruits and vegetables were increased, there was a **48% decrease in antisocial behavior of all types,** including violent crimes, crimes against property, and runaways. This was true for all ages and races. This amazing result was achieved simply by changing the diet with no cost to the taxpayer.

The effect of a tamasic diet of fast and junk convenience foods can cause vitamin deficiencies, which can disrupt the proper working of the brain, not to mention create a disharmonious lifestyle. Our bodies may shift into an imbalanced state, in large part due to vitamin deficiencies, especially of vitamins B_1, B_3, B_6 and B_{12}. A deficiency of these vitamins have been shown to create a number of mental imbalances and nervous system imbalances.

Allergies are often a key symptom suggesting a general breakdown of the body's functioning. As a physician, I find that as a person gets healthier in general, their allergies often disappear. Today there is a tendency for people living a high stress life to compensate for imbalances by megadoses of B vitamins. Used in this way, vitamins become like accepted drug stimulants, helping us cover up the essential rajasic disharmony that is creating the imbalance. These stimulants aid us in the destructive process of self-exploitation. Some lead lifestyles and eat diets which increase exposure to toxic chemicals and heavy metals. Toxins and heavy metals have been associated with hyperactivity, mental retardation, and other forms of nervous system degeneration. Eating organic foods can significantly improve this situation.

Chinese System of Yin/Yang Foods

The interrelating and complimentary principles of yin and yang are key concepts in traditional Chinese philosophy that are used to describe the dynamic nature of the universe. Everything can be potentially described in terms of yin and yang. The principles of yin and yang, though polar opposites, do not exist without each other. According to traditional Chinese thought, even the personality can be viewed from the perspective of yin and yang elements.

Yang attributes are contractive, hot, fiery, dense, heavy, flat, and low to the ground. A yang personality is powerful, strong-willed, extroverted, grounded, outgoing, focused, concrete, active, and prone to getting angry easily. An imbalanced yang personality can be overly aggressive, tense, coarse, and irritable and angry. Excessive intake of yang foods can intensify and amplify these yang mental characteristics. For example, although in India they did not call it yin or yang, they would feed their warriors flesh foods as a way to increase their warlike characteristics.

Yin attributes are expansive, receptive, cool, dilated, light, vertical, and thin. The yin personality is introspective, receptive, self-contained, quiet, mellow, easy-going, reflective, sensitive, and has an expansive, spiritually oriented mind. An imbalanced yin personality may be "spaced out," timid, ungrounded, weak-willed, and passive. An excess of yin foods without other yang balancing factors could cause yin mental imbalances in the mind and body.

Foods are also classified by their predominate yin and yang characteristics. Foods are not all yin or yang. Each food has a combination of yin and yang elements which are complimentary and exist in that food in a dynamic balance. Yin foods are predominantly alkaline-forming, but there are a few yin foods that are acid-forming. Yang foods are predominantly acid-forming, but there are a few yang foods that are alkaline-forming as well. The yin/yang chart helps to visualize this. The following categories of foods are listed in the order of most yin to most yang: chemical additives, processed foods, fruits, vegetables, sea vegetables, seeds, nuts, beans, grains, dairy, fish, poultry, pork, beef, eggs, miso, and sea salt or commercial table salt.

Yin alkaline-forming foods are fruits, vegetables, and honey. Seeds, nuts and beans are acid-forming but slightly yin to neutral. The basic yang foods, such as grains and flesh foods, are acid-forming. Yang alkaline-forming foods are radishes, pickles, miso, and salt. Yin acid-forming foods are sugar, chemical drugs, soft drinks, and alcohol.

Each of these foods has its own yin and yang force and can be said to be an energy in itself which influences the mind toward more expansive or contractive tendencies. Choosing the proper balance of yin and yang food intake is relative to many different factors in a person's life and total environment. A few of these factors are constitutionally determined. For example, a constitutionally hot yang person will be balanced by cooler yin foods. In the Chinese system, the organs and glands of the body are classified by their yin or yang nature or state of imbalance. Appropriate yang or yin foods are given to help balance and heal these particular organs or glands. One's work in the world, environmental conditions, spiritual practices, and level of awareness are all forces that affect the yin/yang balance in a person. Food is one of the main factors influencing yin/yang balance in a person.

Sometimes when eating a very yin food, one may crave some yang foods to balance. For example, wine, which is yin, balances cheese, which is yang. Beer, which is yin, balances salty pretzels, which are yang. Alcohol, which is yin balances meat which is yang. If a diet is too far to one side, it may stimulate cravings of foods from the other extreme in an attempt to achieve some balance. If one eliminates one extreme yang food from the diet, sometimes it is best to eliminate an extreme yin food to maintain the balance. So, if you give up beer, you may better maintain the balance if you also give up pretzels.

Our degree of spiritual awareness and transformation affects how much our mind is shifted by the yin and yang energy of foods in a somewhat different way than the other factors which affect yang and yin. In the spiritual process, because it is expansive, it is my impression that people spontaneously shift to more yin foods to support the lighter, more superconductive needs of the mind and body. The mucous and acid-forming, enzyme-less, yang grains, flesh foods, and other cooked foods, tend to decrease the spiritualizing energy of the body-mind complex. The uncooked, primarily yin foods, support and activate this expansion of consciousness and sensitivity to the Divine. It sometimes happens that spiritual evolution proceeds too rapidly for a person and they become too quickly expanded for comfort. They might find themselves craving yang foods to slow down the process. On the other hand, if a person's awareness is expanded in a way that is grounded and balanced, then yang foods will not be craved. A retrospective research project of mine, on a group of 106 people involved in a spiritual program where there was no emphasis or training on diet, found that 63% of the people shifted to a more yin diet as their awareness expanded over a year's time. It is as if the organism spontaneously shifts to a more yin diet to support the shift in expanded spiritual awareness and sensitivity. The process of eating to enhance spiritual life is to consciously choose a diet that will support the expansion of consciousness so that we are active co-creators of the dietary change process.

As consciousness expands in a mature, balanced way, it is my observation that more and more yin foods can be eaten without developing a yin imbalance. One does not necessarily develop the symptoms of a yin imbalance such as spaciness, lack of motivation, and poor concentration even if one eats primarily yin foods. The power of a shift toward an expanded spiritual awareness of the Divine is often a stronger force than the yin or yang energies of the foods one eats. This does not negate the general observation that the judicious use of yin or yang foods can be helpful when one feels a need to gently counterbalance certain yang or yin mental or physical states. Food is a supportive, rather than the determining, factor in the development of spiritual awareness. It is particularly effective when one chooses a more yin diet to support the development of spiritual transformation.

Enhancing Spiritual Energy and Sensitivity with Diet

Since the body is a condensation of various levels of energy, it is not surprising to realize that within the body there are certain energies that one is able to experience on a subtle, yet sensory, level. For example, most people can experience sexual energy shifts or variations in digestive energies. When the flow and conductivity of the spiritual energy existing within all is awakened, it can also be experienced. This Divine energy transforms the body-mind complex and enables it to withstand more intense and subtler energies involved in the process of spiritual evolution.

If subtle channels of the body are not blocked due to undisciplined habits of eating and an immoderate lifestyle, the spiritualizing energy is able to act with its full force. This is a key connection between nutrition and spiritual life. With an appropriate diet, the transforming and purifying action of the spiritual energy takes place faster and more easily than if one is not on a supportive diet. It is just that a primarily live food, vegetarian diet enhances the awakening of, sensitivity to, and flow of, the spiritualizing process of God's grace and light.

In 1975, God's grace awoke the spiritual energy in me. Among other aspects of grace, I received the message that I needed to understand how to eat to support the awareness of the Divine presence and amplify the power of God's spiritualizing energy. In an attempt to fulfill that transmission of will, since 1975 I have personally worked with more than a thousand people interested in developing a diet to enhance their spiritual lives. A few basic patterns have emerged. The most important observation is that spiritual energies and sensitivity to the sacred and eternal of the Divine are most enhanced by a light, vegetarian diet of live foods. The sensitivity to the Divine presence is most dulled by a diet of flesh foods. An 80% live food, vegetarian diet seems quite sufficient for supporting the development of moral strength, ability to follow God's will, and the activity and power of the spiritualizing energy and sensitivity. Closer to a 95% live food diet and periodic fasting seems to distinctly accelerate this process. Juice fasting particularly seems to have a powerful effect on the awakening and activation of spiritual energy and sensitivity.

Foods have such a strong effect on the process that, when necessary, I even advise the use of certain foods to slow down the energies if people feel uncomfortable or overwhelmed with them. If slowing and dulling is requested, I first recommend 50% or more of cooked grains. This often has a moderate effect in decreasing the sensitivity and the power of the spiritualizing energy. If more slowing than that is needed, I have observed that flesh foods from one to three times a day in large quantities are a powerful numbing force. For all the reasons already mentioned in this book, I hesitate recommending the eating of flesh food, except in rare situations.

Some people come to me complaining that although they have received the grace of spiritual awakening, they have slipped back to a heavier diet, have become less disciplined in their spiritual practices and their focus on God, and feel very little spiritual energy. It has consistently impressed me that time and time again, when people switch to a lighter, high-life-force food regimen, not only does the energy flow significantly better, but they seem to become inspired to intensify their spiritual practices and devotion to God. I have observed this spiritual inspiration to be especially true for people after participation in our spiritual juice fasting retreats.

To conclude, appropriate diet is a powerful aid to awaken and increase overall sensitivity, receptivity, and ability to hold God's grace and light. I want to emphasize that one does not necessarily have to be on such a diet to feel the blessing of God's grace and energy and to be spiritually aware. There are many who eat flesh food who receive grace and grow spiritually. My observation is simply that on a primarily living foods, vegetarian diet, the original diet that was first given to us in Genesis 1:29, it is easier. **Flesh food weakens the moral willpower, weakens the clarity of mind and intellect for understanding the light of God's messages to us, dulls the subtle senses of spiritual receptivity to the light and grace of God, and strengthens the animal tendencies, allowing them**

dominance over our mental and spiritual powers. My finding is not original; it is in alignment with the teachings of Jesus in the *Essene Gospel Book I (p. 36)*:

> "But I do say to you: Kill neither men nor beasts, nor yet the food which goes into your mouth. For if you eat living food, the same will quicken you, but if you kill your food, the dead food will kill you also. For life comes only from life and from death comes always death. And everything which kills your bodies kills your souls also. And your bodies become what your foods are, even as your spirits, likewise, become what your thoughts are....Therefore, he who kills, kills his brother. And from him will the Earthly Mother turn away, and will pluck from him her quickening breasts. And he will be shunned by her angels, and Satan will have his dwelling in his body. And the flesh of the slain beasts in his body will become his own tomb. For I tell you truly, he who kills, kills himself, and whoso eats the flesh of slain beasts, eats of the body of death. For in his blood every drop of their blood turns to poison; in his breath their breath to stink....And their death will become his death."

In my personal and clinical experience, there is an obvious connection between a healthy vibrant body, mind, and intellect and the awareness of the light of God. In the *Essene Gospel of Peace Book I (p. 20)*, Jesus states it clearly:

> " I am sent to you by the Father, that I may make the light of life to shine before you. The light lightens itself and the darkness, but the darkness knows only itself, and knows not the light. I have many things to say to you, but you cannot bear them yet. For your eyes are used to the darkness, and the full light of the Heavenly Father would make you blind. Therefore, you cannot yet understand that which I speak to you concerning the Heavenly Father who sent me to you. Follow, therefore, first, only the Laws of your Earthly Mother, of which I have told you (vegetarian and live food diet as one of the main laws). And when her angels shall have cleansed and renewed your bodies and strengthened your eyes, you will be able to bear the light of our Heavenly Father."

After many years on this diet, as well as much prayer and meditation on God, I have noticed in myself, and with others who have followed this approach, that there arises an experience of an extraordinary, exquisite, gentle flow of the Divine spirit, God's light, and Divine sound filling the body. It is a constant reminder of God's presence and love. Although I often feel it through most of the day, many mornings the Divine presence and light is so intense I simply cannot move. I will just lie there reveling in gratitude and joy for the experience of God as reflected in the mirror of my human body. This is the blessing of a live food vegetarian diet. The energy of God is extraordinary and powerful, and a live food, vegetarian diet helps to build a larger and stronger Divine tuning fork to resonate and amplify God's grace. It is a Divine tuning fork that every one of us can build.

Hypoglycemia and the Mind

Perhaps the most socially significant disruption of brain-mind function is caused by white sugar. Dr. Paavo Airola, the internationally famous nutritionist, naturopath, and author, estimates that the annual intake of white sugar is 125 lbs. per person. One way the cumulative effects of excess white sugar consumption manifests itself is in the form of hypoglycemia (what people commonly call "low blood sugar"). This imbalance seems to affect somewhere between 10% to 70% of the population, depending on whose statistics one uses.

Hypoglycemia, with the exception of the rare occurrence of organic hypoglycemia, is not a disease but a symptom of a generalized physiological endocrine imbalance. A malfunctioning pancreas, as shown by my hypoglycemia research reported in *Hypoglycemia, A Better Approach*, is not the only cause of hypoglycemia. Functional hypoglycemia may also be caused by poorly functioning adrenals, thyroid, pituitary, ovaries, liver, allergies, or a combination of all of these organs and glands. Functional hypoglycemia is caused more from general endocrine stress than being the opposite of diabetes. Other possible causes are chromium, zinc, pantothenic acid, magnesium, potassium, or pyridoxine deficiency. In rare cases, pancreatic tumors, Addison's disease, and pituitary tumors may cause organic hypoglycemia.

Allergies are also a common contributor to hypoglycemia. The allergen is often white sugar itself, but it may be any substance. The major cause of a phenomenon that affects at least 24 million people is most likely not specific vitamin deficiencies, allergies, or tumors, but a self-exploitive, stressful, overextended lifestyle and a diet high in fast foods, white sugar and other sorts of stimulants. One could say that it is a result of living the "all-American dream" of moving faster, wanting more and more things, and living a highly competitive, aggressive lifestyle, which is out of harmony with our inner self and Mother Nature. Hypoglycemia is literally fueled by the preoccupation with convenience and fast foods.

To relieve the pain of this self-exploitation and energize oneself for short periods, people use white sugar, megavitamins, alcohol, cigarettes, coffee, and other caffeine-containing foods. This destructive way of compensating for inner emptiness and a lack of peace is another example of trying to treat a headache caused by banging one's head against the wall. People seem to be willing to do and try anything and everything to treat the headache *except* stop banging their heads!

A stable blood sugar is important for the normal functioning of the brain and nervous system. This is because the blood glucose is the primary fuel for the neurological and brain tissues. I have observed that many meditators seem to increase their desire for sweets after beginning to meditate. It is my impression that meditation has a healing effect on the nervous system and this healing requires more energy input in the form of glucose. The mistake many meditators make is to seek more glucose for the system by eating refined foods with excess white sugar. Unfortunately, this poor dietary choice imbalances the body toward hypoglycemia and produces irregular glucose levels in the blood. A high, complex carbohydrate diet of soaked nuts and seeds, fruits, vegetables, and grains will supply an adequate and gradual release of glucose into the blood, unlike the ups and downs created by white sugar ingestion. I have had the experience of treating many monks and other spiritual aspirants involved in intense spiritual practices who developed hypoglycemia because they did not understand this basic idea. My clinical research has shown that when meditators with hypoglycemia go on a diet to prevent hypoglycemia, their ability to concentrate, meditate, and become steady in their meditation improves.

With meditators, as well as with those who do not meditate, I have found that those who move away from fast foods and other highly sugared foods tend to be more emotionally stable, awake, and aware. It is very common to find those who are suffering from emotional instability, unexplained crying spells, panic attacks, drowsiness in the late morning and mid-afternoon, low energy, and concentration lapses have some degree of hypoglycemia. Mental function seems to improve when one adopts an antihypoglycemic diet comprised of high complex carbohydrates, low protein, with **no sweets, caffeine, alcohol, marijuana, or cigarette intake.**

Specific Healing Qualities of Food

The next step in the specificity of the energy of a food is to understand that each food has specific healing qualities, which is different than a general pitta or vata or yin or yang effect. This is highlighted in Dr. Bernard Jensen's book, *Food That Heals*, and in the classical juice therapy book by Dr. N. W. Walker, *Raw Vegetable Juices*. Jensen's book lists the foods, and Walker's book lists the food juices and their specific healing qualities. The juices in our spiritual juice fast retreats are used according to these healing principles. The different Chinese medical texts also give extensive lists of foods and their specific healing qualities. Herbs are also considered food, and there are hundreds of herbal books that describe the specific healing qualities of herbs. The importance and role of food in the preservation of health cannot be underestimated. Dr. Jensen quotes Dr. Victor G. Rocine in 1930 who said:

"If we eat wrongly, no doctor can cure us; If we eat rightly, no doctor is needed."

Rocine was among the first western doctors to understand that particular foods had particular minerals that our bodies need more of when we have certain diseases. For example, if one had hypothyroid from an iodine deficiency, eating foods that are high in iodine, such as kelp, supply the iodine needed to help correct the condition. He also clarified that there were personality types that could be traced to the dominance of either calcium, silicon, or sulfur in a person's system.

The homeopathic system developed by Samuel Hahnemann over two hundred years ago has shown in daily practice that when certain minerals, herbs, and other plant and animal substances are energetically amplified by way of homeopathic preparation they help to heal specific constitutional types. Homeopaths have discovered that certain personalities respond to specific potentized substances. Sulfur, club moss, calcium carbonate, phosphorous, and arsenicum albumin are just a few of hundreds of substances that are specific remedies for different personality types and medical conditions.

The highly respected spiritual teacher, Paramahansa Yogananda, found that many foods affect specific characteristics of our personality. For example, in *Fourteen Steps to Higher Consciousness,* by J. Donald Walters, Yogananda is quoted as saying that almonds improve "self-control" and "calmness of the mind and nerves;" bananas increase "humility and calmness;" blackberries create "purity of thought;" dates help to remedy an overly critical nature by bringing out the quality of sweetness and tenderness; oranges help to banish melancholia and stimulate the brain; and raspberries enhance "kindheartedness." The Bach Flower remedies developed by the English physician Edward Bach in England in the 1930s, are specifically based on how specific flowers, trees, and herbs can "flood our natures with the particular virtue we need, and wash out from us the fault that is causing the harm." In this way, the Bach Flower Remedies heal specific emotional imbalances.

The book, *Flower Essences*, by Gurudas, goes into depth on the particular energies and specific effects that the different flowers and herbs have on the physical constitution, personality, mind, and spirit of a person. The point is, that in their natural living forms, food, juices, herbs, and minerals are living energies that affect us on every level of our being in very specific ways.

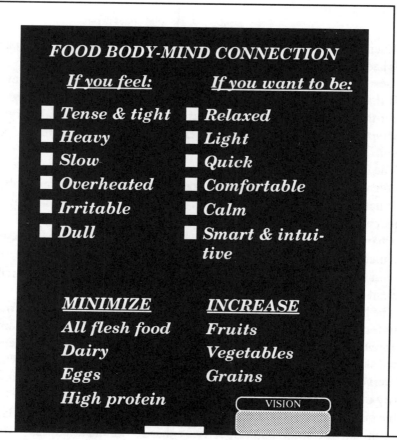

FOOD BODY-MIND CONNECTION

If you feel:	_If you want to be:_
■ Tense & tight	■ Relaxed
■ Heavy	■ Light
■ Slow	■ Quick
■ Overheated	■ Comfortable
■ Irritable	■ Calm
■ Dull	■ Smart & intui-tive

MINIMIZE	_INCREASE_
All flesh food	Fruits
Dairy	Vegetables
Eggs	Grains
High protein	

VISION

BLACKBOARD FOOD FOR THOUGHT

Effects of Overeating or Eating Acid Foods in Excess

Overeating in general, especially of excess protein, and eating late in the evening, are two sure ways to make the mind and body go numb. The body-mind life force becomes drained because it has to divert essential energy to support the overstrained digestive system and compensate for low cellular oxygen from blood sludging and high fats.

By eating too much protein, one not only encourages bowel toxicity, but often tends to become too acidic. The more acidic our system becomes, the slower and less clear becomes our thinking process. When our blood pH moves from its normal pH of 7.4 to even a slightly acid pH of 6.95, the nervous system begins to shut down, one becomes stuporous, and may slip into an acidotic coma. That is one way that excess acidity may affect the mind. If one's pH becomes too alkaline, one may become physiologically and emotionally sensitive and irritable, or in some cases, a "space" case with difficulty concentrating. **A stable acid-base balance of the body is important for maintaining a stable mental state.**

Timing of Eating and the Mind

Paying attention to the natural digestive cycle is also quite important. When the digestive system is not overworked and the body is functioning well, it is easier to maintain a clear mind, which in itself enhances our desire and ability to meditate with increased clarity. According to the Ayurvedic system of medicine, the time of optimal digestive power is 10 am–2 pm. In the Chinese system it is 7–9 am. Eating between 1 pm and 3 pm is also a good time. Nighttime, when most people in the U.S. customarily eat their largest meal, is a slow time for the digestive system. If a big meal is eaten after 7 pm, or less than three hours before going to sleep, undigested food often accumulates, which serves as a breeding ground for food-rotting bacteria. The food then putrefies and consequently adds toxins to the system, both from the rotting food and toxins given off by the putrefactive bacteria. In the morning, instead of awakening refreshed with a clear mind, one may feel bloated, tired, and sometimes just wretched. Because of the toxic feeling, one feels much like a clogged sewage pipe and one finds oneself unable to meditate, pray, or exercise, thereby missing out on activities that are essential to maintain balanced health and spiritual growth.

Because digestion depends also on the emotional and mental peace of the eating atmosphere, some people may not feel comfortable eating the biggest meal at lunchtime and might choose to wait until returning home to a more emotionally friendly space where they feel more relaxed. Though digestive energies may not be optimal at this time, there is some validity to this approach if one's evening meal remains moderate and relatively low in protein.

When it comes to eating high protein meals, I have observed a subtle stimulation when excess protein is eaten. According to Dr. Morter in *Your Health, Your Choice,* the body metabolism speeds up by about 30%. The body may keep this increased rate for 3 to 12 hours. Protein does not actually increase body energy, but stimulates it. A large protein meal, even if eaten several hours before going to sleep, can then act as a stimulant and keep one awake. This excess stimulation may also manifest as "nervous" energy with a variety of "fidgety" mannerisms. For this reason, I suggest eating any large protein meal at breakfast or lunch, depending on what time you feel your assimilation powers are the strongest. For myself, the Chinese observation of eating the biggest and highest protein meal between 7 am and 9 am works best for me.

Discovering the dietary pattern which works best for me is an ongoing experiment linked to my evolving body-mind-spirit complex. Presently, I primarily do not eat after 2:30 pm except for maybe a half cup of water or fresh juice in the evening. Prior to this, I used to take several glasses of fresh vegetable juice in the evening, but I discovered it made me too alkaline and also overhydrated me. Remember, kaphas can easily overhydrate on even less than six glasses of fluid a day. This same amount would leave a pitta underhydrated. Jesus, in *Essene Gospel of Peace Book I* (p. 38), also recommended eating only two times per day.

> "For I tell you truly, he who eats more than twice in a day does in him the work of Satan."

Other spiritual and/or health practitioners have had similar ideas of not eating after 2 or 3 pm. For centuries, Buddhist monks have understood this and have practiced not eating anything after 2 pm. One French healer I met had discovered an ancient system in which one could eat anything one wanted until 2 pm. After that, one would not eat anything for the rest of the day and night until morning. He found that this system was very powerful in helping people regain their health and lose weight. Although this may seem to be an extreme example, it supports the importance of the timing of when one eats. For many people, two meals a day is a major transition. I have found that clients who make the evening meal their lightest meal with the lowest protein also achieve good results.

On this system of not eating after 2:30 pm, I wake up feeling clear and energized in the morning. In the years I have been experimenting with this approach, my weight has remained the same. I especially like it because it gives my digestive system an 18 hour rest each day. Eating by this time pattern and eating so moderately that after each meal I do not feel full and can be fully physically active within an hour, seems to be working out well for my total body-mind health. What is most profound for me about this light eating pattern is the flow of the cosmic energy I feel coursing through my body. Although years of meditation are the primary cause for this, overeating, even of health foods, or late evening eating, distinctly dulls the magnificence of my awareness of this energy. It is a wonderful and spontaneous communion. During the day it feels as if joy is simply running through every cell independent of external factors. This noncausal joy is always there, of course, but light eating, with one's larger meal at the beginning or middle of the day, seems to accentuate these ongoing feelings. **Part of eating consciously is to eat in a way that maintains and supports one's consciousness.**

Fasting as Part of the Diet for Enhancing Body-Mind-Spirit

Fasting is perhaps the most remarkable and simplest self-healing approach related to our food intake for rebalancing and clearing the body and mind and elevating the spirit. Although classically defined as complete abstinence from food and water, in a larger context, it means to abstain from that which is toxic to body, mind, and spirit. Fasting is the elixir of spiritual nutrition. I base this statement on my own experiences of fasting two to four times per year for 7-10 days duration each, my experience of one forty day spiritual fast, and my observation of the awesome body, mind, and spirit transformations of many people on our biannual, seven-day spiritual fasting retreats. Within four days of fasting, participants on the retreats have shared that their concentration improves, creative thinking expands, depression lifts, insomnia stops, anxieties fade, and the mind becomes more tranquil. It is my hypothesis that when the body's toxins have cleared from brain cells, mind-brain function greatly improves. I have also observed that a natural joy begins to make its appearance. It is becoming more apparent to me that the toxic wastes that accumulate in our brain cells have a much more significant effect on our mental and spiritual functioning than has been previously recognized. I still am amazed on each spiritual fast to see how rapidly people's minds clear and what a difference it makes in their spiritual capacity. The fasting retreats also accelerate the spiritualizing process in the following ways: the complete break from one's customary social setting and routine; doing meditation, hatha yoga, and exercise; practicing the Essene communions; holding small group detox healing sessions; doing enemas; doing foot, abdominal, and head massage; and group discussions where people share their feelings. People who normally have trouble meditating or praying for one half hour find themselves going two hours at a time without difficulty. Because the conductivity of the force is so enhanced by the fasting and meditation or intense prayer, more than 90% of the retreat participants often have a spiritual awakening or quickening. Fasting is a powerful part of the live food spiritual nutrition program and an essential part of any nutritional program for spiritual life and health. The mental and physical toxic environment we live in exposes everyone to a toxic buildup that regular fasting at least two times per year helps to unload.

Body Toxins Are Real

Many people think that the phrase "toxins in the body" is just some jargon of food faddists. Research over the last 100 years shows that these bowel toxins actually exist. Not only do they exist, but they have a tremendous negative impact on mental and physical well being. Toxins usually come from a process called intestinal toxemia, an overgrowth of putrefactive intestinal bacteria in the small and large intestine. These toxins are then absorbed into the blood stream and from there affect both our mental and physical functioning. Intestinal toxemia is predominantly caused by a high-protein and low, complex carbohydrate diet. Overeating, eating late at night, and/or a slowing of bowel eliminative function directly contribute to it. Constipation also contributes a lot to this bowel toxemia.

In 1933, Dr. Anthony Basler, a professor of gastroenterology, summarized his 25-year study of 5000 cases by saying:

> "Every physician should realize that the intestinal toxemias are the most important primary and contributing causes of many disorders and diseases of the human body."

Dr. H. H. Boeker, as far back as 1923, said:

> "It is now universally conceded that autointoxication is the underlying cause of an exceptionally large group of symptom complexes."

In general, the research shows that when the intestinal toxemia is removed, general symptoms such as fatigue, nervousness, gastrointestinal conditions, impaired nutrition, skin manifestations, endocrine disturbances, headaches, sciatica, various forms of low back pain, allergy, eye, ear, nose, and throat congestion, and even cardiac irregularities have been healed in hundreds of cases. Excessive amounts of a chemical called indican has also been associated with sacroiliac, upper lumbar, and thoracic subluxations that do not respond to appropriate adjustments. This is not to say that this is the only cure for many of these diseases, but often it is an important factor that is overlooked because we consider the toxemia of our high-protein, overeating habits as a normal state.

Some of the main bowel toxins are: ammonia, indole, indican (a conjugated indole), skatole, clostridium perfringen enterotoxin, gaunidine, phenol, and high concentrations of histamine. I have found that a simple test for indican in the urine is an easy and effective way to diagnose bowel toxemia. The liver is able to detoxify some of these toxins, but when high concentrations are reached, the liver becomes overwhelmed and these toxins saturate the blood stream. Skatole and phenol cannot even be detoxified by the liver at all.

Bowel toxins have more than just a symbolic effect on the mind and nervous system. An increased concentration of ammonia in the blood, for example, increases the cerebrospinal fluid concentration. This seems to interfere with brain metabolism in some way. The results of a high cerebrospinal ammonia are evidenced by clinical reports of neurological and mental disturbances, tremors, brain wave changes, and even coma. Eleven different research laboratories on bowel toxins have reported that schizophrenics have five times more 6-hydroxyskatole in their urine than normal people (a skatole breakdown product from bacterial putrefaction). These findings correlate with the findings of Russian researchers, who, according to Dr. Allen Cott in *Fasting as a Way of Life*, have had excellent success using water fasts to cure 65% of the so-called "incurable schizophrenics." It is interesting to note that one of the main causes of relapse for these "incurables" was a return to high-protein, flesh food intake, which is a diet that stimulates bacterial putrefaction and intestinal toxemia.

Intestinal toxemia not only has been associated with severe mental symptoms, such as psychosis, but with a variety of mental imbalances. As early as 1917, Drs. Satterlee and Eldridge presented 518 cases at an American Medical Association conference that had mental symptoms which were cured by removing the intestinal toxemia. They reported symptoms of intestinal toxemia which are familiar to many people: mental sluggishness, dullness, and stupidity; loss of concentration and/or memory; mental incoordination, irritability, lack of confidence, and excessive and useless worry; exaggerated introspection, hypochondrias, and phobias; depression and melancholy; obsessions and delusions; and hallucinations, suicidal tendencies, delirium, and stupor. Senility symptoms are also common with intestinal toxemia.

Fasting is one of the best and quickest treatments for bowel toxicity. Researchers have found that the urinary indican was "markedly decreased" even after a seven day fast. Phenols, another class of bowel toxins, have also been decreased significantly by fasting. The fasting process allows the bowels to rest and the inflammation to subside. If there are no proteins on which to feed, the putrefactive bacteria will also diminish.

For those who do not want to fast, excluding surgical intervention, a low-protein diet (20-30 grams of protein per day), along with a high complex, high carbohydrate, 80% raw food diet, is a slower but effective cure. When connected with periodic fasting, it is even more powerful. Fats should be kept to a minimum, as heated fats especially intensify the process of intestinal toxemia. Learning to eat in a way that causes no strain on the digestive system is extremely important. This means eating in a manner in which one rises from the table feeling almost as light as when one sits down. If we eat too much or too late, there is incomplete digestion and the process of putrefaction is reinforced. Adding lactobacillus acidophilus (normal large intestine bacteria) culture to the system helps to re-populate the small and large intestine with healthy bacteria, therefore diminishing putrefactive (abnormal) bacteria. Exercise also helps to stimulate the digestive system. Although many will respond to these basic aids to digestion, in the short run, one may need some digestive enzymes and/or digestion-stimulating herbs to help rest and rebuild the digestive power that has been weakened after long years of digestive abuse.

Sweet Mind - Bind Cycle

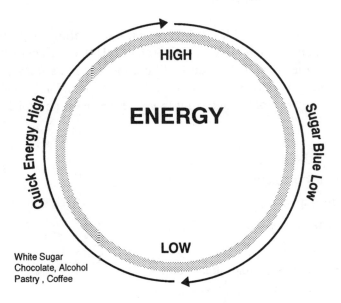

Symptoms of Sugar

- ☐ Spacey
- ☐ Sad without a reason/or too easily
- ☐ Angry without a reason/or too easily
- ☐ Violent without a reason/or too easily
- ☐ Anxious without a reason/or too easily
- ☐ Crying without a reason/or too easily

- ☐ Exhausted
- ☐ Poor Concentration
- ☐ Hyperactive
- ☐ Crave Sweets
- ☐ Low Energy

Sugar is seductive, safe sex—and it's everywhere.
Are you trapped in this cycle?

How to Break the Sweet Mind - Bind Cycle

1. Eat sprouted grains, seeds and/or nuts, seed sauces, sea vegetables, vegetables, or fruits at each meal.

2. Eat three regular meals at constant times.

3. Snack between meals so blood sugar doesn't drop.

4. Stop eating all refined foods, sweets, junk and fast foods, such as anything with white sugar, chocolate, and pastries.

5. Avoid stimulants and other drugs, such as coffee and alcohol.

6. Lead a balanced life.

7. Let go of life in the fast lane.

107

Preview of Chapter 7
Fasting Feeds the Spirit

Fasting is one of the oldest forms of conscious eating. Instead of eating material food, one switches over to the nectar of the Divine energy. Fasting is a deep part of the Judaic-Christian tradition, including the forty day fasts of Moses, Elijah, and Jesus. It is mentioned 74 times in the Bible. The reader is introduced to the physiology of fasting as well as the health and spiritual aspects of fasting.

I.   Spiritual Fasting

    A. Found in many religious traditions

II. Health Aspects

    A. What kind of benefits

    B. Who should not fast

    C. Removing the toxic load in the cells

    D. A way to find real dietary needs

III. Safety of Fasting

IV. Juice Fasting

Chapter 7

Fasting Feeds the Spirit

Spiritual fasting is conducive to rest and rejuvenation on every level of mind, body, and spirit. It allows our physical bodies to turn to the assimilation of Divine or cosmic energy rather than biochemical energy.

In the *Essene Gospel of Peace Book I* (p. 41), Jesus, when talking about fasting one day a week, makes this point quite beautifully.

> "On the seventh day eat not any earthly food, but live only on
> the words of God, and be all the day with the Angels of the Lord
> in the kingdom of the Heavenly Father...let the Angels of God
> build the Kingdom of the heavens in your body...and let not
> food trouble the work of the Angels in your body."

Because fasting accelerates the purification of the body, it enhances the movement of all levels of energy in the body, including the spiritualizing energy. Through repeated fasting, one becomes a clearer receptacle for the assimilation of God's energy into the system. One spiritualizing effect of the fast is that the more we are in touch with the Divine energy, the easier it is for us to be motivated to live in a way that will continue to enhance spiritual development. According to respected teacher Paramahansa Yogananda:

> "Fasting is one of the great ways of approaching God: it releases
> the life force from enslavement to food, showing you that it is
> God who really sustains the life in your body."

When one fasts for spiritual purposes, one goes beyond simply stopping food intake and resting from worldly responsibilities–ideally, one withdraws from everything that is toxic to the mind, body, and spirit. After the first few days of a fast, the appetite usually fades and one's attachment to food diminishes. In this larger, biospiritual context, the mind becomes free to merge into higher states of God communion. Fasting is supportive to anyone's spiritual life because until one reaches a certain level of spiritual development, the desires of the body-mind complex are often stronger than the desire of God communion. Because of these and other beneficial effects of spiritual fasting, many of the great spiritual teachers fasted, including: Moses, Jesus, Elijah, Plato, Aristotle, Pythagoras, Hippocrates, Zarathrustra, Confucius, Leonardo da Vinci, Gandhi and the Essenes, some of who were known for doing yearly, 40-day fasts. The 40-day fast was also practiced by Plato, Aristotle, and Pythagoras. Pythagoras actually required his disciples to fast for 40 days before he would initiate them into the mysteries of his teachings. He felt that only through the power of a 40-day fast could the minds of his disciples be sufficiently purified to understand the profound teaching of the mysteries of life. In more recent history, Mahatma Gandhi told people to fast and purify their bodies, and regardless of their circumstances, they would find peace and joy on earth. Gandhi is quoted as saying:

> "Fasting will bring spiritual rebirth...the light of the world will illuminate you when you fast and purify yourself."

Jesus also advocated fasting for physical, mental, and spiritual transformation. In the *Essene Gospel of Peace, Book I,* (p.14) he teaches:

> "...the word and power of God will not enter into you, because all manner of abominations have their dwelling in your body and your spirit; for the body is the temple of the spirit, and the spirit is the temple of God. Purify, therefore, the temple that the Lord of the temple may dwell therein and occupy a place that is worthy of him....Renew yourselves and fast. For I tell you truly that Satan and his plagues may only be cast out by fasting and prayer (also in Mark 9:29). Go by yourself and fast alone....The living God shall see it and great will be your reward. And fast til Beelzebub and all his evil spirits depart from you, and all the angels of our earthly Mother come and serve you (harmony with nature). For I tell you truly, except you fast, you shall never be free from the power of Satan and all the diseases that come from Satan. Fast and pray fervently, seeking the power of the living God for your healing."

Effect of Fasting on the Vital Force

Fasting also has a powerful effect on the body. It allows the vital force within to rebuild and recharge. Overall mind-body organization is increased with fasting. It is this curative force which throws off the accumulated toxins, clears the dead cells, and rebalances and rejuvenates the body. Hippocrates said:

> "Everyone has a doctor in him, we just need to help him in his work."

According to American health teacher and author of *The Miracle of Fasting*, Paul Bragg, who was a great tower of natural, healthy living in the world:

> "The greatest discovery by modern man is the power to rejuvenate himself physically, mentally, and spiritually with rational fasting."

Most people can receive benefit from fasting. The exceptions are those people more than ten pounds underweight, those with severe wasting diseases, such as neurological degenerative diseases and certain cancers, and pregnant and lactating women. Diabetics should have medical supervision. I generally do not recommend that people with severe hypoglycemia fast until their hypoglycemia has been stabilized, but even hypoglycemics can fast under supervision. Prolonged fasting has completely healed some people with hypoglycemia.

Fasting has been known to alleviate many diseases. It has withstood the test of time for over 5000 years as the one sure and healthy way to lose weight. My experience with weight loss is that periodic fasting is extremely effective over time when alternated with a progressively lighter raw food diet or simply fruits and vegetables. Raw food is excellent in helping people lose weight because it gives more utilizable nutrients with less volume of food intake. The high enzyme content of the raw food helps with assimilation, and there are no detrimental heated fats. A single fast is not nearly as effective as repeated fasts because it helps the person adjust to a progressively lighter food intake after the fast, as well as helps to become accustomed to a new set point in health. The periodicity over time allows the person to gently reprogram the body and mind to a new relationship and experience with food.

The need for supervision is greater when there is a larger toxic load. A person on a typical American diet will have more to detoxify than someone who has been on a raw-food, vegetarian diet. Fasting is an excellent method of helping people overcome addictions to food, cigarettes, and other drugs. Fasting helps because what is sometimes metaphorically called "cell memory craving" for the addictive substance is erased when toxins are removed. It usually takes 5-7 days to eliminate these strong cell memory cravings. The elimination of these toxins from the body during the fast increasingly makes it easier for people to overcome their addiction to a poisonous substance. After the fast, it seems to be easier for them to eat foods that are closer to their original biophysiological needs, namely, fruits, vegetables, sprouts, seeds, and grains, et cetera.

With the toxic cell memory diminished or removed by the fasting process, one is able to get in touch with real dietary needs. The end of a fast provides a special opportunity to reorganize one's habits around a higher quality diet. Fasting helps erase past deleterious habits and serves as an opportunity to begin a dietary program and lifestyle that is more conducive to optimal health. As Paracelsus, the great medieval physician, once said, "Fasting is the greatest remedy."

Fasting is Safe

With all of its good points, one wonders why fasting has not caught on here to the extent that it has in many countries in Europe. In America there seems to be an irrational fear centered around fasting. Perhaps this fear is associated with the overabundance of food in our society. In the United States there are more people suffering from diseases of overeating than of malnutrition. It is estimated that in the U.S. there are over 80 million people who are overweight. The U.S. Congressional Joint Nutrition Monitoring Committee reported that 28% of Americans (32 million) between the ages 25 to 74 were considered overweight. This includes 11.7 million who were considered severely overweight (more than 20% overweight).

Many people have created a variety of ego defenses against experiencing their feelings through their addiction to food. For many, the mere mention of fasting becomes a threat. We have become a nation dependent on, and addicted to, excess. Even the natural cycle of seasonal scarcity seems threatening and unnatural to us. But the fact is, one can live healthily a long time on juices or even on water. The great fasting experts, such as Airola, and the fasting clinics in Europe, point out that we can go 40 days on water and 100 days on juices without danger. At the major European clinics where hundreds of thousands have fasted, 14–21 days are considered therapeutic and 7–10 days are considered completely safe for almost anyone.

The fasting process actually begins after two to three days when the body goes into autolysis. Autolysis is the process of the body digesting its own cells. In the body's wisdom, it selectively decomposes those cells and tissues which are in excess, diseased, damaged, aged, or dead. World renown fasting expert, Dr. Buchinger, with whom I personally studied, describes fasting as "the burning of rubbish." The appropriate time for a fast to stop is when this autolysis process is completed and true hunger returns. Because autolysis is the key mechanism which produces the beneficial effects already mentioned, I define fasting as any process in which the body is encouraged to begin the process of autolysis. This usually also occurs on a juice fast.

Juice and Water Fasting

Juice fasting is a form of fasting in which living food juice supplies enzymes which further aids this cleansing process. Although there is some debate about whether juice or water fasting is better, I prefer the overall effect of the juice fast because there tends to be fewer healing crises. Since juices are high in minerals, vitamins, and enzymes which help with the rejuvenating process of the body, the juices are assimilated directly into the body without stimulating digestive enzymes. The alkalizing properties of the juices helps to neutralize the acid condition from which many people suffer, as well as the toxins being released by the body. The alkaline component of the juices helps to reestablish the alkaline reserve needed for rebuilding health in the body. Also, most people have more energy for meditation on juice than on water. The famous Max Bircher-Brenner, M.D., whose raw-food clinic is the oldest in Europe, felt that raw juices contain an unidentified factor which stimulates the function of the cells to absorb nutrients and excrete toxins. Paavo Airola, Ph.D., one of the top fasting experts in America and one of my teachers, much prefers juice fasts for many of the above-mentioned reasons.

The Buchinger Clinic in Germany has supervised over 250,000 fasts, more than any other clinic in the world. Dr. Buchinger, with whom I also studied in Germany, feels strongly that juice fasts are the "safest and give the best recovery."

Fasting as a Form of Youthing

During a fast, digestive enzymes are relieved from their digestive role and are mobilized for the cleansing and rejuvenation of the body. This happens on both water and juice fasts. As was mentioned, on the physiological level, fasting works by rapidly removing dead and dying cells and toxins. But fasting also stimulates the building of new cells. Aging occurs when we have more cells die than are being built. "Youthing" happens when more new cells are produced than are dying. After fasting, the experience of "youthing" abounds. Senses get sharper, food tastes better, there is more energy, meditation is easier, and the communion with the Divine is enhanced. Paul Bragg describes it several ways:

> "Fasting clears away the little things which clutter the heart and mind. It cuts through the corrosion, renewing our contact with God."

> "When you fast you are working with nature. God and nature will not perform a miracle until we are willing to bring our lives and our habits into conformity with nature's laws."

Athenaeus, a Greek physician, once said:

> "Fasting cures diseases, dries up bodily humors, puts demons to flight, gets rid of impure thoughts, makes the mind cleared, the heart purer, and the body sanctified, and raises man to the throne of God."

Rumi, the reknown Sufi poet and mystic, wrote a beautiful poem about fasting in a book called *Open Secret*, which expresses it all:

> *"There's hidden sweetness in the stomach's emptiness.*
> *We are lutes, no more, no less.*
> *If the sound box is stuffed full of anything, no music.*
> *If the brain and belly are burning clean with fasting,*
> *Every moment a new song comes out of the fire.*
> *The fog clears, and new energy makes you run up the steps in front of you.*
> *Be emptier and cry like reed instruments cry.*
> *Emptier, write secrets with the reed pen.*
> *When you are full of food and drink,*
> *Satan sits where your spirit should,*
> *An ugly metal statue instead of the Kaaba (a Muslim holy rock).*
> *When you fast, good habits gather like friends who want to help.*
> *Fasting is Solomon's ring.*
> *Don't give it to some illusion and lose your power,*
> *But even if you have, if you have lost all will and control,*
> *They come back when you fast,*
> *Like soldiers appearing out of the ground, pennants flying above them.*
> *A table descends to your tents,*
> *Jesus' table.*
> *Expect to see it, when you fast,*
> *This table spread with other food, better than the broth of cabbages."*

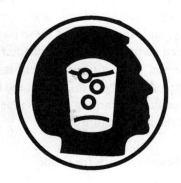

"Spiritual fasting is a mystical sacrifice of body and mind that opens the heart to God."

Preview of Chapter 8
Acid-Base Balance

This information about acid-base balance is relatively new for the general, health-conscious public. A proper acid-base balance of the system is intimately and critically related to good health. Although for some this may seem like complicated material, I have tried to compensate by illustrating the difficult and important concepts with pictures that capture the main points. In this chapter you will get a full practical education on acid-base theory, the role of alkaline and acid food balancing, alkaline and acid foods and supplements, symptoms of excess acid and alkalinity, and how to correct these imbalances. If you are not scientifically inclined, then go to the end of the chapter where a simple home approach for measuring and correcting your acid-base balance is offered. Spending time on this chapter so that you do understand is another way of taking responsibility for your health and learning to individualize your diet. Are you ready to take this part of the responsibility?

I.   Importance of acid-base balance for health

II. Acid-Base research findings

   A. Vegetarians are not always alkaline

   B. Meat eaters are not always acid

III. Acid- and alkaline-forming foods and supplements

IV. Symptoms of excess acidity or alkalinity

V.   What is a healthy body pH

VI. How to measure your own pH

VII. How to balance acid or alkaline conditions

VIII. Summary of three easy steps for achieving acid/alkaline balance

Chapter 8

Acid-Base Balance, a Basic Key to Health

The acid-base balance of the body is critical to good health. **One cannot seriously think about individualizing a diet without considering how the diet affects one's acid-base balance.** We are constantly generating acid waste products of metabolism that must be neutralized in some way if life is to be possible. Humans, therefore, need a continual supply of alkaline food to neutralize this ongoing acid generation. **Our very life and health depends on the ability of the body's physiological power to maintain the stability of blood pH at approximately 7.4.** This process is called homeostasis, or physiologic balance system.

The term pH means the "potential" of "Hydrogen." It is the amount of hydrogen ions in a particular solution. When there are a lot of hydrogen ions, the pH indicates an acid solution. When the amount of hydrogen ions is small, the pH will indicate an alkaline solution. The pH is measured on a scale from 0.00 to 14.00. Anything above 7.0 is defined as alkaline and anything below 7.0 is considered an acid pH. A pH of 7.0 is defined as neutral. The pH of pure water is 7.0.

The normal pH for all the tissues and fluids in the body, except the stomach, is alkaline. The following diagram shows the approximate pHs in the digestive system. In addition, the digestive secretions from the liver and liver bile range between 7.1 and 8.5. Bile from the gall bladder ranges from 5.0 to 7.7. If any of these pH systems are not at the optimal pH range, the digestive and metabolic enzymes in those areas and organs will function sub-optimally and we will suffer from decreased health. With the exception of the blood, all of these systems have a wide range of pH, in part so they can shift pH to maintain a balance of the blood pH, which must be maintained between the narrow range of 7.35 and 7.45.

Because the healthy pH of the blood exists in such a narrow range, the body gives a very high priority to maintaining the homeostasis of the blood pH at 7.4. Although all these tissues and fluids have their optimal enzymatic functioning in the alkaline part of their range, they will shift to less optimal acid range if they need to release alkaline minerals to keep the blood from becoming too acidic. For example, if the system becomes too acidic, the blood will take alkaline-forming elements from the digestive enzyme systems of the small intestine. What may happen then is that the pancreatic and liver digestive enzymes, which are designed to function maximally at the proper alkaline pH of the small intestine, do not have an alkaline pH strong enough for them to function properly and our digestion suffers. **A balanced blood pH, therefore, is intimately and critically related to good digestion** (see fig. 1).

The second priority of the delicate homeostasis system is to maintain the digestion so that nutrients will be assimilated and transported to various parts of

ALKALINE BLOOD

If the blood is too alkaline, the body shifts acid elements from the stomach to the blood to compensate.

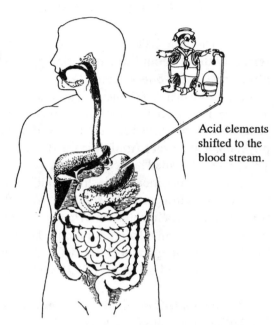

Acid elements shifted to the blood stream.

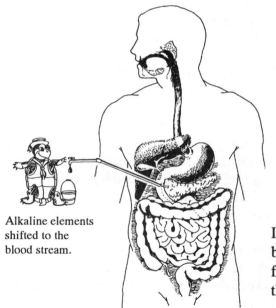

Alkaline elements shifted to the blood stream.

ACID BLOOD

If the blood is too acid, the body shifts alkaline elements from the small intestines to the blood to compensate.

Fig. 1

the body to maintain the proper acid-base balance of the blood and body in general. Proper digestion of nutrients supplies the essential electrolyte and other nutrients needed for optimal balance in the fluid surrounding the cells. This important fluid around the cells is called the extra-cellular fluid (ECF). If there are digestive imbalances, there will usually be electrolyte imbalances, particularly of sodium, potassium, magnesium, and calcium ions. These electrolyte imbalances affect the fluid transport system, which can be likened to ECF "inner oceans" in the body that carry nutrients and wastes in and out of the body. Electrolytes and other nutrients are necessary to carry on cellular oxidation and other metabolic functions necessary for the life of the cell. The ECF is able to absorb acid and other waste products from the cells. Poetically speaking, this inner ocean of the ECF reflects the outer ocean which once surrounded the single cell organisms which first lived in the ocean. Once organisms became more multicellular and more complex, they had to develop an inner ocean to continue to cleanse and supply oxygen and other nutrients to the cells which were no longer in direct contact with the outer ocean (see figs. 2 & 3).

The total fluid in our bodies is approximately 70% of our body weight, about the same percentage of water to land of planet earth. The fluid within the cells of our body accounts for 55% of our body weight. The ECF accounts for approximately 15% of the body weight. Five percent of the ECF is blood and 10% is the fluid in the tissues that bathes the cells.

If the fluid transport system or ECF has imbalanced concentrations of minerals, insufficient nutrients, or insufficient oxygen, then the cells cannot function appropriately and they begin to die. A basic teaching of modern physiology is that for the cells of the body to function properly and to thrive, there is an important requirement, and that is that the extracellular fluid which bathes the cells must have its composition controlled exactly throughout the day so that no single important element of the ECF varies by more than a few percentage points. **Maintaining correct acid-base homeostasis in the blood and the extracellular fluid is another key to health** (see fig. 4).

A healthy ECF is supported by properly functioning eliminative organs, such as the kidneys, liver, large intestine, and skin. These organs not only eliminate waste products and toxins, but are a main way the body eliminates excess acid or alkaline elements in its quest to maintain the blood pH and ECF pH in their normal ranges. By studying what is eliminated in the urine, one can see a reflection of the body's electrolyte and acid-base buffering mechanisms. For example, if the system is too acid, the kidney will eliminate acid through the urine. In this case, the urine pH is acid because acids are eliminated in the urine in an effort to make the blood more alkaline. The urine is a preventative health indicator. Its pH may vary from 4.8 to 8.4 on a day to day basis. The urine pH values guide us in the direction we need to go to maintain health. Significant blood pH changes are usually an indication of disease.

A healthy extracellular ocean which nurtures the cells.

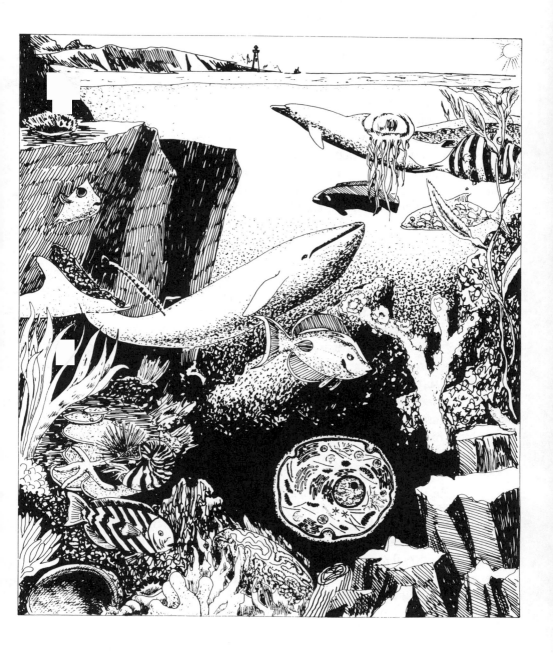

Fig. 2

An unhealthy toxic extracellular ocean which leads to cell misfunction and early cell death.

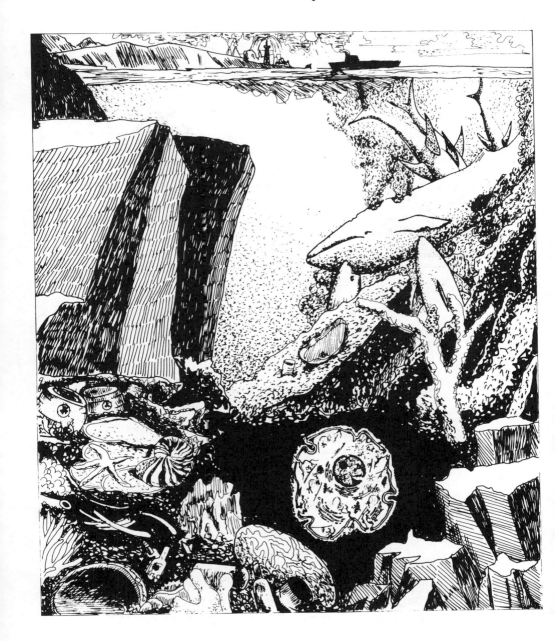

Fig. 3

ACID-BASE LINK TO HEALTH

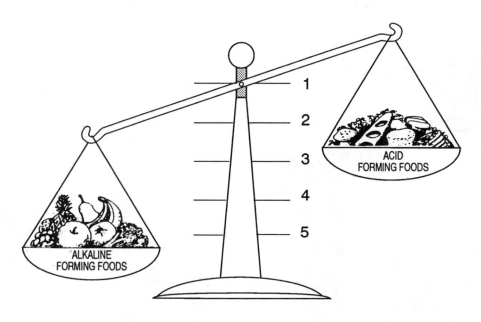

ACID-BASE LINK TO HEALTH

Appropriate acid/alkaline balance of food intake

⬇

Homeostatic blood pH at 7.4

⬇

Digestive enzymes throughout body
working at optimum pH

⬇

Electrolyte balance

⬇

Optimal extracellular fluid for cells to bathe in to absorb
nutrients, discharge toxins, and function at
maximum energy levels

Fig. 4

Importance of Diet for Balancing Acid-Base

There is a limitation, however, as to how much the body can compensate for acid-base imbalances if we do not change our diet to balance the acid and alkaline components coming into the system through our food. **Therefore, food intake plays a critical role in acid-base balance of the body.** If the body is not able to adequately compensate for an imbalanced diet, the body's internal environment becomes sub-optimal and eventually reaches a condition in which the cells cannot live. Many diseases are the result of the body's attempt to rebalance this internal environment. Some people feel that cancer is a condition that is accelerated by an acid condition of the body fluids. Cancer cells are able to live better than normal cells in an acid and low-oxygen ECF.

There are a variety of causes of acid-base imbalances, but the diet is the major factor in either balancing or unbalancing the pH. Generally, if our dietary intake includes too many acid-forming foods, such as high amounts of flesh foods, grains, pasteurized dairy, most beans, lots of fats, white sugars, and excess proteins in general, we will become acidic. If we eat too many alkaline foods, such as mostly fruits, vegetables, sea vegetables, and miso, we may become alkaline. Researchers around the world have suggested that the optimal ratio of alkaline-acid intake of foods is approximately 80% alkaline-producing foods and 20% acid-forming foods. This is a generalization that may turn out to be misleading in view of my following research which indicates each individual must find their own proper balance of acid and alkaline intake of food. In other words, **there is no single intake ratio of acid to alkaline foods which applies to everyone.**

I used to have the impression that all animal product eaters were acid, and vegetarians, especially raw food vegetarians, were alkaline. However, preliminary research I have conducted on one hundred and seventy-two new clients did not support this generalization. Much to my surprise, I found that 28.5% of the vegetarians had acid urines and 17% of the flesh food eaters had alkaline urines. Closer to my hypothesis was the finding that 46% of the flesh food eaters had acid urines and 28.5% of the vegetarians had alkaline urines. A higher percentage of vegetarians than flesh food eaters had what is conventionally considered a balanced urine pH between 6.3-6.9 (see fig. 5).

The system of urine pH I use is the 24-hour urine collection. I use this as the standard for this research and as my reference for discussion of urine pH values in general. This approach has two advantages. The first is that random urine pHs taken through the day are quite variable since the body pH usually cycles over 24 hours. The 24-hour urine gives the total amount of acid or alkaline elements that are eliminated in 24 hours, so it gives an average. The second advantage is that everyone can do this test on their own urine. The results of the measurement of the pH of these patients' 24-hour urine samples before beginning any treatment are on the chart. Alkaline was considered 7.0 or above. Acid was considered 6.2 or below. The flesh food eaters with a pH between 6.3 and 6.9 were often those people who ate meat just one or two times per week rather than daily. It seemed that the pH status of those who ate flesh foods less than one time a week resembled vegetarians more than flesh food eaters. My impression is that daily flesh food eaters generally have a higher percentage of acidity than the occasional flesh food eaters. Due to the way my data was collected, I was not able to sort the actual difference in pH between occasional flesh food eaten and daily ingestion of flesh food.

These results suggest, regardless of the diet, that there are other additional variables operating. One possible explanation is that some people have a constitutional tendency to be either acid or alkaline in their metabolism regardless of their diet. Rudolf Wiley, Ph.d., in his book *BioBalance,* has documented the same thing. Wiley's research also suggests, as does my preliminary work, that acid or alkaline levels of a person may vary with the cycle of the day. In women, Wiley reports that acid-alkaline cycles may vary either way during the premenstrual, preovulatory, and menses cycles. Much research needs to be done in this area. This means that females especially need to check their pH values during these three times to understand how to vary their diets to balance their rhythmic pH changes. The idea of a genetic predisposition to become either acid or alkaline is also supported in the Ayurvedic system, which has three physiological body types. The pitta type particularly tends to go into acid imbalance.

I suspect that some of the meat cravings that occasionally are observed when a person makes a transition to a vegetarian diet are a result of the person having an alkaline constitutional tendency and the vegetarian diet accentuating this tendency. The craving for flesh food is the organism's effort to bring the system into balance by acidifying the body with flesh food. The flesh food supplies the strong acids which bring the pH back to the familiar pH zone.

The critical point for those committed to a vegetarian diet for health, social, moral, economic, ecological, political, and spiritual reasons is that it is simple to acidify the system with vegetarian foods, apple cider vinegar, or with the specific use of live plant digestive enzymes. One does not have to resort to extreme measures like eating flesh foods to balance out the body. **It is possible on a vegetarian diet to bring the body into the proper acid-alkaline balance no matter what one's constitutional acid-base tendency is.**

The other major explanation for my results is **one cannot assume that complete digestion simply occurs automatically.** For example, if a vegetarian has an acid pH on a diet of alkalinizing foods, it suggests that the person's body is not properly breaking down the complex carbohydrates so that alkalinizing minerals are properly released into the system. If the digestion of the person were normal, these alkaline minerals would be making the system alkaline. A

ACID / BASE RESEARCH

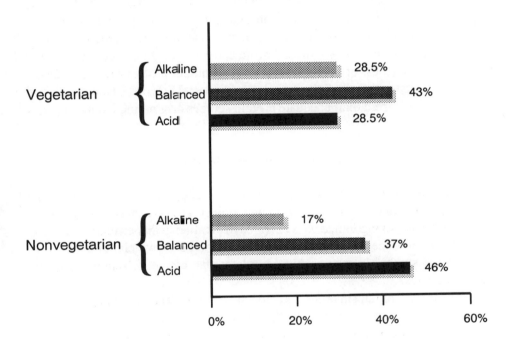

Fig. 5

vegetarian who has poor protein digestion would tend to be more alkaline than another vegetarian who has good protein digestion and who is eating the exact same diet. This is because effective digestion of protein acidifies the system.

The mental state of the person also plays an important role in the pH observed in the urine. I've observed vegetarians whose diet would normally make them alkaline, but because of their negative thinking they were instead acid.

All of the above explanations help us understand why we cannot automatically assume that all vegetarians will be alkaline and that all flesh-food eaters will automatically be acidic. My research results, however, also support the view that certain diets generally move the pH in one direction or the other.

One's constitutional tendency to be more acid or alkaline can be balanced by paying attention to one's mental state and ability to digest protein or complex carbohydrates. This, of course, cuts through the argument that there are some people who "just need to eat meat." More correctly, they just need to have the right plant enzymes, or take apple cider to stimulate protein digestion and to directly decrease the alkalinity to help them reestablish proper digestion and release of acids from their adequate protein sources originating from a vegetarian diet.

Acid Production is Normal

Our normal body metabolism is always producing acids. In the animal kingdom, alkaline is changed to acid and almost all of our waste products are acid. In the plant kingdom, acid is changed to alkaline in that primarily acid soil conditions produce primarily alkaline plants, some of which humans use as food. This symbiotic relationship completes one of nature's most exquisite natural cycles.

The human organism produces acid whenever one exercises; lactic acid and carbon dioxide are produced. In the intracellular fluid, the carbon dioxide released as a waste product from the cells is converted to carbonic acid. The sulfur and the phosphorous in our acid and protein foods are converted by oxidation to sulfuric acid and phosphoric acid. The complete digestion of protein foods makes hydrogen ions available to the system, which makes the body more acidic. The metabolic breakdown of proteins also produces uric acid which further acidifies the system. Urea is another protein by-product. It increases the fluid excretion of the kidneys in a way that causes the loss of much-needed, alkaline-forming minerals (see fig. 6).

Fats as a general class are slightly acid-forming or neutral because fat slows digestion, which makes for more putrefaction and hence more of an acidifying effect. Fat metabolism also produces acetic acid. The incomplete breakdown of fat produces ketones which also make the body acidic. Diabetic acidosis is an example of a severe form of this type of acidic condition.

126

NORMAL CELLULAR ACIDS

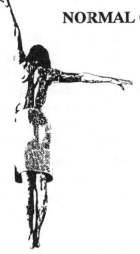

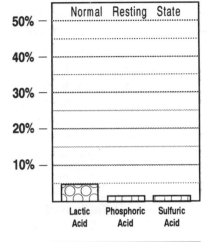

Normal Resting State

50% —
40% —
30% —
20% —
10% —

Lactic Acid | Phosphoric Acid | Sulfuric Acid

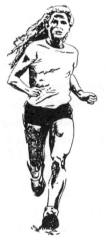

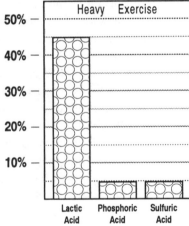

Heavy Exercise

50% —
40% —
30% —
20% —
10% —

Lactic Acid | Phosphoric Acid | Sulfuric Acid

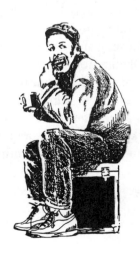

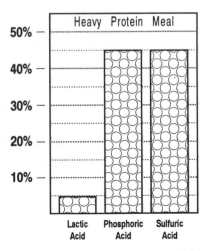

Heavy Protein Meal

50% —
40% —
30% —
20% —
10% —

Lactic Acid | Phosphoric Acid | Sulfuric Acid

Fig. 6

127

Simple carbohydrates, such as white sugar, are slightly acid-forming because they enter the system too quickly and metabolize too rapidly. This includes both monosaccharides (glucose) and disaccharides, such as sucrose (cane sugar), lactose, and maltose. The result of this is the production of lactic, butyric, pyroracemic and acetic acid. Due to their processing, these refined, simple carbohydrates are devoid of alkaline minerals. This further increases the acidity because the body must use up its alkaline minerals to buffer the slight acidity of the organic acids produced by the fast-burning, simple sugars. The complex carbohydrates, such as the grains, metabolize more slowly and evenly and do not produce these organic acids. Because of their alkaline minerals, complex carbohydrates that have more alkaline minerals than acid minerals in them create an alkalinizing effect. Millet and buckwheat are examples of slightly alkalinizing grains.

Definition of Acid- and Alkaline-forming Foods

It is important to understand that one cannot tell which foods are acid or alkaline by the taste of a food. There are several factors that determine whether a specific food renders the body more alkaline or acid. For example, a ripe, organic lemon, which is a food that contains high concentrations of organic acids, tastes acidic, and is classified as an acidic fruit, is actually an alkaline-forming food. This is because its high concentration of alkaline minerals has an overall effect of increasing the alkaline reserve of the body, thereby making the body more alkaline. The lemon's mild organic acids act as cleansing agents in the stomach. In the process of digestion these acids are oxidized into carbon dioxide and water, and therefore do not create an acid condition in the system.

Calcium, magnesium, sodium, potassium, and iron are the main alkalinizing minerals. Foods which have high concentrations of these minerals are considered alkaline-forming foods. Foods which are high in sulfur, phosphorous, iodine, and chlorine are acid-forming foods. Most natural foods have both acid- and alkaline-forming minerals in them. If the acid-forming minerals are greater in concentration, then the food is considered acid-forming and vice versa. One major way to determine the degree of the acid- or alkaline-forming power of a food is through chemical analysis in a medical laboratory. To determine the acid- or alkaline-forming potential of a food, it is first burned to its mineral ash and then dissolved in neutral pH water. The pH of this water is then tested to see if it is alkaline or acid. Because we can measure the exact alkalinity or acidity of a solution, we are able to rate just how acid-forming or alkaline-forming a particular food is (see fig. 7).

Acid- and Alkaline-formingChart
(for selected foods)

Very Acid-forming	Acid-forming	Neutral	Alkaline-forming	Very Alkaline-forming
Unripe cranberries	Unripe fruit		Sweet/sour cherries	Figs
Watermelon seed	Prunes		Ripe fruit	Ripe lemons
Yellow dock herb	Plums		Most vegetables	Chaparral
Walnuts	Yeast		Tomatoes	Carrot / beet juice
Peanuts •••	Kelp		Millet	Vegetable juice
Raw apple cider vinegar	Pasteurized/raw yogurt		Buckwheat	Miso
Sauerkraut	Pasteurized milk		Kelp	Vitamin K
Fermented foods	Cheese		Raw cow's milk ••	Calcium ascorbate
Eggs •	Pasteurized butter		Raw goat's milk	(Vitamin C)
Flesh foods •	Animal fat		Beansprouts	
Vitamin A	White sugar		String beans	
Ascorbic acid	Most beans		Azuki beans	
(Vitamin C)	Lentils		Soy beans	
	Kidney beans		Lima beans	
	Soy sauce		Onions	
	Soft drinks			
	Medical drugs			
	Alcohol			
	Most cooked grains: (rice, oats, etc.)			
	Soaked sprouted grains			
	Soaked sprouted wheat		Wheatgrass	Wheatgrass juice
	Most nuts: Soaked sprouted nuts		Sprouted almonds	
			Brazil nuts	
	Most seeds: Soaked sprouted seeds			
	Soaked sprouted alfalfa seeds		Alfalfa sprouts	
	Soaked sprouted sunflower seeds		Sunflower sprouts	
	Raw butter*	Honey**		
* between neutral and acid	Avocado*			
** between neutral and alkaline	Vegetable oils*			

- *Included for completeness, but not recommended.*

•• *There is no total agreement whether raw milk products have an acid/alkaline effect on the body. For example, clinical research by Dr. Crowfoot on urine pH after ingesting raw milk suggests that raw milk has an alkalizing effect. On the other hand, Dr.Morter feels that the recent increases in protein in the diet of dairy cows has resulted in a higher protein in milk, and therefore a higher acid ash that creates a more acid effect in the body.*

••• *Dangerous, high, pesticide residue on non-organic peanuts are the most pesticide-saturated food in the American diet. A mold aflatoxin,which is carcinogenic,often grows even on organic peanuts. Sundried organic peanuts may prevent aflatoxin growth and are without high peanut toxic residues. Arrowhead Mills has such a peanut product.*

Fig. 7

Yin / Yang   Acid - base
Qualities of Food

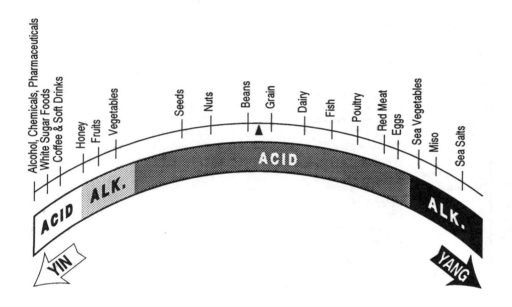

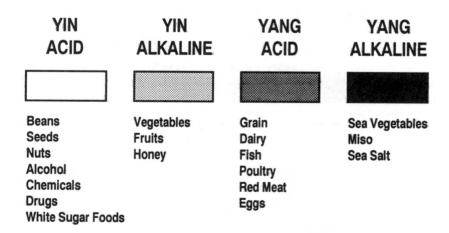

Fig. 8

Acid- and Alkaline-forming Foods

Using the above system, scientists have made tables of acid- and alkaline-forming foods. The following acid-alkaline chart was compiled by myself and Dr. Harold Krystal, an experienced clinician in this specific area. It was developed from a wide variety of sources, including our clinical experience of how food actually affects people. Flesh foods are acid-forming. Most grains are acid-forming, except millet and buckwheat. Most dairy products are acid-forming, especially if they are pasteurized and soured such as yogurt. Raw goat, human, and cow milk are slightly alkaline-forming. Hard cheeses are acidic. Butter is neutral to acidic. Most oils are slightly acid-forming or neutral. Most nuts, beans, peas, simple sugars, and vegetarian proteins are acidic to some extent. Soybeans are slightly alkaline, as is tofu. String, lima, and azuki beans are also slightly alkaline-forming. Almonds, brazil nuts, and sesame seeds are slightly alkaline. Peanuts are strongly acid-forming.

There is considerable confusion about the acidity or alkalinity of fruits. Almost all vegetables and fruits which are **ripe** are alkaline-forming. Fruits and vegetables grown in inorganic, commercially prepared soils are less alkaline-forming because they are grown in mineral-depleted soils. Prunes, plums, and cranberries have benzoic and other acids which make them acid-forming (see fig. 7).

Most fruits which are **not ripe** are acid-forming. One can even test these ripe or unripe fruits or vegetables with a special type of pH meter and see a difference between the two stages of the same fruit. For example, in a freshly ripened banana with a moderate amount of black spots, the pH was 6.4. On an almost ripe banana with a few black spots, the pH was as acid as 5.7. The acidity of cranberries is due largely because they are typically harvested and prepared in an unripe, sour state. Cranberries that are left to ripen are sweeter and alkaline-producing. Generally, one can say that fruits and vegetables and certain herbs will be the most alkalinizing of all food substances. Proteins, especially flesh foods, are the most acidifying. Flesh food protein produces a lot of urea which also causes a loss of alkaline-forming minerals through the urine. Fats, which are slightly acidifying, increase their acidifying effect because they clog the arteries and decrease circulation so that cells do not get enough oxygen. Decreased oxygen to the cells causes increased cell toxicity and death. Dead and dying cells further acidify the system.

Generally speaking, the yin acid and yang acid foods create the most acidity. These, unfortunately, reflect the high-protein flesh food, high-fat, high-sugar, low-complex carbohydrate, all-American diet. Fortunately, the various Congressional reports, such as the McGovern Committee on Diet and Health, brought some awareness regarding the hazards of such a diet. The general tendency in Western cultures is to eat an acidic-producing diet. This is perhaps becoming true of the affluent classes of third world cultures who want to mimic

Sugar   Cane

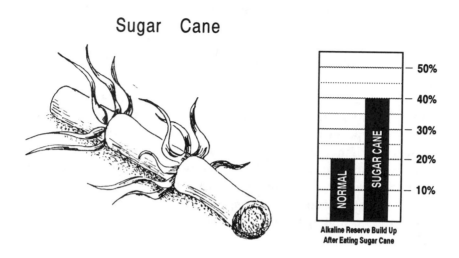

Alkaline Reserve Build Up
After Eating Sugar Cane

Unprocessed Whole Sweet Food Contains Alkaline Elements

Candy   Bar

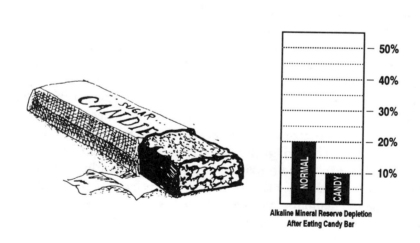

Alkaline Mineral Reserve Depletion
After Eating Candy Bar

Processed Sweet Missing Alkaline Minerals

Fig. 9

the United States by following a high flesh food diet as a prestigious sign of affluence (see fig. 8).

Other foods which have some acidifying effect are the yin acid foods, such as: white sugars, white flour, synthetic vitamins, saccharin, chemical additives, colorings, preservatives, refined and heavily processed foods, prescription and psychedelic drugs, soft drinks, and other synthetic drugs. These products are acid-forming because they either never contained alkaline-forming minerals or the minerals were leached out during chemical processing. Compounded by this is that most of these foods have a slight acidifying effect of their own, which is then further compounded by the fact that the alkaline minerals have been leached out by the refining process. The net result is the alkaline mineral reserves of the body are used up in the remineralizing of these refined foods and chemicals for assimilation. This depletes the body stores of alkaline-forming minerals and thus creates a shift toward acidity in the body (see fig. 9).

In order for the body to excrete metabolic acids, such as sulfuric acid or phosphoric acid, from the system without hurting the kidneys or the bowels, it neutralizes them with the alkaline-forming mineral salts such as calcium, magnesium, sodium, and potassium. When these alkaline reserves are diminished or used up in the system, the body shifts toward becoming more acidic. The body then begins to draw the calcium, magnesium, sodium and potassium from the nerve cells to help buffer the blood. The result is that the nervous system begins to malfunction. Mental clarity begins to diminish. The mind slows and eventually coma occurs below an acid blood pH of 6.95. A slow mind and decreased mental clarity are typical of those whose diet is too acidic. This is why it is important to maintain high alkaline mineral salt reserves to neutralize emergency situations in which the body becomes acidic. This is done by eating a diet high in fruits and vegetables (see fig. 10).

In my clinical observations on myself and my clients with closely monitored urine pHs, the sprouting of nuts, seeds, beans, and grains turns them closer to a neutral or alkaline pH. Most sprouted seeds and grains eventually become alkaline because they turn into vegetables, which are alkaline. There still is not sufficient data on the question of the effects of sprouting on seeds and nuts to make a definitive statement.

Effects of Supplements and Medicines on Acid-Base Balance

Another common cause of acid-base imbalances are the supplements or medicines people take. Most synthetic vitamins are acidifying. One of the most acidifying of all is ascorbic acid. Its very name reveals that it is acid by nature. People who are acid and taking ascorbic acid (the synthetic form of vitamin C separated from its natural components) should consider switching to another, more balanced form of vitamin C if their urine pH is less than 6.3. This is because this form of vitamin C will tend to make them even more acidic. Vitamin C in

EFFECTS OF ACIDITY ON NERVOUS SYSTEM

In order to preserve the health of the body and keep the pH of the blood from being acidic, the body will take alkaline minerals from the nervous system and put them back into the blood stream.

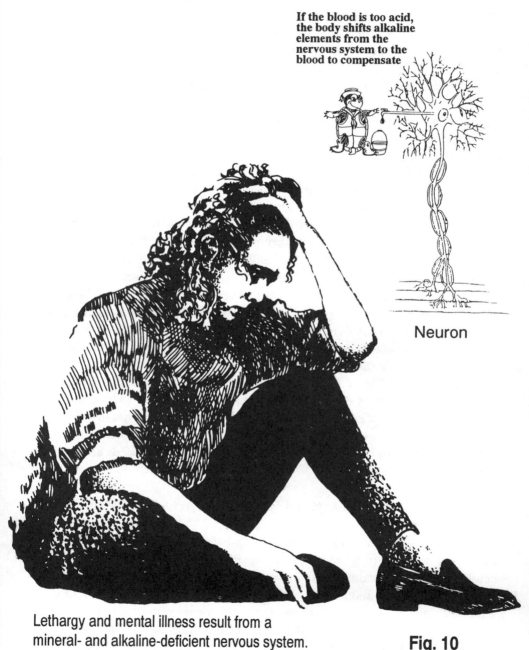

If the blood is too acid, the body shifts alkaline elements from the nervous system to the blood to compensate

Neuron

Lethargy and mental illness result from a mineral- and alkaline-deficient nervous system.

Fig. 10

the form of calcium or sodium ascorbates, or in the form of buffered C on the market, are all alkalinizing. Vitamin A, whether synthetic or not, is also acidifying. This does not seem to be true for beta-carotene. If someone needs to become more acid, one could use ascorbic acid C and vitamin A in moderation to achieve this effect. Vitamin K is alkalinizing and it helps to keep calcium, one of the main alkalinizing minerals, in its ionizable form in the blood serum. The ionizable form of calcium is the utilizable form in the blood. The intelligent use of supplements requires a thorough understanding of their effects on the acid-base balance of the organism.

Symptoms of Excess Acidity

Most authorities agree that an overacid body is a precondition for the onset of either acute or chronic disease. The world-famous nutritionist Paavo Airola feels that acidosis is one of the basic causes of all disease. An acidic system is fertile ground for disease for several reasons. The more acidic a system becomes, the less the alkaline biochemic buffers are able to maintain the blood's healthy pH of 7.4. One way the system compensates in order to preserve the blood pH is to deposit excess acid substances in the tissues and joints. This is one reason Airola feels that an acid body greatly contributes to the development of arthritis.

As the cytoplasm (protoplasm of a cell surrounding the nucleus of the cell) becomes more acidic due to an acid ECF and acidic blood, there is a decrease in the bioelectric potential that exists between the naturally acidic cell nucleus and the alkaline cytoplasm that surrounds the cell nucleus. These two poles serve essentially as a cell battery that maintains the bioelectric potential that is needed to drive cell function and life force. The degree of bioelectric vitality is a measure of cell vitality. The less bioelectric potential, the less vitality and function. When there is no bioelectric potential left in a cell, cell death occurs. The more acidic we get, the less bioelectric potential there is in the cells and the less life force there is. It is interesting that raw foods seem to be exceptional in their ability to restore the bioelectrical potential to the cells (see fig. 11).

There are several contributing factors that make us acidic aside from flesh foods and/or grains, simple sugars, fats, and highly processed and refined foods. These factors are listed on pages 146-147.

The major consequence of systemic acidosis is a depression of the central nervous system. **An acidic person often experiences dulled mentality, slower thinking processes, headaches, and depression.** Fatigue and muscle stiffness are other major symptoms. Pain in the lower back and generalized muscle stiffness is secondary to a low calcium state. The calcium loss of other alkalinizing minerals are used up in buffering the acidity. The more acidic a person becomes, the more irritable he or she becomes as the calcium, magnesium, potassium, and sodium are lost from the muscle and nerve cells. Tension in neck and shoulders, arthritis, and

135

FULLY CHARGED BATTERY

Alkaline Cytoplasm,
Acid Nucleus –
has a charge between poles

A healthy cell is like a battery fully
charged with bio-electricity!

Healthy Cell

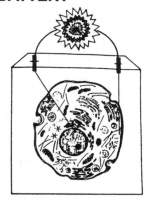

BATTERY WITH NO CHARGE

Acid Cytoplasm,
Acid Nucleus–
has no charge between poles

An unhealthy acidic cell is like
a dead battery!

Unhealthy Cell

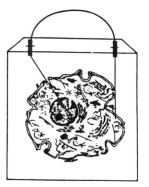

LIVE FOODS CHARGE CELLS

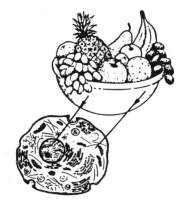

Fig. 11

ACIDITY SYMPTOMS

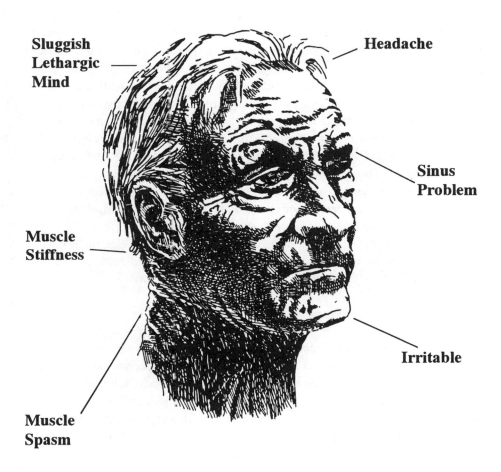

Sluggish Lethargic Mind

Headache

Sinus Problem

Muscle Stiffness

Irritable

Muscle Spasm

Fig. 12

osteoporosis are also typical problems. Muscle spasm and twitching also occur from the low calcium. There is a general sense of fatigue and weakness from a toxemia that develops because the kidneys are working so hard to excrete the acids that they do not function as well in eliminating other types of systemic toxins that continue to build up in the course of everyday life (see fig. 12).

Stomach aches, nausea, vomiting, and chest pain are also common in overly acidic people. People who are acidic may have an irritation in the gastric linings of the small and large intestines. Gastritis and ulcers occur more frequently. Even the urethral lining may begin to burn from too much acid irritation. Because of the irritation of the mucous linings, the food moves through the digestive system too fast for the body to fully absorb and assimilate the necessary nutrients. This fast digestion may leave undigested food coating the intestines, which has the effect of impairing assimilation. Minerals are often leached out because of the increased gastric motility. Constipation is another symptom that sometimes occurs. Fat, protein, and carbohydrate digestion are often compromised because the body is not able to maintain the proper alkalinity needed for the pancreatic enzymes to function properly in the small intestine. Some researchers feel that cancer growth is stimulated by an acid system, since cancer cells, and not normal cells, are able to thrive in an acidic, anoxic ECF.

If the urine pH of a 24-hour urine collection drops below 6.3, the body can be said to be abnormally acidic. It is at this point that the acidity begins to negatively affect the function of the body's enzyme systems.

Symptoms of Excess Alkalinity

The major symptoms of alkalosis in vegetarians that I have observed directly is an overexcitablity of the nervous system. Usually the peripheral nerves and muscles are affected first. The first sign of this is muscle twitching, especially in the face or forearm. There is an increased general tendency for muscle spasm and cramps. Although I have never seen it happen, this supposedly can progress to a full scale spasm of all the muscles, which is called tetany. Some osteopaths and chiropractors report that muscle and joint adjustments do not hold when the body is too alkaline. Central nervous system dysfunction may also manifest as extreme nervousness. Another tendency of excess alkalinity is to become "spacey," with its accompanying decrease in one's ability to concentrate. One can also become slightly euphoric with a high alkaline pH. Many people enjoy this effect, but for some it may be threatening. In people susceptible to epilepsy, simply overbreathing can increase their alkalinity and predispose them to convulsions. One reason for this increased nerve sensitivity is that there is a decrease in ionized calcium. The acid-forming, hydrogen positive ions from the protein are used to try to buffer the alkaline system. The positive ions of the calcium then are drawn out of their ionic state in the ECF and become protein-

SYMPTOMS OF EXCESS ALKALINITY

Anxiety / excitability

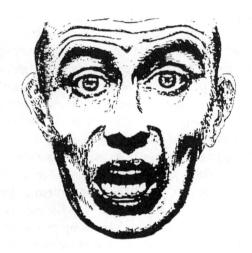

Muscle spasm

SYMPTOMS OF EXCESS ALKALINITY

1. Anxiety & excitability; overexcitability of central nervous system

2. Muscle spasm, tetany, low tolerance of physical stimulation & muscle tension

3. Slow injury recovery, physical adjustments don't hold well

4. Muscle pain

Fig. 13

bound. In this protein-bound state, calcium is much less available to the nerve and muscle cells. This tendency toward hypersensitivity and a euphoric spaciness are the two symptoms I have seen in vegetarians who become too alkaline. In my clinical experience, these symptoms may happen more often at urine pHs of 7.5 or higher. Fortunately, these symptoms and the excess alkalinity are relatively easy to correct with intelligent dietary changes that take into account acid/alkaline factors (see fig. 13).

Slowed intestinal peristalsis or activity and constipation are other symptoms that have been reported. This symptom may occur in both types of alkalinity, but I do not see it commonly in vegetarians who are a urine pH of 7.2 or less. Because of the increased alkalinity, acid is taken away from the stomach's secretions in an attempt to buffer the alkaline blood. This results in a consequent decrease in protein digestion in the stomach because there isn't enough HCL available for protein digestion. If the pH of the urine goes above 8.0, it is possible to have more acute indigestion and an inflamed descending colon because of the incomplete protein digestion and clogging of the colon. These sort of symptoms may also occur when the system is too acid and when there is ammonia in the urine. With a high alkalinity there may also be a decreased assimilation of protein. This contributes to problems with hypoglycemia because, normally, when there is adequate digestion of protein, 56% of all digested protein is slowly metabolized to glucose in a way that helps balance the blood sugar. Decreased protein assimilation has also been associated with bleeding gums and pyorrhea.

A lack of hydrochloric acid may also compromise part of the immune system because there is not enough HCL in the stomach to digest parasites and bacteria. As in acid conditions, there is also an increase in colds and flus with excessive alkalinity. My very consistent clinical observation is that people on a high percentage of raw food in their diets become strongly resistant to colds and flus if their urine pH stays equal to, or less than, 7.2.

What is a Healthy 24-Hour Urine pH?

It seems possible that vegans and raw food vegetarians whose diets tend to make them more alkaline, may undergo a slight physiological shift in what constitutes normal pH values as compared with a mixed sample of flesh food eaters. I believe, based on preliminary research on clients, that vegans and raw fooders may undergo a physiological shift of .1 to .2 urine pH points toward more alkalinity and still have normal physiological functioning and good health. This hypothesis is suggested because those who have stabilized on a primarily raw food, vegetarian diet are usually in excellent health, without any symptoms of excess alkalinity even though their urine pH may be 7.2. This is a hypothesis based on my own self-observation and clinical monitoring of some of my clients who fit into this category of nondairy vegetarian and raw fooders. My general observation is many 80-95% raw food vegetarians feel, and are, healthy at a pH of 7.2.

Dr. Theodore A. Baroody, Jr., author of several health books and a person involved in studying spiritual evolution, has suggested, based on his own personal and clinical experience, that as one evolves spiritually, the body becomes lighter and transforms physiologically to become more alkaline. In my work with myself and clients who are 80% or more raw food vegetarians and also on a spiritual path, I too have observed this phenomenon: **that people who are evolving spiritually become lighter, more alkaline, and still maintain improved, if not good, health.** In time, perhaps, these clinical impressions will be substantiated with more documented clinical research.

Dr. Morter, another researcher in this field, and author of *Correlative Urinalysis* and *Your Health, Your Choice,* in a personal communication with me, stated the average urine pH range which is compatible with optimal health is approximately between 6.8 and 7.2. He has even seen people be quite healthy at pHs of 7.8. He does not feel it is possible for people to have too much alkaline reserve. This is because the body is always producing acid which balances the excess alkaline reserve built up from a vegetarian diet. The body, on the other hand, does not produce alkalinity. Alkaline mineral reserve comes from a dietary intake of alkaline foods. Dr. Loomis, who has much clinical experience in this area, in a personal communication, supports the idea that between 6.3 to 6.8 for non-vegetarians or lactovegetarians seemed within normal ranges and that around 7.0 was safe for vegetarians eating mostly fruits, vegetables, or raw foods.

One of my long-term, 90% raw food clients, who keeps close watch of her urine pH, has noticed becoming spacey and suffering from a lack of concentration at a urine pH of 7.5–7.8. Just taking some acid food like a piece of bread is enough to bring her pH closer to a urine pH of 7.2–7.3 where she feels healthy and strong. At a 24-hour urine pH of 7.2–7.3 she is feeling healthier and more vital than she has in years. The fact that she feels excellent at a urine pH of 7.3 raises the question as to how alkaline can one become and remain healthy. I had another patient who had been chronically ill, weak, and mentally confused for more than 5 years. Her initial 24-hour urine was acidic. When her pH reached 7.1 in the treatment program, all her symptoms went away and she felt filled with her old energy. Some vegetarians, especially raw food vegetarians, feel excellent at pHs as high as 7.2. Above 7.2 seems to be the area in which the pH starts to become too high for optimal health. **It's pivotal then, to find the 24-hour urine pH which makes one feel the best, and then determine the correct ratio of acid and alkaline foods to keep it at the right pH for you.**

Is alkalinity part of an evolutionary process as suggested by Dr. Baroody? In answer to this important question, I feel that it is possible for some people to become too alkaline and develop symptoms at urine pH levels of 7.5 and above. Urine pHs of 6.8 to 7.2 seem to be quite healthy, particularly after the person has spent a period of time on a vegetarian diet in which the body has slowly shifted its physiology toward a more optimal state of health. The final determination is how one feels and whether there are any symptoms of "alkalosis" after an extended period of time at a particular alkaline pH.

A 24-hour urine pH below 6.3 is generally considered acidotic by myself and most researchers using the 24-hour urine system.

How to Measure Your Own Acid-Base Balance

Measuring the acid-base balance of the body at your own home is easiest done by collecting all urine which is produced in 24 hours, usually the second urine of the morning through the first urine of the next day. Then shake the total collection a few times and dip in some pH paper and read it. **Don't be shy, get to know yourself—test your urine; it's sterile!** The least expensive and most accurate pH paper I've found for my clients is pHydrion paper by Micro Essential Laboratory, Inc., Brooklyn, N.Y. 11210. The range is from 5.5 to 8.0.

> **For nonvegetarians and lactovegetarians (vegetarians who eat dairy) a generally good pH range is 6.3 to 6.9. For vegetarians who do not eat dairy and for raw food vegetarians, 6.3 to 7.2 is within a safe range** (see fig. 14).

In addition to the urine pH, I also like to have a saliva pH. It is thought that the saliva pH is an indicator of alkaline reserve in the body and the condition of the pH of the cells. **A normal saliva pH taken before eating in the morning and before meals is 6.8 to 7.5.** It should become more alkaline after meals, up to a pH of 7.2. Dr. Morter's clinical research indicates that if the morning saliva pH is below 6.2, it suggests an acid system with an inadequate amount of alkaline minerals, but with some alkaline reserve. If the saliva pH is between 5.5 and 5.8 with no rise in pH after a meal, it means the body is extremely acid and there are no alkaline reserves left.

Although more research needs to be done on this question of optimal body pH for vegetarians, and especially raw food vegetarians, there are guidelines that go beyond laboratory results. Perhaps the best way to ascertain whether one is functioning at an optimal pH for oneself is by the following characteristics.

Optimal pH Function Indicators

1. Good energy
2. A calm nervous and muscle system
3. Bowels are moving regularly and the digestion is effective
4. Doesn't catch colds and flus
6. General feeling of physical, mental, and spiritual vitality and clarity

URINE - may not be pleasant to smell or look at, but checking your urine to learn about your own acid/alkaline chemistry helps you understand yourself. It gives information about your healthy ratio of acid- and alkaline-forming foods and how your acid/alkaline balance shifts with your monthly cycle or stress.

VISION

BLACKBOARD FACTS

My overall impression is that one's physiologically healthy pH shifts more toward the alkaline as one becomes more spiritualized and the diet contains more and more raw food. As with diet, the pH change reflects both the cause and effect of one's overall, improved health.

How to Balance pH

Our bodies are simultaneously both alkaline and acid at the same time. These two tendencies become one in a dynamic equilibrium. Striving to give the body the optimal percentage of acid- or alkaline-forming foods helps to maintain this balance. One can check the pH of one's 24-hour urine. Based on the pH results, one can begin to organize one's diet toward an alkaline-acid balance of foods that brings the pH to normal. At the same time, I suggest that there are some individual variations. I also try to explore if the pH changes before, during, and after menses, as well as pre-ovulatory. Men may also have monthly cycles with their pH, but the times to check are not so obvious. If the body tends to shift toward more alkaline or acid on certain days, then the appropriate approach is to adjust one's acid-alkaline food intake on those days to compensate for the body's own shifting. For example, if during premenstrual time one becomes acidic, then it's appropriate to eat more alkaline foods during this premenstrual time.

At the normal range of pH, all the enzymes and electrolytes of the different digestive systems, organ systems, and glandular systems function optimally. When the enzymes and electrolytes are optimally functioning, the cells of all the glands and organs also begin to work at maximum function. Consequently, the body begins to reorganize back into a stable, healthy homeostasis. I am not saying this is a cure for all diseases. Bringing the urine pH back into the normal range is a preventative measure. It is an attempt to reestablish homeostasis. When the body has become so deranged that the blood pH is no longer at 7.4, usually deeper structural levels of pathology have been reached that take a lot more skill in reversing. The urine pH imbalances tell more about the body on a preventative level. Blood pH abnormalities reflect body pathology.

There are two primary and complementary approaches to balancing the pH. One is eating foods and herbs that keep one healthy and help one reestablish one's acid-base balance. This, of course, assumes that one is digesting the foods one is eating. The second major approach is to use live plant digestive enzymes to help digest the foods that were not being digested. For example, if one is too alkaline, it is beneficial to eat more protein because when protein is fully digested, it brings acid elements into the system. This only works when one is able to properly digest protein. Without full digestion there is not an acidifying effect by eating the protein. Plant protein digestive enzymes are indicated for

144

solving this problem. The same issue exists if one is too acid and is unable to fully digest complex carbohydrates. The appropriate plant enzymes are needed to activate full complex carbohydrate digestion so that the alkalinizing minerals of the complex carbohydrates can fully be released into the system to build up the alkaline reserve and alkalinize the system.

Incomplete digestion of fats tends to release acid by-products, such as ketones, into the system. Enzymes are needed that will give us a complete digestion of fat so there will not be a metabolic acid build-up.

There are other factors which tend to make the body system acidic. One is poor breathing habits. The deeper and better one breathes, the easier it is to remove acid from the system by blowing off carbon dioxide and thus decreasing the carbonic acid in the blood. One reason most people are slightly acidic in the morning is that during sleep our breathing decreases in depth and rate. This results in the retention of carbon dioxide and hence the build up of carbonic acid in the blood. Heavy exercise without proper breathing or ventilation builds up both a lactic acid and a carbon dioxide. Poor oxygenation of the cells creates poor cellular oxidative metabolism and eventually cellular death. Ninety percent of our oxidative metabolism is supplied by the oxygen we breath. Deep breathing exercises in the morning, throughout the day, and before and after exercise, will reduce acid build-up. Repressed emotions, excessive anger, "acid" thoughts, and other emotions can also increase acidity. I've documented that people with normally balanced pHs become acidic after negative "acidic" thoughts. In the Ayurvedic system, the pitta constitutional type tends to be acid. They become particularly acid with anger. The stress of an excessive lifestyle also contributes to acidity.

The converse can happen as well. For instance, in one case, when a client of mine let go of her "acid" negativities without any dietary change, her urine pH, which had been previously acid, became balanced. One patient, after a major psychological breakthrough from negativity, had her acid urine go to an alkaline pH of 7.5.

Ways to Alkalinize the System

1. Decrease or stop the intake of flesh food.
2. Decrease protein intake in general.
3. Decrease the intake of fat.
4. Decrease intake of pasteurized dairy.
5. Minimize yin acid foods such as white sugar.
6. Eat more raw fruits and vegetables and their juices.
7. Eat more raw, biogenic foods, such as sprouted greens, grasses, and certain alkaline-forming nuts, seeds, and grains. All sprouted nuts, seeds, beans, and

grains shift from their acidic-forming tendencies to either neutral or slightly alkaline-forming. Protein taken in this sprouted form is an excellent way to fulfill one's dietary requirements without making the system excessively acidic.

8. Take specific alkalinizing foods and herbs that have been proven clinically to alkalinize the body, which are: juice of fresh lemon at least two times per day, chaparral tea or herbal extract, apricots, and vitamin K foods. The outer leaf of cabbage is high in vitamin K. Wheatgrass juice is an excellent alkalinizer.
9. Use plant digestive enzymes to improve poor digestion of complex carbohydrates.
10. Use plant enzymes to improve poor fat digestion and therefore prevent the production of extra acids from incomplete metabolic breakdown.
11. Keep emotionally balanced and avoid creating acid emotions.
12. Live a balanced, low-stress lifestyle.
13. Detox and heal the kidneys, liver, and bowel.
14. Breath deeply all day long.
15. Avoid heavy, prolonged, and strenuous exercise.

Ways to Acidify the System

1. My first choice in balancing the tendency to become alkaline is the use of raw, organic, apple cider vinegar. In addition to its pH balancing affect, I agree with Dr. Paul Bragg, who espoused the use of vinegar many years ago as a great tonic. Use only apple cider vinegar which is organic and has not been pasteurized or filtered. It is a real food "with a mother lode" still in it. If the apple cider is clear, it is probably acetic acid, synthetically produced from coal tar, or distilled apple cider vinegar. This type should not be used. The truly "living" apple cider vinegar comes directly from the juice of fermented apples. It has many enzymes in it and is extremely high in potassium, as well as phosphorus, chlorine, natural organic sodium, magnesium, sulphur, iron, copper, silicon, and other minerals. It also contains the organic acid called malic acid which is helpful in dissolving body toxins. Paul Bragg has found that apple cider vinegar has been beneficial for "softening the arteries," clearing crystal deposits out of the muscle tissue, supplying much-needed potassium to the body, and helping to heal a variety of ailments, such as sore throats, bladder infections, and prostrate disorders. Apple cider vinegar stimulates digestion if taken five minutes before meals. If held in the mouth for thirty seconds, it stimulates ptyalin secretion for starch digestion as well as stimulates gastric enzyme secretion. The amount may vary from a few drops in water before meals to two tablespoons with meals or in salad dressings. Although often recommended to be taken with honey in a ratio of two teaspoons of apple cider vinegar with one of honey in a glass of water before meals, according to Patricia Bragg, and in my own experience, using honey is not necessary to produce the beneficial effects.

2. Improve protein digestion with plant enzymes.
3. Increase protein intake with nuts, seeds, and grains; walnuts are particularly acidifying, as is corn. I have one client who is able to regulate her acid-alkaline balance by eating varying quantities of walnuts and adjusting the percentage of the soaked nuts and seeds she takes in.
4. The herb yellow dock is another excellent acidifier.
5. Watermelon seeds also have an enzyme that is very acidifying.
6. Fermented foods, such as sauerkraut, which is high in lactic acid, support the growth of healthy intestinal flora and are also good acidifiers.
7. Cranberry juice is also good. Onions and garlic have been cited as acidifying as well.
8. Vitamin A from animal sources.
9. Ascorbic acid.
10. Exercise strenuously.

I want to emphasize that the above-mentioned foods and herbs really work in actual practice. If we know how to use Mother Nature's gifts, she will serve us well.

The ultimate balancing of the acid and base is to integrate the duality in our diet, as well as in our lives. In this way we do not polarize out of fear in a senseless acid versus alkaline diet debate. Cultivating this sort of attitude toward dietary oneness helps lead to a larger sense of spiritual wholeness rather than the fear and separation created by duality. In this basic way we take "the acid" out of our lives.

Summary of Practical Steps for Acid-Alkaline Balance
1. Take 24-hour urine at appropriate times during the month.
2. Shift the balance of acid/alkaline-forming foods to make the 24-hour urine reach 6.3–7.2 if vegetarian and 6.3–6.9 if a flesh food eater.
3. If more approaches are needed, refer to acid or alkalinizing charts.

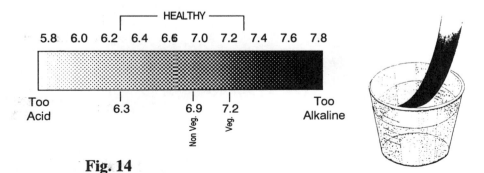

Fig. 14

Preview of Chapter 9
A New Paradigm of Nutrition

In order for me to relate the subtleties of the human organism and the subtleties of our food to the wonderment of spiritual life, I had to develop a new theory of nutrition which included God as the ultimate source of all nutrition. This theoretical chapter gives the reader a framework for understanding the physical and nonphysical meaning of the word nutrition. It allows us to understand certain spiritual phenomenon and recent nutritional research which the old model of nutrition cannot even begin to adequately explain. It is a conceptual model that helps us become more conscious about what we eat and how it affects us. Are you ready to take this addition step of awareness in your conscious eating program?

   I. Spiritualization of the body

  II. Foundations of new nutritional theory

    A. God is the ultimate source of nutrition on every level

    B. Subtle organizing energy fields (SOEFs)

    C. Why material-mechanistic theory of nutrition is not complete

 III. SOEFs in food

    A. Processed food depletes SOEFs

    B. Fresh, raw, live food most energizes our SOEFs

Chapter 9

A New Paradigm of Nutrition

Perhaps the most important way to understand and to commune with Mother Nature is to develop a nurturing relationship with her. Without the nutrients she supplies us we could not survive. In a basic way, what we eat and how we care for ourselves affects how we relate to the ecology issues of the planet. Ecological reform starts with ourselves. How can we possibly come into a meaningful harmony with the rest of nature if we pollute ourselves? If we do not take care of our own inner rivers and streams (circulatory system), our own inner atmosphere (lungs), and our own soil (skin and tissues) in a way that brings us into harmony with ourselves as a glorious manifestation of nature, how can we believe that we can take care of the planet? As we change our attitudes about our own bodily ecology, we will begin to change our attitudes about the larger ecology of the planet. Our own insensitivity to our inner nature begets insensitivity to the outer world of nature. Conscious eating doesn't exist separately from the planet.

Our spiritual development is also linked to the quality of our nutrition. Presently we are part of what I perceive as a rising spiral of planetary consciousness that is bringing about an ever-increasing amount of spiritual awareness among the people of the world. In this process of awakening, if the body is not able to raise its vibration rate to keep up with the rest of the spiritualization process, it is possible to slip into a state of imbalance. There needs to be a corresponding spiritualization of the body that keeps us in harmony with our expanding mental and spiritual awareness.

By consciously building the type of physical body that is able to be sensitive to, attract, conduct, nurture, and hold, the higher spiritualizing energies, we become more capable of holding the full power of God's Light. This approach is what I refer to as "full body enlightenment" in which we experience ourselves as the body rather than simply *in* the body. In this context, the body is not separate from spirit, but is the manifestation of spirit. Spiritual development is an essential building block of the foundation with which to attain a full nutritional understanding.

Perspectives on Nutrition

All comes from God and is nourished by God. The energetic power of God is the ultimate source of all nutrition.

> "...that He might make thee know that man doth not live by
> bread only, but by everything that proceedeth out of the mouth
> of the Lord doth man live." (Deut. 8:3)

> "In the beginning was the Word, and the Word was with God,
> and the word was God." (John 1:1)

This Divine cosmic force, manifesting at various levels of density, is the most basic and primary nutrient on which our organism can nourish itself. From the perspective of these preceding two biblical quotes, we can consider all levels of energy available to us as nutrients. This includes the pure, nonmaterial, cosmic force, or virtual energy, as some quantum physicists call it. Sunlight is also a major nutrient, as well as radiation from the other stars (stellar) and moon (lunar) energies, oxygen, electromagnetic radiation from the earth, and the densest, and most tasty condensation of energy, our material food from the vegetable kingdom. The expansion of our understanding to include the wide spectrum of the nutrients that nature gives us broadens our understanding of what, in fact, qualifies as a nutrient. The aspect of this new nutritional paradigm that food is not only material, but also energy, is fully acknowledged in the Chinese, Tibetan, and Indian Ayurvedic systems of health. In our Judaic-Christian heritage there is also such a tradition that energy is the original, essential nutrient. In *The Forgotten Books of Eden*, in the section of the *Secrets of Enoch*, Enoch was said to have ascended alive for 33 days and then returned to share his teachings to his children. He said:

> "Hear, child, from the time when the Lord anointed me with the
> ointment of his glory, there has been no food in me (material
> food), and my soul remembers not earthly enjoyment, neither
> do I want anything earthly."

Two famous examples of living on the direct, nonmaterial, nutritive energies of the divine are that of Moses, who spent a total of 80 days on Mt. Sinai without food or water, and Jesus, who spent 40 days and nights in the desert without food or water. In John (4:31), when Jesus' disciples said "Rabbi eat," he said to them, "I have food to eat which you do not know...." Two major inferences from these examples can be made. One is that these great ones reached a level of spiritual transformation on a cellular level which allowed them to assimilate enough of the cosmic energy of the Divine directly into their bodies so that they could survive solely on the energetic "manna from heaven." The other implication is that there is a relationship between the energetic density of our nutrition and our spiritual transformation. As we transmute spiritually on the physical, mental, and spiritual planes, we are more and more able to partake of the feast of God's Divine sustenance on the primary level of the cosmic energy.

A nutrient, in this context, is what we absorb into our overall body-mind-spirit from the different density levels that have precipitated from the

cosmic force. Material food is the densest, sunlight is the least dense on the material plane, and pure cosmic energy is the most subtle nutrient.

Subtle Organizing Energy Fields

Now that we understand that a nutrient can be energy as well as material, we are ready to take the next step in developing a functional hypothesis for understanding how to work with our nutrition in a way that brings us into harmony with Mother Earth. A key concept for understanding health and nutrition is what I call the Subtle Organizing Energy Fields (SOEFs), a concept that is developed extensively in *Spiritual Nutrition and the Rainbow Diet.*

The SOEF concept is built on a synthesis of both intuitive and scientific knowledge, yet rooted in cultural, historical, and spiritual traditions. The existence of SOEFs is founded on the idea that all living systems are surrounded and permeated by an energy pattern that determines the functioning of that system on every level.

The book *The Secret Life of Plants*, has helped to popularize the idea that plants have distinct energy fields that possess specific patterns. The work by Rupert Sheldrake on morphogenic fields of living organisms, *A New Science of Life*, also helps to support the thesis of the SOEFs. These morphogenic fields correspond to the potential structural forms of a developing system that is present before it materializes into its physical form. They are the template for the form. The SOEFs are similar to the architect's plans that determine the form and function of a building. They can be correspondingly understood as the thought before the words which culminates in the physical action.

The state of the SOEFs reveal the state of our functioning on all levels. SOEFs are reflected in the strength of our cellular emanation in the subtle force field that surrounds the body, called the aura, and the even more subtle force field called the mind, which exists prior to the physical seat of the mind called the brain. The SOEFs exist prior to the physical levels of our existence and are reflected in the subtle vibrations of our physical, mental, and spiritual levels.

The hypothesis of the existence of the SOEFs fundamentally differs from the current 200-year-old theory of nutrition which I call the material-mechanistic theory, which from now on we'll call the M & M theory. It proposes that food is material only, composed of proteins, carbohydrates, fats, vitamins, minerals, and other material factors. In the M & M theory, the value of a food's usefulness is measured on the basis of the amount of protein, carbohydrate, or fat it contains and the food's caloric value. The energy content of food in this old way of thinking is measured only in calories. A major limitation of this theory is that it does not account for the fact that humans are multi-leveled organisms that operate on a mind-body-spiritual level and that we take in a variety of subtle

151

energies that support life function. The M & M theory does not acknowledge that our physical food has an energy field that is associated with the living plant.

According to the M & M theory, it would have been impossible for Jesus, Moses, and Enoch to have gone without water or food for 40 days or more. The SOEF theory uses these examples to make the point that when our organism has been sufficiently spiritualized it is able to be nourished directly from God's Divine energy. If a theory cannot account for all unusual phenomena associated with it, it needs to be challenged and changed. The SOEF theory does not throw out the material-mechanistic theory, but incorporates it in its overall body-mind-spirit approach.

What is important to understand about the SOEFs is that they exist prior to the existence of physical form and are the blueprints or templates for biological forms and structures. This means they do not emanate from the physical form of an organism like the magnetic lines of a bar magnet might. In the SOEF theory, the physical form, function, and energy is the result of a preexisting energetic form or SOEF. Some recent evidence for the existence of SOEFs has been supplied by Marcel Vogel, one of the world's top crystal experts. Vogel was able to take video photographs of the crystallization of cholesterol esters. What he observed was that just before the physical crystal appeared, there was the existence of a blue energy form that revealed itself a fraction of a second before the unstructured liquid cholesterol melt entered a structured crystalline phase.

SOEFs exist as the maintaining template for all living organisms. The dynamic interaction of the SOEFs of the plants, which we take in as food, with the SOEFs of our human organism, is an important aspect in understanding this new paradigm of human nutrition.

The SOEF theory also relates to what some physicists feel is the general theory of how material existence comes into being. Such great thinkers as Einstein and Nikola Tesla, an electrical engineering genius and inventor who made alternating current practical, theorized that matter is the concrete condensation out of the vibrating universal subtle energy. This vibrating universal energy has been given names such as virtual energy, vacuum state, or zero point energy. These are all names for what scientists call a perfectly orderly, unmanifest state out of which comes the manifestation of the physical universe. Spiritual terms used to describe this state of energy are cosmic energy, pure consciousness, or cosmic prana. The SOEF theory is an attempt to describe how this precipitation from God's subtle, faster-than-the speed-of-light, zero point energy manifests as material form. The term I will be using for this potential energy which fills the universe is zero point energy. It is that energy which exists prior to the materialization of a physical object. Through a personal interview with Adam Trombley, astrophysicist and expert in zero point technology, it was explained to me that the energy used for the materialization of an object from one cubic centimeter represents one quadrillionth (1×10^{15}, which is 1000 times greater than a trillion) of the energy available in that volume of space. In other words, there is essentially an unlimited amount of potential energy available at the zero point level. All we need to do is learn how to tap in to it. Dr. Trombley estimates that in one cubic centimeter there is energy available equal to a million, million tons of uranium.

Bob Toben, in his book *Space, Time, and Beyond*, points out how Einstein, in his unified field theory, repeatedly stressed the view that the energy field precedes and creates the form. The SOEFs originate out of the zero point energy and serve as organizing templates for every level of a living organism's structure from the RNA/DNA structure to the cellular and organ system levels, and to the overall shape and energy of the totality of a living system. A key understanding is that the SOEFs resonate with the zero point energy and help transduce this energy down into the energy fields of the human body. The SOEFs resonate with, and energize, the body-mind-spirit complex. The body in this paradigm is a form stabilized by the SOEFs.

One important aspect of the SOEFs is that the zero point or cosmic energy is omnipresent and we are always resonating with it to some extent through the SOEFs. At certain times in our spiritual evolution we become more in tune with the SOEFs and consequently, the zero point energy. These positions of greater awareness with the cosmic force or zero point energy may first be experienced in special moments of meditation, prayer, or even in those peak experiences that may occur in sports. The more we are transformed spiritually, the more we become resonant with the zero point and Divine energy, and the more the mind begins to merge with, and identify with, this unchanging truth of who we are. The more we exist in this Divine resonance, the more it becomes part of the conscious awareness of our everyday existence. Eventually we become transformed by the continual experience of this energy flowing through us so that we become one in awareness with this energy. This is known as cosmic consciousness. This is conscious nutrition at its most sublime level. Experiencing the continual flow of the cosmic energy through the physical vehicle, no matter where we are, even when taking our children to an amusement park and riding upside down in a roller coaster, is extraordinarily supportive to the maintaining of an unbroken state of Divine awareness. **The awareness of the cosmic energy flowing through our bodies links us with the heavens and the earth. We become like The Tree of Life, with our branches reaching to the heavens and drinking in the heavenly energies, and our roots experiencing the energies of the earth.**

These SOEFs have form and also can gain, retain, or lose energy. Because of this, they are different than Rupert Sheldrake's brilliant description of organic forms or morphogenic fields which are concerned only with form and are neither a type of matter or energy. Once the body has materialized, it becomes a focal point for the SOEFs in the realm of time and space.

An important understanding in this new nutritional way of thinking is that when the SOEFs are energized they become more structured and a clearer template for our total organism. This in turn enhances the form and function of the organism on the physical plane. Practically speaking, this means an improved functioning of the RNA/DNA system, better protein synthesis, enzyme function, and cellular function and division, as well as an improved glandular, organ, and total system functioning of the organism. In short, when the SOEFs are energized, there is better form and structure on every level of an organism, and the total health of the living organism is improved. When the energy of the SOEF's are dissipated, just the opposite occurs and the total health of the organism degenerates.

SOEFs in Food

All living members of the vegetable kingdom have SOEFs. The food we eat is a specific way that SOEF energy from nature is transferred to we humans to build the energy of our SOEFs. Food with more structured SOEF energy transfers more of this energy into our own SOEFs and consequently enhances our form and function. Whenever food is cooked or processed in any way, it loses the strength of its SOEFs. **Fresh, raw, live, or unprocessed food most enhances our SOEFs and therefore is the healthiest for us.**

The concept of the importance of structure in food regarding health is supported in research by Professor Israel Brekhman of the Far East Scientific Centre Academy of Sciences in Vladivostock, Russia. He found that the structural integrity of a food affects the overall energy of the food in a way that goes beyond the simplistic concept of calories as the only measure of the energy a food carries. He developed a measurement called Significant Units of Action (SUA). SUAs measure how long an animal can carry out a certain amount of physical work when fed a specific food. He discovered that live, unprocessed foods had significantly more SUAs than the same foods that had their structural integrity compromised by any cooking or other form of food processing. The animals could work longer when fed the "highly structured" raw foods in spite of the fact that the cooked or processed foods had the same number of calories. Cooked foods have less structure because the application of heat through cooking disrupts the physical structure and ultimately, their SOEFs. This finding challenges the traditional M & M theory of nutrition which assumes that foods, whether cooked or raw, carry the same amount of energy. It supports the SOEF paradigm because it suggests there are additional levels of energy associated with a food. If the structure of these fields is disrupted, the energy and quality of health the food transmits to the organism is also diminished.

We see the similarity of the processed versus live food effect working on several levels in the nutritional spectrum. For example, chromium, which normally comes in whole, unaltered wheat, is processed out in the making of white bread. Nature puts the chromium in wheat because we need it to metabolize the carbohydrates in the wheat. In order to compensate for this lack of chromium in the white bread, our bodies use our up own chromium stores. Eventually our bodies become depleted in chromium. Another example of this depletion phenomenon can be understood with enzymes. Live foods also come with their own enzymes, which aide with the digestion when we ingest them. If the food is cooked, then these enzymes are inactivated. In order to compensate, our bodies must use more of our enzyme stores to digest the incoming food. The result is an accelerated enzyme depletion. This will be explained further in the chapter on enzymes. The point of these two examples is to show that cooked and processed foods actually take energy from our own bodies in order to properly assimilate them. Theoretically, at the SOEF level, this same type of depletion of energy also happens. Cooking or otherwise processing foods disrupts the SOEFs. Our body then needs to use some of its SOEF energy to reorganize the SOEFs of the incoming food. The result is a subtle depletion of energy and structure on every level. This is a theoretical, energetic explanation for Dr. Brekhman's findings that animals on live foods have more endurance and energy, and for the energetic depletion that may be happening in general when cooked or other forms of processed foods are taken into the system for an extended period of time. In the chapter on live foods a further discussion will help to deepen the understanding of this point.

The ability to energize the SOEFs enables us to reverse the aging process to some degree. This occurs because the body becomes more organized in its functioning. The more organized our bodily functioning is, the less aging occurs. Aging is the progressive disruption of the functioning of the living organism. Aging is an increase in entropy or level of disorganization. Energizing the SOEFs reverses the entropic process of aging. As a physician I see this reversal of aging all the time in clients who have come to me to improve their level of health. Those who change their eating habits and lifestyles toward more harmonious and SOEF-energizing ones seem to get younger.

These natural laws are no mystery. They are described in many spiritually based healing systems such as in Ayurveda and the Essene "Tree of Life" tradition. When natural law is followed, people have a tendency to feel more flexible and energetic, clearer mentally, and have an improvement in all their overall bodily functioning. Just to make this point a little clearer, there was a study reported at the *American Geriatric Association* in 1979. The study involved 47 participants whose average age was 52.5 years. It found that people who had been meditating more than 7 years were approximately 12 years younger physiologically than those of the same chronological age who were not meditating. Meditating is a very powerful way to increase the energy of the SOEFs.

A simple, physical experiment with a glass of brown sugar in water can help to metaphorically illustrate how energy and order are complimentary. If the water in the glass is not stirred, the brown sugar lies in a lump on the bottom of the glass. When the water is stirred, which adds energy to the system, a vortex swirl of water is formed which is analogous to adding energy to the SOEFs. In this vortex is also the brown sugar, which is swept into the vortex of water and takes a well-defined physical shape corresponding to a well-organized body function. However, when we take the spoon out, the vortex swirl of water immediately starts to become diffuse because energy is no longer being added to the system. Corresponding to this fall in energy, the brown sugar shape loses the clarity of its form. This is similar to what happens when we live in ways that deplete the SOEFs, with the result that we create by our lifestyles a disorganization in the body and mind (see fig. 15).

Although this new nutritional way of thinking, like the old M & M theory, has not been conclusively proven by rigorous scientific standards and may not be until the necessary scientific instrumentation is developed, the SOEF model provides a useful way to understand the processes of health, disease, and aging. It gives us a new and more complete way to experience and think about how we take in our nutrition from nature.

BROWN SUGAR DIAGRAM

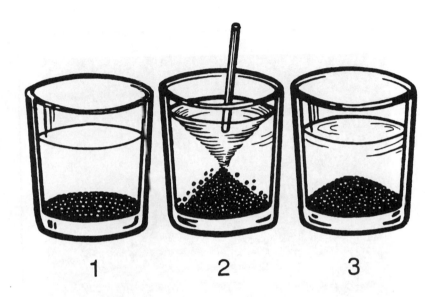

1   2   3

1. In the SOEF theory, adding energy to a system creates order.
2. This diagram is a metaphor for the relationship of energy to order.
3. By stirring the water, you are adding a vortex of energy to the system, which in turn creates order out of the brown sugar (step 2).
4. When the stirring action is stopped, as in step 3, the brown sugar becomes lumpy because it loses its order.
5. In the same way, our health becomes "lumpy" when we don't put sufficient energy in (live food and good health habits) to maintain the SOEF.

Fig. 15

The wonderful thing about this new paradigm is that we do not have to be a physicist to put it into practice.

We just have to accept God's gifts of nature in their original form.

It is no accident that fresh, raw, live, or unprocessed food most enhances our SOEFs and therefore is the healthiest for us.

VISION

BLACKBOARD FOOD FOR THOUGHT

Part II

Vegetarianism as a Choice

In making the choice to become a vegetarian many subtle personal resistances and cultural and religious doubts often arise. There is also a great deal of pseudo-scientific rumor and fear which has been created in the public mind about vegetarianism. This section is specifically designed to address those questions. Contrary to current mainstream thinking, vegetarianism cannot be conveniently labelled and discounted as a health food or new age fad. It is part of a spiritual and cultural tradition that goes back thousands of years.

The Judaic-Christian tradition and many of the oldest religions and spiritual paths of the world have strong traditions of vegetarianism: Hinduism, Jainism, Zoroastrianism, Buddhism, the Yoga tradition, Pythagoreans, and the Essenes are but a few. Currently, it appears, that the Judaic-Christian tradition does not support vegetarianism, but there is ample evidence that in the original purity and simplicity of the Judaic-Christian tradition, there is a strong tradition of vegetarianism. The point of this section is to help people let go of what they perceive as religious traditions that do not support vegetarianism so they can feel comfortable in their particular tradition and with their vegetarianism. Once given this information, people are then in a position to make a more educated choice.

Preview of Chapter 10
General Guidelines for a Healthy Diet

In this chapter we will explore some basic guidelines for a healthy diet. The most healthy gifts of life, according to the scientific evidence, is food in its organic, whole, natural form just as God has given us, and the healing power of the sun, water, and earth from which we draw sustenance. In short, if it is not broken, don't try to fix it. Are we ready to accept God's gifts as they are given to us?

I.   Critera for judging dietary recommendations

II. General guidelines to healthy eating

    A. Eat natural foods

    B. Eat whole food

    C. Eat organic food

    D. Eat primarily fresh, live food

    E. Eat a high complex carbohydrate, low protein and fat diet

III. Sunlight and health

IV. Breathe, bathe, and work the earth

V.   Quality of thoughts affect nutrition

160

Chapter 10

General Guidelines for a Healthy Diet

A conscious eating approach for a healthy diet includes going beyond our personal biochemistry to understanding diet as a way of consciously relating to the world. I call this the harmony of wholeness. It is understanding diet from the perspective of its impact on the topsoil, water supplies, air, animal population, human population, and its effect on peace in the world. Unfortunately, it now must also include the new art of learning how to live in a polluted, radioactive environment and in a society that is estranged from nature. The more artfully we can adapt ourselves, despite the nonsupportive culture we live in, the more we will be able to enhance our communion with the Divine. The fruits of our efforts will be increased harmony with our own evolution and the world.

The general diet that best fits with the harmony of conscious eating is vegetarian. A vegetarian diet allows us to follow all the general health guidelines that I will be discussing in this chapter, especially suggestions one through five. This recommendation does not contradict the concept of individualizing our diet because within the realm of vegetarianism it is completely possible to individualize a diet that accounts for: constitutional type; acid-base balance; heating or cooling; yin or yang balance; the seasonal changes; work; meditation, prayer, and other spiritual needs; digestive power; state of health; and all other factors associated with developing an individualized diet. Although there will always be exceptions to this suggestion of vegetarianism, just remember I am asking you to explore the question with me from many different aspects.

In presenting the dietary recommendations contained in this book, the information has had to pass three basic criteria. The first is: Does it fit with economically and politically unbiased research conducted to date? For this research I look to such organizations as the International Society for Research on Nutrition and Diseases of Civilization (ISRNDC). Founded by Albert Schweitzer, M.D., the ISRNDC is comprised of several hundred top researchers, physicians, natural healers, and scientists from over seventy-five countries. The organization is not supported by any industry, profession, or vested economic interests.

I also have looked to the documented experience of authoritative teachers and natural healers of great integrity, such as Paavo Airola, Ph.d., Dr. Bircher-Benner, Dr. Max Gerson, and Dr. Edmond Bordeaux Szekely. In the case of Dr. Szekely, over a thirty year period at Rancho La Puerta, Mexico, he had greater than a ninety percent recovery rate with over 123,000 patients with all types of health problems, including cancer, using what was an essentially 80–100% live food, vegetarian diet. If people were very ill they would be put on a 100% live food diet and then go back to a maintenance 80% live food diet.

The second criterion for considering dietary recommendations is: Are my health recommendations in accordance with the historical evidence of thousands of years of actual practice in various cultural settings?

For example, nowadays vegetarianism is considered by some a novel and radical way of eating; but vegetarianism is not a new idea nor is it radical. Vegetarianism is recommended in the ancient Persian *Zend Avesta* of Zoraster, which predates the Bible by thousands of years. The Essenes, who were reported by several historians to have an average life span of 120 years, followed vegetarianism and the principles espoused in this book. My general recommendations are also consistent with what I believe to be the diet recommended by the Greek spiritual teacher and mathematician, Pythagoras.

Studies of some of the healthiest cultures in the world, such as the Hunzas, Vilabamban Indians, Mayans, and various other groups which have a much higher number of centenarians, found that they all followed diets that are very similar to the vegetarian diet which I suggest you explore in your process of conscious eating. Of course, not all these cultures ate exactly the same diet. For example, in South America, the primary grain is corn. In Hunzaland, the primary grain is wheat, et cetera. Most were completely vegetarian, although some, such as the Hunzas, ate a trace of flesh food on a monthly basis or for celebrations.

The third criterion for considering dietary recommendations is: Do my recommendations fit with my own personal and clinical experience as a physician working with clients since the early 1970s? Consistently, I have observed that the basic vegetarian pattern of diet and lifestyle recommended in this book has worked to bring health, joy, and spiritual inspiration for thousands of clients I have seen in the last 20 years of my practice.

The points I make for a general program of good health and conscious eating are essentially those made by the International Society for Research on Nutrition and the Diseases of Civilization. The following is a list of these points.

1. Eat natural foods.

These are foods grown under natural conditions on organic and fertile soil. These foods are consumed in unprocessed form in their natural state. Food is not natural if it is grown in depleted, chemically treated soil. These unnatural products of unnatural soil are sprayed with herbicides or pesticides. They often are picked prematurely and processed by heat or irradiation. This unnatural produce is sometimes genetically altered so that it can withstand long shipping distances and still look good cosmetically.

Commercial methods of growing foods have significantly altered the natural growing process. The appearance of commercially grown foods may sometimes look better than organically grown products, but the quality and nutritive value of these synthetically grown fruits, vegetables, nuts, seeds, grains, and legumes have been greatly reduced. The nutritive value of organically grown foods is usually significantly superior to those foods grown commercially in the same local soil. One major study at Rutgers University found that organic produce had an average of 83% more nutrients in it. Of course, even the nutritive value of organic foods will vary from soil to soil. Because of this, I recommend eating a variety of vegetables, fruits, nuts, seeds, legumes, and grains so that one is assured of getting the full spectrum of nutrients. In other words, rotate and vary plant intake, and if possible, buy foods from a variety of organic sources.

The entire world food supply depends on the quality of the soil. According to *Topsoil and Civilization*, every great nation has risen and fallen according to the quality of its topsoil. The sustenance of all animal life comes primarily from the vegetable life that is grown on this soil. The health of humanity depends on the health of the soil. Nutrition begins with the topsoil. This crucial understanding has not been significantly appreciated by the commercial food producers or by most dietetic schools. We can no longer speak about a beet or a carrot as if they had a static nutritional content. The nutritional content of a food can vary tremendously, depending on the quality of the soil and the growing methods.

There are several other major problems with commercial growing. The use of synthetic fertilizers in the short-term might produce what appears to be abundant growth and large-sized produce, but in the course of this process commercial growers add chemicals which upset the soil's ecological balance. These chemicals upset the natural harmony between the plants and the soil. The plants become overstimulated and hurried in their growth. When the plants are forced to grow too rapidly, the natural rhythm of their metabolisms are disrupted so that they fail to fully transform their starches and acids into their normal plant sugars. They also fail to absorb valuable minerals. This problem is compounded by the common commercial practice of picking the fruits and vegetables before they are ripe so they can be shipped with minimal loss of produce. Because of this, most commercial fruits and vegetables are not ripe when they reach our kitchen tables. Not only does the produce have less taste, but some of the produce tends to be acid- rather than alkaline-producing in the body. These foods usually are deficient in nutrients and their resistance to disease is decreased. When humans eat these less vital plants, we also become less vital and more prone to disease.

Not only does synthetic, commercially grown produce give less nutritive value, but it requires the use of pesticides and herbicides to eliminate insects and fungal growth on these less resistant plants. Many of these herbicides, fungicides, and pesticides are also very poisonous to humans. These poisons seep into the interior flesh of the plant from both the surface and through the roots. No matter how much they are washed, they still contain these poisons because they have been absorbed on a systemic, cellular level. These human-made poisons also kill the normal soil bacteria and the earthworms which help form the humus which is so important for the plant's optimal growth. Unfortunately, even if some of these more toxic sprays are banned in this country, they are used in other countries whose produce we import, so that they come back to us in a roundabout way. In my own organic garden, I do not even spray with organic pesticides. I let the insects take their share and there is always plenty left for my family.

Unless we pay attention to our harmony with the topsoil, we humans, who are created out of the dust of earth, will return much sooner to personally re-fertilize it. The overall quality of our nutrition begins with the topsoil and continues through the normal development and harvesting of the plant. When these factors are considered, a healthy diet is more likely to be created, with its corresponding health dividends for us.

The best ways to assure maximal nutrition is to either grow your own organic produce or buy only organic produce to supply your needs. A nice way to buy organic produce is to locate a farmers' market where organic produce is sold. These markets can be found in many cities as well as the country. Introduce yourself directly to the farmers and find out about their farming methods. By doing this, your food and the person who grows it are no longer anonymous. In this way you become part of the food cycle process.

Health and longevity are in a direct relationship to the degree of naturalness of the foods you eat. Dr. Airola points out in *Are You Confused* that the nutritional researchers, such as Dr. Weston A. Price, Vilhjamur Steffansson, Dr. McCarrison, and Arnold DeVries, all studied the dietary habits of many "primitive" cultures and found that when their diets were comprised of natural, unprocessed, locally grown foods that the people had "no disease or tooth decay." When these same cultures began to use denatured, processed foods, such as white flour and white sugar, canned foods, and insufficient amounts of uncooked foods, these researchers found the "primitive" populations began to suffer from dental decay and the degenerative diseases of modern civilization.

Arnold DeVries studied the historical records of the North and South American Indians; Eskimos; Asian, African, and Australian aboriginals; and New Zealand Maoris. He found that all of them enjoyed excellent health, fertility, no tooth decay, fast and relatively painless childbirth, and minimal degenerative disease at comparable ages to those in our culture. As soon as processed foods of any sort were introduced into their culture, general health began to decline, childbirth became painful, and tooth decay became prevalent.

2. Eat whole foods.

Whole foods are those that have not been fragmented or adulterated in any way. Whole foods contain all their original nutrients. They have neither been refined nor enriched. Every time a chemical or nutrient has been added or subtracted from a food, the natural balance is disrupted. As described earlier, the yin/yang balance of the food and the proper synergy of all five elements is disrupted. After thousands of years of eating natural and whole foods, our bodies have become biologically programmed to utilize them in their natural state. When the composition of the foods is altered with additives, preservatives, dyes, microwaves, irradiation, or even cooking, the body is only partially able to readjust. The eventual result is an early onset of chronic degenerative diseases, as suggested by the cultural studies.

Recent history serves as evidence of the importance of eating whole foods. During World War I, Denmark suffered serious food shortages. In order to compensate, the government increased whole grain production and consumption, as well as limiting livestock production and putting quotas on the sale of meat. Grain processing was stopped and only whole grain products were allowed to be sold. Farmers were directed to produce more grain, green vegetables, fruit, and dairy products instead of meat. After one year of this program the death rate dropped 40%. According to Paavo Airola, diseases that affected other European countries, including an influenza epidemic, only minimally affected Denmark. Denmark became the healthiest nation in Europe.

The use of fresh juices is one exception to the whole food guideline. Minimal processing by juicing is only marginally disruptive because all of the live factors are left intact. Raw juices contain all the elements of live food, such as the enzymes, minerals, and vitamins, in a more concentrated form that is more readily assimilated into the cellular system with less digestive energy required. The primary part of the whole food that is missing is the fiber. The energy that is saved by not having to process the fiber goes toward the healing and repairing of the body. Dr. Walker, who lived to age 116 on raw juices and primarily raw food, in his book, *Raw Vegetable Juices,* states that raw food is the nourishment intended for human beings. He qualifies this by pointing out that the transition to raw foods is a big switch and the raw juices taken as part of the transition give a person many of the advantages of the raw food diet without necessarily being on the 80% or more raw food diet. Juices furnish the body with the live enzymes and bioactive vitamins, minerals, trace minerals, and other unknown factors which are destroyed when the food is cooked. The juices bring an alkaline force into the body which helps to neutralize the toxic acidity from which most people suffer. These alkalinizing minerals help to restore the alkaline and mineral balance in the cells. They speed the recovery from disease by supporting the body's own healing activity and cell regeneration. Airola points out that raw juices contain an unidentified factor which improves the micro-electrical tension in the tissues and improves the cell's ability to absorb nutrients and excrete metabolic wastes. The use of raw juices has been a major part of many healing programs. For example, they are a major part of Dr. Gerson's therapy approach to cancer, a program which has been very successful over the last thirty or more years. Almost all European biological clinics that I am familiar with use raw juices as part of their rejuvenative program.

It is Dr. Walker's feeling that when a food is juiced and the fiber is separated out, most of the toxins are eliminated with the fiber. If this is true, then this is another advantage of live juices. The combination of the live fiber in the whole food, and the high concentration of enzymes, vitamins, and minerals of the live juices make an excellent dietary program. Even though live juices are not totally whole in the strictest sense, because they are so high in live enzymes, I classify them as biogenic (high life force), rejuvenating foods. Paavo Airola calls them the "internal baths of health and youth."

Many questions arise about the quality of different juicers. The Norwalk juicer or other types of expensive hydraulic press juicers are considered the best types available. This is primarily because they breakup the cellulose walls more effectively and make available more minerals and vitamins to be pressed out into the juice. The hydraulic press juices are also substantially more expensive.

Other juicers, such as the Champion, are also excellent. Centrifugal juicers, which are usually round in shape, are equal to the Champion as a juicer in efficiency and pressing ability, but are less versatile in that one can use the Champion to make other types of food preparations. Regardless of what juicer one uses, as Dr. Walker points out, the most important thing is to drink juices fresh and on a daily basis, regardless of the manner in which they have been extracted.

The freshness of one's juice is vitally important. Some recent research by the Flanagans, as reported in their book, *Elixir of the Ageless,* suggests that the bioelectric, colloidal potential of most juices diminishes significantly overnight and is usually gone within twenty-four hours after they are juiced. Other health practitioners estimate that the enzymes in the juices are destroyed within a few minutes up to an hour or so. Similar to herbs, vegetables and fruits have specific healing properties that are beneficial for specific organs. The principle of food relating to certain disease conditions is a well-established clinical finding in Western naturopathic systems, as well as in both the Chinese and Ayurvedic systems. In the western natural healing tradition, Dr. Walker's book, *Raw Vegetable Juices* elaborates how specific juices are good for certain health conditions and organ systems. Since each juice has its own particular properties and is rejuvenative for different parts of the body, I try to vary my juice intake, especially during fasts. Some of the main juices that I use are carrot, beet, kale, wheatgrass, alfalfa, sunflower and buckwheat sprouts, celery, parsley, spinach, apple, watermelon, orange, and zucchini. It should be briefly mentioned that for certain people with autoimmune diseases where the immune system starts to attack itself, such as rheumatoid arthritis and lupus, the consumption of copious amounts of alfalfa sprouts in juice or in their whole form has been associated with the worsening of these conditions. This information came from only one informal study and further research must be conducted to further confirm this finding and to ascertain what in alfalfa sprouts may be responsible for making certain autoimmune diseases worse (see page 372).

There is so much we do not understand about the subtleties of nutrition that we are essentially shooting in the dark when we start to alter and process our foods. Whole foods contain not only whole nutrition, but also the enzymes and other factors needed to digest and assimilate these foods. They also contain a specific balance of natural forces that are programmed to affect the body in a particular way. Plant foods have a wholeness and integrity that is more than just the collection of proteins, minerals, and vitamins found within them.

We have yet to improve on what Mother Nature has given us to eat. Plant foods simply cannot be artificially duplicated in the science laboratory. **What are touted as improvements so one can prepare food and eat it more quickly, or so commercial growers and processors can make more money, can hardly be considered an improvement in terms of health and longevity.** As with everything else in life, when one "sacrifices the eternal for that which dieth in an hour," one's well-being is often sacrificed in the process. When it comes to food, it is not worth it to make cheap compromises with our health by selecting sub-standard building materials with which to nourish our bodies, minds and spirits. **There is no necessity to sell out our health and shorten our life so that someone else can profit from marketing so-called "longer shelf-life," modern, "convenience foods."**

There is no short-cut to health and happiness except by following the natural laws of life to the best of one's ability and present knowledge. Humanity and all sentient beings are sustained by the same radiating light of the universe within and without us. If we are to be in harmony with this light as it comes to us through the natural interplay of earth, water, air, and fire via the vegetable kingdom, then it is essential to choose to eat as much organically grown agricultural products that are grown in the fullness of this light. We should be very cautious when we attempt to tamper with nature.

When it comes to nature and live foods "if it's not broken, don't try to fix it." This is especially true since so few, if anyone, are even close to fully understanding the subtle energetics, biophysics, and biochemistry of Mother Nature's offerings to us.

3. Eat primarily living foods.

Natural and whole foods are by definition, living. Living or raw food means it has not been processed in any way, including cooking. Because of this none of the heat-sensitive micronutrients have been destroyed and the full life force and energetic pattern of the living plant is best preserved so that it can transfer the highest amount of its life force to us. Its SOEFs can most fully transfer their energy to our SOEFs so that we may live more vibrantly and healthier for a longer time. A further discussion of live foods will be given in the stage IV presentation. The minimum of living foods one can eat to get the full benefits of living foods is approximately 50% (if they are eaten at the beginning of the meal).

4. Eat only organic, poison-free foods.

Aside from radiation, the poisons on and in our foods from the thousands of herbicides, pesticides, fungicides, et cetera, is one of the greatest dangers to health today. According to Paavo Airola, there are over one thousand chemicals used in the food processing industry. Even if the food is organically grown, it is good to wash off the surface parts of the plant because of incidental radiation fallout, migrated aerial sprays, lead from automobiles, and other industrial pollution in our air. One exception to the thorough washing off of organic produce is root vegetables, which are somewhat protected from incidental airborne pollution because they grow underground. Another reason that one might not want to thoroughly scrub root vegetables such as carrots, beets, turnips, et cetera, is because B_{12}-growing organisms are often plentiful on the surfaces of these vegetables. Simply rinsing off the soil from root vegetables is sufficient. However, in the case of commercial vegetables and fruits, the oil-soluble sprays and waxes that are present on the surfaces of the produce requires that some vegetable cleaning soap be used with the wash water.

5. Eat a high, natural carbohydrate and low-protein diet.

This is the general dietary pattern of all healthy, long lived cultures. This theme has been developed in depth in other sections of the book. For those who need to acidify their system, by improving protein digestion with digestive enzymes, eating moderate levels of protein, and using other suggestions from the acid-base chapter, one can still operate within the high end of this recommendation about protein intake.

6. To maximize your nutritional assimilation, be conscious of the various subtle sources of energy.

A broader definition of a nutrient is anything which enhances the SOEFs. In this context, it is useful to include the cosmic energy we bring into our system from prayer and meditation, as well as the nutritive energies we bring in from natural sources like the sun, air, water, and earth. In addition to absorbing these forces into our organism through our food, absorbing each of them directly is also important.

168

Sunlight

The sun's rays (contrary to recent "bad press") are not necessarily a deadly enemy that automatically causes skin cancer. Without the sun, all life would die. The UV rays of the sunlight on the skin react with ergosterol (a pre-vitamin D substance) to form much-needed, natural vitamin D. The sun also balances the biorhythmic hormonal cycles of the body. Research done on people with vision-blocking cataracts, shows many hormonal irregularities. Most, if not all, of these hormonal imbalances disappear when the cataracts that block the flow of sunlight into the eyes are removed. The Egyptians, Romans, and Greeks made significant medical uses of light. Herodotus, the father of heliotherapy (sun therapy), felt that sunlight was very necessary for people whose health needed restoring. Dr. Hufeland, in 1796 in his book, *Macrobiotics,* wrote:

> "Even the human being becomes pale, flabby, and apathetic as
> a result of being deprived of light, finally losing all his vital
> energy...."

Recently medical doctors have begun to recognize a problem called seasonal affective disorder (SAD) which occurs when people do not absorb enough sunlight into their eyes. Jacob Liberman, O.D., Ph.d., points out in his book *Light: Medicine of the Future:*

> " The medicine of the future is light—we are healing ourselves
> with that which is our essence."

Although our airborne pollution has burned holes in the protective ozone layer of the atmosphere and thus has upset our natural harmony with the sunlight, recoiling in fear from the sun only further confuses the issues. We still need a certain amount of light on the bare skin and through our eyes to be healthy. According to Dr. Ott, the foremost light expert in the world, as well as Dr. Liberman, daily light exposure should be between thirty to sixty minutes per day of direct or indirect light. Neither recommends extensive outdoor time in the noon hours during the summer. One important way to get light into the system is to not wear anything but full spectrum glasses or contacts. Wearing regular contacts, glasses, or sunglasses when one is outside will block our reception of the full spectrum of sunlight and keep it from entering into our eyes. Full spectrum light is so essential to proper hormonal function that Dr. Ott cites four cases of women who previously were unable to get pregnant who became pregnant when they stopped wearing sunglasses.

Excessive ultraviolet light may create a problem, but a certain amount seems to be needed for health. Both Drs. Ott and Liberman cite research that suggests that completely blocking UV light may actually suppress the immune system. Research in Dr. Liberman's book indicates UV light increases the cardiac output in a high percentage of people, improves EKG readings and blood profiles of individuals with atherosclerosis, reduces cholesterol, helps with weight loss, and is helpful for treating psoriasis, tuberculosis, and destroying infectious bacteria. Light therapy is used by Russians and Germans to treat black lung disease. Adequate exposure to natural light increases the level of the sex hormones, and activates the skin hormone called solitrol. Solitrol is believed to be a form of vitamin D_3 which works with melatonin to generate changes in mood and circadian rhythms.

There are hundreds of studies which prove the health-promoting effects of UV light. *Light Therapy*, published in 1933 by Dr. Krudsen, cites 165 different diseases which were treated by UV light. In Australia, some interesting recent research by Helen Shaw in the British Journal, *Lancet,* found that people working outdoors, and even at high altitudes, which increases exposure to the sun, had one half the skin melanoma than those working indoors under florescent lights. Perhaps we would do well to look at all the factors associated with skin cancer rather than just myopically focusing on the dangers of UV light.

The key point regarding sunlight and its UV radiation is "moderation." It is true that an imbalance has been created by our poking holes in the ozone layer. This does not mean, however, that we have to compound this imbalance by completely avoiding the sun, the very source of life on this planet. This radical and fearful relationship to the sun illustrates how much our society is out of touch with the natural harmony with nature that has sustained life on the planet for millions of years. Sunlight is the nutrient of life on this planet. The sun is an outer manifestation of our inner light. Although the destruction of the environment alters the natural and normal balance, we should use intelligent moderation when it comes to exposing our bodies to the sun's rays. We must cultivate a healthy balance with the sunlight and not hide fearfully in darkness.

Breathe, Bathe, and Work the Earth

Less controversial health-enhancing practices are: deep breathing, thera-peutic use of water (using various baths), and working with the earth.

Deep breathing brings in the healing forces of the oxygen to help cleanse our system of carbon dioxide waste. The oxygen we take in supplies ninety percent of the fuel for our metabolism, whereas food only supplies ten percent. Vitamin O, or oxygen, is the most important nutrient there is. Without it we would be physically dead within just a few minutes. Presently, many people have so little oxygen in their system that dark field analysis of the blood often demonstrates that within a high percentage of people there is red cell clumping. Often the cause of this condition is inadequate oxygen, a situation which is alleviated when deep breathing exercises or the habit of deep breathing is cultivated.

Air bathing, which is the practice of exposing one's skin to the air and sun with a minimum of clothing on, is another way that toxic waste in the form of gases leave the skin.

According to Dr. Szekely, a daily water bath has powerful healing and cleansing effects. Daily bathing is considered by yogis to be beneficial for health and spirit.

Spending time in contact with the earth, such as gardening and taking long walks in nature, helps us absorb the health-promoting magnetic radiations of the earth. This is a little-known practice that seems to bring many health benefits. This is particularly important if one is spending a full work day in a high-rise, city setting where earth contact is very limited.

Sunning, breathing, bathing and earth time are all forms of more subtle, but nonetheless important, sources of nutrition that Mother Nature offers us. Being in harmony with these natural forces of sun, air, earth, and water provides a subtle nutrition that is essential to true health. This type of health is not simply the absence of disease that typically passes as health nowadays.

One additional aspect of our nutritional intake is the quality of our thoughts. If our thoughts are in harmony with the natural and spiritual laws, then we will be more able to live and eat in a healthy, harmonious way. Although the types of foods we eat affect our thoughts, eating a totally "pure" diet does not necessarily mean our thoughts will be harmonious and pure. Because of this, it is important to limit our exposure to negative or violent inputs that come from some types of T.V. programs, movies, and "negative thinking" people. It is important to spend as much time as possible in an uplifting environment with people who are generating positive and uplifting thoughts. **The key to being able to generate positive thoughts is to start every thought with love. This means to feel, or try to feel, love in your heart with every act in life. The food of love is the most powerful nutrient we can eat.**

Preview of Chapter 11
Vegetarianism: A Step Toward Health and Harmony

The practice of eating flesh food is not only inhuman, but directly detrimental to our physical health. This chapter directly dispels the high protein myth created by the early protein need research done by the livestock and dairy industry that has scared people into a high flesh food diet. Current research indicates that not only do we get more than sufficient protein on a vegetarian diet, but that a vegetarian diet is generally healthier, increases longevity, and increases physical endurance. It is even a prime preventer of osteoporosis to the extent that vegetarian women have less osteoporosis than meat-eating men. A vegetarian diet is a way of loving yourself. Are you ready to let go of your fear of not getting enough protein when shown the evidence that a low protein diet is better for your health? Are you ready to start loving yourself by eating healthy food?

I.   Problems of eating flesh food

    A. Cruelty to animals

    B. Danger to your health

II. Difference between plant and animal nutrition

III. Myth of the need for a high protein diet

    A. High protein need based on fear not science

    B. Vegetarian diets have twice the required protein

    C. Overconsumption of protein contributes to diseases such as osteoporosis

    D. High protein may accelerate the aging process

IV. Vegetarian diet increases endurance

    A. Endurance increased 2-3 times

    B. A higher percentage of world class athletes are vegetarian rather than nonvegetarian

V.   Long life span and better health with a vegetarian diet

Chapter 11

Vegetarianism, a Step Toward Health and Harmony

The late Paul Bragg, a great advocate of healthy natural living and vegetarianism, used to go to the meat market before certain press conferences and get a freshly killed chicken. He was a master at dramatically and cleverly confronting people with the reality of eating dead flesh. He would bring the dead chicken to the conference and as he held it up in front of the reporters he would describe the horrible living conditions of the chicken; or he would describe how it was filled with antibiotics, arsenic, and a variety of other dangerous substances, i.e. often being infected with salmonella, tuberculosis, or cancer. Then he would point out that if humans were naturally carnivorous, we would act like carnivorous animals and eat the chicken by biting into it raw. And if we were truly carnivorous, we would bite into the guts as carnivorous animals do to their prey. Then he would swing the chicken around his head, throw it into the crowd, and laugh as the people would scatter. It is not surprising that no one would pick up this free chicken.

The word flesh, in the context of the Bragg story, has a certain dramatic connotation, but in its general usage it best defines the meaning of vegetarianism. A vegetarian is one who does not eat any red meat, fowl, or fish. Often people define themselves as vegetarian if they do not eat "meat" because meat for them is defined as red meat, and not fish or fowl. People who eat fish or fowl are not classically defined as vegetarian. The word "flesh" is not meant to shock the reader as much as to help us operate from a common definition of vegetarianism. Secondarily, it does serve to cut through the subtle denial system that is created when euphemistic terms are used, such as "meat" or "red meat" (for cows, oxen, goats, lambs and other such animals), "broilers" (for fowl), and "sea vegetables" (for fish).

Many things are done to keep us from being aware that we have participated in the killing of Mother Nature's animals to satisfy our appetites. Rather than letting the public be numbed out and anesthetized, Bragg boldly challenged his audiences with such demonstrations. He tried to awaken people from the lulling effects of background Muzak at the supermarket where they bought dead animals for food or awaken them from the quiet sophistication of a fancy restaurant, with Mother Nature's flowers artfully placed on a candle lit table where flesh foods are further disguised under delightful sauces.

In today's world, even more so than in Bragg's day, we have escalated the level of abuse that we subject animals to on a daily basis. Animals are routinely and systematically treated as "things;" as simply raw materials of the agribusiness; as stock in the market like gold and silver coins or computer microchips; or as "livestock" rather than living creatures which have a spark of God in them. The outstanding book, *Diet for A New America*, by John Robbins, discusses these issues in detail. For example, we do not even call chickens by their names any more. They are called "broilers" if they are going to be eaten or "layers" if their industrial purpose is to lay eggs. The living conditions for chickens are so inhumane, according to Dr. Virginia Livingston-Wheeler, a top cancer researcher, a great many chickens develop microscopic or identifiable cancer before they are one year old. She says in her book, *The Conquest of Cancer:*

> "I consider the potential for cancer in chickens to be almost one hundred percent. That is, most of the chickens on the dining tables and barbecue grills of America today have the pathological form of the PC (Progenitor Cryptocides) microbe, which I contend is transmissible to human beings."

She reports that:

> "Many of the chickens processed for human consumption already display tumors both visible and invisible to the human eye but because of hurried processing techniques have sped by inspectors on the production lines."

Dr. Rous, Nobel Prize winner and long-time researcher at the Rockefeller Institute for Medical Research, states that 95% of the chickens for sale in New York City are cancerous. He also concurs with other researchers, stating that the chicken cancer is transmissible. I have to also point out that the transmissibility of these chicken cancer viruses to humans has not been conclusively proven, but as consumer advocate Ralph Nader points out on this issue, there is no proof to show that the cancer is *not* transmitted.

Rarely do these chickens live a normal life span of 15-20 years. The health conditions of the chickens by the time they are used for food are so horrible that a leading poultry worker union official in a private communication said that he would never eat chicken knowing what he has seen. Flesh eating, particularly as it is practiced today, rather than returning us to harmony with Mother Nature, increases our alienation from nature.

The Difference Between Plant and Animal Nutrition

Plant nutrition, which we have already understood as condensed sunlight in various rainbow forms, is distinctly different from animal nutrition. Without plant nutrition we could not even have a "Rainbow Diet."

Plants have two mouths through which they gather energy and nutrients to share with us. In their leaves, they store and give us the energy of the sun in a direct transfer of light energy in a way that both stimulates our inner light, as well as brings sunlight-activated electron energy to our whole system. A tree is a good model for us because the branches move in every upward direction to gather in the light. The plant or tree stands between the earth and the sun in gathering in the sunlight. Without the tree, the earth would not be able to draw sustenance from the sun. The plant kingdom also connects us to the unrevealed cosmic forces which rain upon the plant and soil day and night.

The plant also burrows with its other mouth in the form of a root into the soil of the Mother Earth to bring us nutrition directly from the earth. The roots keep growing into the unknown depths of the earth to gather nutrients. Alfalfa, which is exceptionally rich in minerals, may send its roots deeper than 60 feet into the mysterious force field of the earth. The food we take in from the plant is permeated with a synthesis of the earth, sunlight, rainwater, and cosmic forces from the stars and planets. This is entirely different than what we can get from animal nutrition. The stellar and other cosmic forces taken in by the plants stimulate our harmony with the universe and accelerate our spiritual development.

According to Rudolf Steiner, plants supply us with their store of the outer light of the sun, which stimulates our inner light during the process of assimilation. Rudolf Steiner was an extraordinary philosopher who lived in the early part of this century and developed biodynamic gardening, the Waldorf school system, and anthroposophical medicine, among other contributions. In the system of anthroposophical medicine, the light released by the plant world helps to stimulate, form, and maintain our nervous system. In an exquisite, divine way, the taking in of plant food makes a cyclic connection of our inner light with the outer light of the solar system and plant world. One benefit of eating vegetarian food is that the light of plants is directly released into our bodies in a way that stimulates the inner light and the nervous system. This benefit is lost when we eat a primarily animal diet. When we take in animals as food rather than plants, we have to work harder to overcome the energy of the animals' considerably developed and individualized nervous systems. Because of this, the anthroposophical system of medicine suggests that those with nervous system disorders will do better with vegetarian foods. Dr. Swank, an eminent multiple sclerosis physician, has observed that his patients do better by avoiding flesh foods, particularly from four-legged animals.

To digest vegetarian food requires more inner spiritual light and digestive power than it does for meat digestion. Just as we lose our muscle tone and endurance when we do not exercise much, in the same way, by eating animal products, we indirectly weaken our ability to take in plant food. This is one reason why a transition to vegetarianism often needs to be gradual. Some of us need to overcome generations of heavy meat-eating behavior in which we have lost some of our subtle digestive power and may initially have difficulty assimilating the living plant forces of a vegetarian diet. One person told me it

175

took him ten years to stabilize into a vegetarian diet and feel healthy. Most people are able to make the transition comfortably within one or two years.

Our relationship with plants also reveals a natural harmony with nature in that we have a reciprocal exchange of gases with the plant kingdom. The animal kingdom, of which we are a part, takes in oxygen from the plants and breathes out carbon dioxide as a waste product. Our plant friends metabolize the carbon dioxide and with the help of sunlight, convert it to complex carbohydrates and give off oxygen. Plants also supply basic alkalinizing nutrients when we eat them—nutrients we need to balance an acid-generating metabolism. In return, when our acid bodies return to the soil, they nourish plants.

A vegetarian diet avoids the disharmony connected with the poor treatment and killing of animals. This is particularly important because of the inhumane way animals are treated today. In what amounts to animal concentration camps created primarily to maximize profits, euphemistically called livestock farming, we have turned animals into victims. When an animal is about to be killed, there is a release of adrenaline into the tissues of the soon-to-be-slaughtered animal. This fear-released adrenaline is then absorbed by the eater of the dead animal. **Since animals are victims, when we eat animals, we also partake in their victim consciousness. When we eat animal flesh, we too, take on their fear and pain of death, which permeates every cell.**

An additional perspective of the harmonious animal kingdom–plant kingdom cycle is that the plant kingdom (according to the Old Testament), was given to us for food. The consuming of plant life for food is in harmony with nature's cycles in that the fruits and vegetables we eat are harvested in their seasonal cycles in synchrony with their own life and death cycles.

Each plant, as a form of condensed sunlight, releases specific energies into our systems which help balance our various subtle energy centers as well as our glands and organs. Bircher-Benner, a world famous European physician who made prominent use of raw foods, felt that the closer our food was to the natural sun energy, the higher it was on all levels of nutritional value for the human organism. In this context, plant food is at the top of the nutritional scale and animal food is at the bottom. Rudolf Steiner asserted the belief that nothing clouds the nervous system when nourishment comes from the plant realm, and that on a vegetarian diet humanity can more easily delve into the cosmic interrelationships which take people beyond the constricted limitation of the mundane personality.

The Myth of a High Protein Need

The need for high protein is centered more around the issue of fear rather than based on fact. The initial research on which this myth was based was done in Germany around the turn of the century. The research, for the most part, was

176

financed by the meat and dairy industry. They decided 120 grams of protein per day was needed. Today, modern research shows something entirely different. Research from around the world shows that a more accurate protein need is between 20 and 35 grams for men or nonpregnant women. The *Journal of Clinical Nutrition* states that we need approximately 2.5% of our total calories to be protein. This is approximately 18 grams of protein per day. The World Health Organization suggests 4.5% of our calories, or about 32 grams per day. Mother's milk has about 5% of its calories as protein.

In 1981, Frances Lappe stated in her revised edition of *Diet for a Small Planet,* that as long as one is getting enough healthy calories in the diet, one will automatically get enough protein in a vegetarian diet. In her *original* edition of *Diet for A Small Planet,* she popularized the idea of combining protein foods as a way to maximize protein intake. In doing so, she indirectly perpetuated fears concerning not getting enough "complete" protein. In her *new* edition, she skillfully corrected the inadvertent scare she had created when, after further research, she found out that protein complementarity at each meal is unnecessary. In addition, as the physiologists have known all along, humans are able to store protein, so that just as long as there is some semblance of a variety of foods in the diet, there is really no need to worry about protein food-combining in the first place.

According to the American Dietetic Association, pure vegetarian diets in America usually contain twice the required protein for one's daily need. Harvard researchers have found that it is difficult to have a vegetarian diet that will produce a protein deficiency unless there is an excess of vegetarian junk foods and sweets. The well-known British medical journal, *Lancet,* said that vegetarian protein is no longer considered second class. In fact, if the vegetarian protein is consumed in its live state, even less protein intake is needed because research shows that one-half of the assimilable protein is destroyed by cooking. The Max Planck Institute has found that the complete vegetarian proteins, those with all eight essential amino acids, are superior to, or at least equal to, animal proteins. They showed these complete proteins were available in various concentrations from almonds, sesame seeds, pumpkin seeds, sunflower seeds, soybeans, buckwheat, peanuts, potatoes, all leafy greens, and most fruits. Many fruits have been found to have the same percentage of complete protein as mother's milk. Paavo Airola, who was one of the world's most respected nutritionists, stated:

> "It is virtually impossible not to get enough protein, provided
> you have enough to eat of natural, unrefined foods."

High-protein Versus Low-protein Intake

Paavo Airola points out that the overconsumption of protein contributes to the development of many of our most common and serious diseases, such as arthritis, pyorrhea, schizophrenia, atherosclerosis, heart disease, cancer and kidney damage. Airola's research shows that a "high-protein diet causes premature aging." Other researchers have linked high meat consumption with tissue, organ, and cell degeneration and the consequent premature aging that follows. A high-protein intake creates amyloid deposits (a by-product of protein metabolism) which are deposited in the connective tissues and cells and cause tissue and organ degeneration. Dr. Schwartz, a professor of pathology at Frankfort University and one of the leading experts on amyloid, feels that amyloid build-up could be one of the most important contributors to the aging process.

The metabolic combustion of excessive protein is also associated with creating an overly acid system because of the accumulation of toxic protein metabolic wastes, such as uric acid, purines, and ammonia by-products. This results in what I call autotoxemia. Along with the excess protein in the system is a putrefaction process of the partially digested protein that results in the stimulation of unhealthy bacterial growth in the colon. These bacteria give off toxins that are absorbed into the blood through the colon. Ammonia, which is a breakdown product of a high flesh food diet, is directly toxic to the system. It has been found to create free radical damage, cross-linking (a process associated with skin wrinkles and aging), as well as depleting the body's energy. I have seen alcoholics with liver disease be admitted to the hospital after ingesting a steak because they went into ammonia toxicity. Their damaged liver was not able to detoxify the excess ammonia and they became so ill they needed to be hooked up to life support machines.

An excess protein diet has been shown by the U.S. army to cause a deficiency of B_6 and B_3. Protein has also been found to leach out calcium, iron, zinc, and magnesium from the system. In treating "incurable schizophrenics," Alan Cott, M.D., in his book, *Fasting as a Way of Life*, points out that the Russians have had some success with water fasting and a follow-up, low-protein, vegetarian diet. Relapses were reported to occur often when some patients began to eat meat again.

Over the past 30 years, a family of research physicians, the Wendts, has developed evidence to show that those who ingest too much protein actually develop a generalized protein storage disease. The Wendts showed, through the use of electron microscope photography, that excess protein results in clogging the basement membranes. Basement membranes are the membranes through which nutrients and oxygen are filtered into the cells from the capillaries and through which the waste products of the cells are filtered out of the cells back into the blood to be eliminated. The more excess protein there is in the diet, the more protein there is stored in the basement membrane. Eventually the basement membrane becomes so clogged that nutrients and oxygen are not able to pass into the cells and waste products are not able to be eliminated. Contrary to the clogged and thickened membrane of an excess protein eater, a baby's basement membrane has wide-open pores through which nutrients easily pass.

This clogged membrane results in cellular anoxia (decreased oxygen in the cell) and cell malnutrition. In the Wendts' observations, the protein builds up in such a way that it contributes to hypertension, atherosclerosis, cardiovascular disease, and adult onset diabetes. The Wendts coined the term "capillogenic tissue degeneration," meaning degeneration at the capillary level of circulation. By fasting and through following a low protein diet, they were able to reverse this process of basement membrane clogging, cellular stagnation, malnutrition, and anoxia. Excess protein in the system, which is almost always the case with a high flesh food diet, results in a protein storage disease which slowly chokes off the cellular system. This clogging of the basement membrane is reversed and prevented by a low-protein, vegetarian diet. As our diets get progressively lighter, our basement membranes become more porous, like a baby's, and our cellular assimilation improves.

A Danger of the High-protein Myth

We have a dietary epidemic of osteoporosis (loss of calcium from the bones) in the U.S. Approximately one out of three women will sufficiently demineralize her bones to cause at least one fracture in her lifetime. These fractures are significant because more women die from osteoporosis-related fractures than from cancer of the breast, cervix, and uterus combined. The toll due to these fractures is about 200,000 deaths per year. One to two million fractures occur per year. **The evidence is overwhelming that the most important single dietary change one can make to prevent osteoporosis is to decrease the amount of protein in the diet.** The clinical evidence from several major studies shows that **vegetarians have significantly less bone loss than those who have a flesh-centered diet.** The *Journal of Clinical Nutrition,* in 1983, reported in the largest study of its kind ever made, that by the age of 65:

- Female nonvegetarians had an average measurable bone loss of 35% as compared to only a 7% bone loss in female vegetarians. In other words, female vegetarians had fives times less bone loss by the age of 65 as those on a flesh-centered diet.
- Male vegetarians had a 3% bone loss as compared to males on a flesh food diet with 18% bone loss.

Their statistics showed **female vegetarians had 2.6 times less bone loss than nonvegetarian men and five times less bone loss than nonvegetarian women.**

In 1984, the *Medical Tribune* reported that vegetarians had significantly stronger bones. A study in 1988 of 1600 women, reported in the *American Journal of Clinical Nutrition,* showed that by the age of 80, those who had been vegetarians for at least 20 years had 18% bone loss as compared to a 35% bone loss of women on a flesh-centered diet. Note the following information:

Reasons Vegetarians May be Protected from Osteoporosis

1. A vegetarian diet brings us into more general harmony with nature and closer to the way our physiologies are meant to function.
2. Vegetarians consume less protein. The result is that vegetarians tend to be slightly alkaline rather than acidic as are many meat eaters. One way the body compensates to buffer against acidity is to pull calcium out of the bones to make alkaline salts in the blood which act as a buffer against the acidity. Research shows that a protein intake of greater than 75 mg per day results in a negative calcium balance in which calcium is lost from the bones.
3. Flesh foods are considerably higher in phosphorous as compared to plant foods. The high phosphorous draws the calcium out of the bones. This produces a loss in bone density.
4. A high flesh food diet causes more osteoporosis in that it is high in fat. This fat blocks the calcium uptake by actually forming biochemical soaps with the calcium which are then excreted by the system. Poor digestion is also a possible cause of low calcium. Low stomach acid is associated with poor calcium absorption.

The research also shows that high calcium supplementation does not seem to make a significant difference in the prevention or treatment of osteoporosis. For example, the Bantus, an African tribe, get about 350 mg of calcium per day, almost one fourth of the National Dairy Council recommendation of 1200 mg. The Bantu women, however, do not suffer from osteoporosis and rarely suffer from bone fractures. Although there may be some genetic component helping the Bantus, it is significant that the genetic relatives of the Bantus in the U.S., who are eating the standard American diet, have bone loss percentages that are about the same as the Caucasian population. Eskimos who have an intake of calcium of 2000 mg per day, but a high protein intake of 250-400 grams per day, have a high rate of osteoporosis. The Eskimo diet again points to the fact that a high protein diet is a more powerful force in causing osteoporosis than a high calcium diet is in preventing it. A two-year study of postmenopausal women reported in the *British Medical Journal* in 1984 showed that 2000 mg of calcium in the diet, as compared to a diet with 500 mg per day, showed no difference in the demineralization process. A study in the *New England Journal of Medicine* also demonstrated that calcium supplementation has no effect on the rate of osteoporosis as compared to women who took no supplementation. Not only does a high calcium intake not help prevent osteoporosis, but a world expert on vitamin D, Hector DeLuca, PhD., has pointed out that large amounts of calcium in the diet tend to turn off the body's production of vitamin D hormone and thus stops the bone rebuilding process. Excess calcium also seems to reduce copper and zinc absorption in the bone. These are minerals essential for proper bone formation.

There are also certain vitamins and minerals which are important in the biochemistry of bone formation. One of the most important is **vitamin D,** which in its hormonal form facilitates calcium absorption into the system and into the bone. By staying in the sun for at least 20 minutes we get enough vitamin D to meet all our calcium metabolism needs. Unfortunately, perhaps because of sedentary lifestyles of older house-bound people, the average vitamin D levels in older subjects is 47% lower than in younger subjects.

Vitamin C, which is found in higher concentrations in a vegetarian diet than in a meat-centered diet, is another important vitamin for bone development and reformation. **Folic acid** and **pyridoxine (B₆)** are also important.

One of the most important minerals is **silicon**. It stimulates the growth and formation of bone and teeth. Silicon increases the much-needed collagen in the bone which is the reason it has such an important effect. Silicon is found in mother's milk, in the fiber fraction of brown rice, in leafy greens and bell peppers, and in the herb called horsetail grass. These are primarily vegetarian sources. I have also found that horsetail grass, an herb grown in the U.S., is extremely high in silicon and very good for bone repair, regenerating finger nails, and improving hair strength and vitality in my patients. Only organic silicon helps to do this. The inorganic form doesn't seem to have this effect.

Magnesium, although comprising 0.1% of bone as compared to calcium being 20.2%, plays an important role in fixing calcium into the bone and also converting vitamin D to its active hormonal form. Magnesium is found in high concentrations in leafy greens, whole grains, legumes, seeds, almonds, black-eyed peas, curry, mustard powder, alfalfa sprouts, avocados, apples, bee pollen, beets, dates, dulse, figs, garlic, lentils, most green vegetables, grapefruit, kelp, eggs, and liver. Vegetarians get more than enough magnesium in their diet.

Manganese, copper, potassium, strontium, and zinc are other minerals that are important in bone and cartilage formation. Plants that contain magnesium also contain these minerals.

Boron, a little-known mineral, is needed in small amounts for proper bone metabolism. It could be one of the most important minerals in the prevention of osteoporosis. A study done in 1986 on postmenopausal women found that adding 3 mg per day of boron reduced the urinary loss of calcium by 44% and significantly increased the serum concentrations of natural estrogenic hormones. The boron increased the blood 178-estradiol levels (the most biologically active estrogen in humans) to concentrations equal to those found in women on estrogen replacement therapy. Boron has been found to be essential for the production of the active form of vitamin D. This increase in estrogen also helps prevent bone loss. This boron stimulation of natural estrogen levels is important because of the controversy around the use of estrogen supplementation. As pointed out by the National Institute of Health Consensus Development Conference on Osteoporosis in 1984, the risk of endometrial cancer increases with the use of estrogen therapy. The April 1991 issue of the *Journal of the American Medical Association* contained an article showing there was a direct linear relationship between the duration of the use of menopausal estrogens and the risk of breast cancer. This article reviewed the major studies on the subject and is considered by some as one of the most thorough epidemiological studies analyzing the relationship between menopausal estrogens and breast cancer. If all the studies were used, regardless of the quality of the study, the statistics showed if the estrogens were used for 15 years, a woman had a 30% excess risk of breast cancer. If used for 25 years, there was a 50% increased risk of breast cancer. If the five studies with the highest scientific quality were used, an increase of 60% incidence of breast cancer was found in the 15-year use group and 100% percent increase in breast cancer incidence in the 25-year use group. Another piece of this osteoporosis controversy is a recent 14-year study reported in the *Journal of the American Medical Association* in 1984, which showed there was no significant difference of hip fractures between women who did or did not have estrogen replacement therapy. These researchers found no association between fracture risk and hormone replacement therapy.

Boron may make a significant difference in our thinking about osteoporosis for its effect on estrogen alone, as well as its role in improving the metabolism of calcium, phosphorous, and magnesium and decreasing the calcium, magnesium, and estrogen losses. The two best sources of boron are kelp and alfalfa. Kelp is also high in silicon. Spinach, snap peas, cabbage, lettuce, apples, leafy greens, and legumes are also good sources of boron. Since boron is found primarily in vegetarian foods, this may be an additional reason why vegetarians have less osteoporosis. If you are growing your own garden, you may want to put borax in the soil to increase the boron concentration in your fruits and vegetables. The studies show a large margin of safety with boron. Dogs and rats were safe on more than 35 times the 3 milligram dosage. There are areas in the world where people naturally take in 13 times the required amount of boron in their food without any apparent side effects.

One can see that the prevention of osteoporosis is greatly enhanced by a low-protein, vegetarian diet. Such a diet provides an adequate-to-high source of calcium, boron, and other essential minerals and vitamins needed for optimal bone function. The low protein of a well-balanced vegetarian diet does not leach calcium from the bones. One study found that vegetarian women even stop having bone loss after the age of seventy. In addition, leading an active, balanced life with emphasis on a regular communion with the angels of exercise and moderate sunshine helps prevent osteoporosis. One study showed that women in their seventies, who exercised moderately, increased their bone mass by 1% per month as compared to the controls who did not exercise and continued to have bone loss. An optimal level of exercise for the maintenance of bone mass is essentially similar to the activity of a young adult. The best exercises are antigravity ones in order to create healthy bone stress and stimulation. Walking is one of the best antigravity exercises, but there should also be some exercise for the upper shoulder girdle and arms. Hatha yoga is an excellent activity for the upper body, as are mild to moderate traditional exercises like push-ups, et cetera. Betty Kamen, PhD., who has written an excellent booklet on osteoporosis, points out that we need to stand about three hours a day in order to prevent osteoporosis or do antigravity exercises continuously for at least 20 minutes five days per week. A life in balance brings a calcium balance.

Vegetarian Diet Increases Endurance

It has been a well-kept secret that a vegetarian diet increases endurance. Modern athletes are just beginning to discover what Dr. Irving Fisher first reported in the Yale Medical Journal in 1917, and what at least four more recent studies have shown: **A vegetarian diet helps the body function at an endurance rate that is approximately twice that of a flesh-centered diet.** He found that even sedentary vegetarians had more endurance than meat-eating athletes. In a study confirming this finding, Dr. Joteyko of the Academy of Medicine in Paris compared vegetarians and nonvegetarians from all walks of life and found that vegetarians had 2-3 times the endurance and took one fifth the time to recover. In a Danish study in 1968, the performance of the same people on three different diets showed that on a strictly vegetarian diet they averaged 167 minutes on a bicycle endurance test as compared to 57 minutes on a high meat and dairy diet. In Belgian research comparing handgrip strength, vegetarians averaged 69 squeezes as compared to a weaker 38 squeezes for nonvegetarians. They also found that vegetarians had a faster recovery time. Dr. Chittenden, another researcher in this area, and Dr. Fisher, felt that one of the reasons meat-eaters had less strength and endurance is that the protein breakdown products such as uric acid, urea, and purines, poison and interfere with muscle and nerve function. This immediate factor, plus all the other factors we have been discussing, make a difference when one is interested in endurance.

There are several world-class athletes that were vegetarian at the time they won their world records and performed their greatest athletic accomplishments. Dave Scott was a lactovegetarian when he won the Hawaii Iron Man Triathlon an incredible six times! He won it three times in a row, while no one else has ever won it twice in a row. Vegetarian Edwin Moses was an Olympic Gold Medalist for eight years in the 400 meter hurdles without losing a race. Murray Rose, who as a teenager became one of the world's greatest swimmers and later starred as Tarzan, was a vegetarian. Paavo Nurmi was another vegetarian. The "Flying Finn," who set 20 world records and won nine Olympic gold medals, found a vegetarian diet the best for endurance. Gayle Olinekova, a premiere women's long distance runner and longtime vegetarian, told me that she ran the Boston marathon after a seven-day water fast and had one of her best times. Vegetarians have been able to develop strong bodies as well as endurance. For example, there is Andeas Cahling, a raw food vegetarian who won the Mr. International award in 1980. Roy Hilligan won Mr. America. Stan Price, another vegetarian, set a world record in the bench press.

Population Studies Validate the Health and Longevity Effects of Vegetarianism

Of the 154 centenarians in Bulgaria, only five ate meat regularly. It is a well established fact that the longest-lived people throughout the world, such as the Hunzkuts, Bulgarians, East Indian Todas, Russian Caucasians, and Yucatan Indians, are either complete vegetarians or eat meat infrequently. They eat between one third to one half the protein that we eat in the U.S.

In a study of Seventh Day Adventists, the largest single group of vegetarians in the U.S., it was found that their colon cancer rate was 1.0 as compared to 2.7 for those on a flesh-centered diet. They were also found to have 40% less coronary disease than flesh eaters. In a comparison study of strict Seventh Day Adventists versus those of the same religion who ate meat three times per week, they found the strict vegetarians had one half the mortality from breast cancer. The general mortality rate of Seventh Day Adventists was 50-70% less than the U.S. population at large.

The *Journal of the American Medical Association* in 1961 estimated that 97% of heart disease could be prevented by a vegetarian diet. Research statistics show that a high flesh food diet causes ten times more heart attacks in the 45-65 year-old population than a diet of fresh vegetables, fruits, nuts, seeds, and grains. Twenty-six percent of meat eaters have hypertension as compared to two percent of vegetarians. Flesh eaters have 2.3 times more colon cancer, 4 times more breast cancer, 3.6 times more cancer of the prostate, and 10 times more cancer of the lungs than do vegetarians.

Because the animals whose flesh is eaten are higher on the ecological chain, there is a higher concentration of radioactive materials from fallout as well as higher amounts of pesticides, fungicides, and many other environmental toxins. This undoubtedly adds to a decrease in vitality and quality of health. Vegetarian women have been found to have between one third to one half the pesticides in their tissues as compared to meat eaters There is approximately 14 times more pesticides in flesh foods than in vegetarian produce. Flesh eaters also have to face the threat of the disease toxoplasmosis in pigs and cattle and trichinosis in pigs. There is also the threat of salmonella poisoning, especially from chickens. It is estimated that approximately one third of commercial chickens carry salmonella. Over one million cases of food poisoning are reported yearly. Most of these are salmonella.

The social costs of these self-induced, dietary-related illnesses are enormous. The National Heart, Lung, and Blood Institutes estimate that the cost of heart attacks alone in 1983 was 60 billion dollars in medical bills, lost wages, and productivity. Mordecai Ben-Porat introduced a bill in the Israel parliament that would outlaw flesh eating because it was estimated it would save 4,266 billion pounds of money from the improved health that would result from a vegetarian diet. The bill did not pass, however.

Wartime epidemiological population studies of vegetarian diets have brought some fascinating results. In 1917-1918, when little meat was available in Denmark due to the war, the death rate of civilians dropped 34% as compared to the yearly average for the previous 18 years. In the same sort of wartime situation during world War II in Norway, with little meat available, the death rate from circulatory disease dropped significantly. The effect of the nonflesh diet was confirmed when, after the war, the meat consumption rose and the death rate also rose correspondingly. In Great Britain, where there was also a decrease in flesh food in the diet, infant and postnatal deaths dropped to their lowest rates ever. Dental health improved in children. The amount of anemia decreased as did the rate of cardiovascular diseases. In general, overall quality of health statistics improved in England with less meat in the diet.

A recent Cornell-China-Oxford Project on Nutrition, Health, and Environment, which began in 1983 and tracked the health of 6,500 Chinese in sixty-five counties throughout China, has provided some interesting preliminary results. This study offers some particularly potent epidemiological evidence of the superior health benefits of a primarily vegetarian diet. According to Nathaniel Mead of the *East-West Journal*, some scientists are calling this study the "Grand Prix of epidemiology." Although this study may go on for decades, a preliminary release of data available in 1990 has already made several important points.

Preliminary Data
Cornell-China-Oxford Project on Nutrition, Health, and Environment

- Diets for children that are high in protein, fats, calcium, and calories promote early growth, but higher breast cancer rates among women.
- A vegetable-based diet is more healthy than an animal-based diet.
- The healthiest percentage of fat intake is 15-20%, which is easy to achieve on a vegetarian diet.

185

- The body gets adequate amounts of calcium from plant sources and does not need dairy to prevent osteoporosis.
- A vegetarian diet reduces the risk of nutritionally related diseases.
- The study suggests that if flesh-centered societies were to switch to a vegetable-centered diet, it might be a greater factor in improving world health than all the doctors, health insurance programs, and pharmaceuticals that are present approaches to improving world health.

There is an overwhelming amount of evidence, from the microcosmic cellular level to the macrocosmic global cultural level of research, that makes a single point: **a vegetarian diet, and especially a low-protein, vegetarian diet, improves the general health of the body and is superior for one's health in almost every way as compared to a flesh-centered diet. A vegetarian diet is a way of loving yourself and your body.**

In 1983, 60 billion dollars was lost on medical bills, lost wages, and productivity due to heart attacks in the U.S.

Compared to flesh food eaters who are 45-65 years old, lacto-vegetarians have three times less heart attacks. Vegetarians have ten times less heart attacks.

Flesh eaters stab themselves in the heart with their forks.

Is this a way to love yourself?

VISION

BLACKBOARD FACTS

Preview of Chapter 12
Do Vegetarians Get Enough Vitamin B$_{12}$?

In this chapter you will discover that healthy vegetarians get enough B$_{12}$. Because there is so much concern and mythology about B$_{12}$, I chose to make this chapter more scientific in format. It covers the physiology of B$_{12}$ and causes and signs of B$_{12}$ deficiency in a way to empower the reader with enough understanding to take responsibility for choices on this subject. At the end of the chapter there is a clinical summary which synthesizes the information in a simple way. Are you ready to give up your B$_{12}$ fears?

I. Vegetarians and vegans do get enough B$_{12}$

    A. B$_{12}$ studies

    B. B$_{12}$ deficiencies are rare among healthy vegetarians

II. Physiology of B$_{12}$

III. Why vegetarians do not become B$_{12}$ deficient

IV. Causes of B$_{12}$ deficiency

    A. Disease causes

    B. Pregnancy and lactation

    C. Tests for B$_{12}$

V. Summary of B$_{12}$ discussion

    A. Vegetarians do not need vitamin B$_{12}$ supplement

    B. Highest B$_{12}$ is in live foods

Chapter 12

Do Vegetarians Get Enough Vitamin B_{12}?

The often-heard health question raised by nonvegetarians and vegetarians alike is whether vegetarians get enough B_{12}. The answer is an important one because B_{12} deficiency can cause nerve degeneration and even death. I will speak more about the symptoms of B_{12} deficiency later. The answer to the B_{12} question is not one which can be answered merely by a simple recounting of the results of one or two laboratory studies or theoretical discussions. In order to answer this question to my own satisfaction I had to look at my own clinical experience and review a lot of the clinical studies on lactovegetarians and vegans. Vegans are those who do not consume any animal products, including dairy.

As pointed out by Dr. Alan Immerman in his review of vitamin B_{12} status on a vegetarian diet, many studies of vegans have appeared in the literature in the last 30 years. Of those suggesting an apparent B_{12} deficiency in vegans, none of these studies fulfilled the full scientific criteria for a legitimate B_{12} deficiency diagnosis. According to Dr. Immerman, all of the scientifically complete studies on vegans showed no evidence of B_{12} deficiency. Such studies include: 1. Harding and Stare in 1954, who examined 26 vegans and found no B_{12} deficiencies and general good health; 2. Ellis and Montegriffo who also studied 26 vegans and found no evidence of B_{12} deficiency. Four of the vegans had been on the diet for over 13 years with no supplements and had normal B_{12} levels; and 3. A study by Sanders in 1978 on 34 vegans, all of whom had normal blood and physical exams. They divided the subjects into two groups. One group who had been taking some sort of B_{12} supplement (six of these were taking regular B_{12} supplements) and one group who had absolutely no supplements. The average B_{12} serum level was higher in vegans who were taking some sort of food or vitamin B_{12} supplements. Their serum level was 421 picograms/cc (pg/ml) as compared to 253 pg/ml for the vegans not taking any supplements. No subject had a serum B_{12} less than the 80 pg/ml which was defined as indicative of deficiency by the World Health Organization in 1968. Some private laboratories now use 115 pg/ml as the indicator of deficiency. **These major studies, plus other studies, suggest that dietary B_{12} deficiency is rare among healthy vegans and all other types of vegetarians, whether they be lactovegetarians or lacto-ovovegetarians.**

Like the "high protein" myth, the B_{12} scare aimed at vegetarians also dissolves in the face of scientific studies of population subgroups. In studies of Indian villagers in southern India who are vegetarian, B_{12} deficiency was also found to be a rare occurrence. Dr. Baker, who has studied some populations in southern India, has found people with serum levels below 140 pg/ml who were what he considered healthy subjects with no clinical evidence of B_{12} deficiency.

189

This suggests that low serum levels, without neurological, hematological or any other clinical evidence of B_{12} deficiency, is not necessarily an accurate way to diagnose B_{12} deficiency. If serum B_{12} were used as the sole criteria, it would be necessary to categorize much of the population of India and other third world countries as deficient in B_{12}.

My observation, however, is that the serum B_{12} level in vegetarians and in vegans in particular, is lower than that of those on a flesh-centered diet. Instead of thinking of these levels as inadequate, it seems more accurate to broaden the range of acceptable normals based primarily on serum levels of nonvegetarians to include averages for vegetarians, which do run lower.

In general, I have begun to find that the physiological profiles for vegetarians and, particularly vegans, are different than those of nonvegetarians. For example, vegans will have lower cholesterols and triglycerides than flesh eaters. If we used vegan physiology as the standard, more flesh eaters would be considered to have high cholesterols rather than just high normal cholesterols. Broadening the range of normals for B_{12} levels to include healthy vegans gives us a much clearer framework from which to assess health. It also forces us to look at our cultural biases.

Live food vegetarians also exhibit different baseline normals of nutrient levels than other dietary sub-groups, including cooked food vegetarians. Raw food people will have less enzymes in their digestive secretions because their bodies have adjusted to the high enzyme concentrations that come in the raw foods. If large amounts of cooked food were added to their diets, we could expect that within a week the enzyme contents of their secretions would shift back to that of the regular cooked food population. I have also observed that as the health of a person improves and their diet includes more live food and less protein, they seem to need less food and have more vitality. This positive physiological shift is a fairly consistent observation. This may also explain why the cultural studies of those primarily vegetarian populations which abound in good health and longevity find they are able to live healthily on between one third to one half the protein and calorie intake.

The question that needs to be asked is: "Why is it that healthy vegans routinely do not suffer from B_{12} deficiency, despite fears, mythologies, and some 'scientific' prognostications to the contrary?" To answer this, it is helpful to understand a little about the physiology of B_{12}.

Physiology of B_{12}

1. B_{12} is only available from bacterial production. B_{12} is not made by plants or animals. All B_{12} found in plants and animals is from bacteria growing in or on them. Animals are a better source of B_{12} than plants because they have more bacteria growing in them. Not all the B_{12} produced by bacteria are the

same. Some are very useful to humans and others are called analogues, which are similar to B$_{12}$ in chemical structure but are not utilizable by human vitamin metabolism. Some theorize that these analogues may even block the utilizable B$_{12}$ uptake by occupying some of a limited number of B$_{12}$ uptake sites. For example, in a human's stool there are approximately 100 micrograms of B$_{12}$; 95% are analogues, which are not utilizable, and 5% is the true B$_{12}$ that is active for humans (see fig. 16).

2. Humans have B$_{12}$-producing bacteria throughout the body. It is estimated by Doctors Thrash and Thrash that the microorganisms between the teeth and gums, around the tonsils, in the tissue at the base of the tongue, and in the nasopharyngeal passages produce about .5 micrograms per day. Dr. Baker and his associates have shown that there are bacteria in the small intestine which produce utilizable B$_{12}$ which is also assimilated into the system through the lower end of the small intestine (the ileum). Colon bacteria also produce 5 micrograms of utilizable B$_{12}$, but B$_{12}$ doesn't seem to be absorbed from the colon.

3. B$_{12}$ absorption begins in the stomach where gastric secretions of proteases and hydrochloric acid split off the B$_{12}$ from the peptide bonds that attach it to the food. To continue, the proteases from the pancreas also disconnect from the food whatever B$_{12}$ has not been separated out. A healthy pancreas, as well as strong gastric secretions, are needed for maximal B$_{12}$ absorption. Once the B$_{12}$ is disconnected from the food, it binds to the intrinsic factor. It then goes to specific receptor sites in the ileum part of the small intestine and is then absorbed into the system. About one percent of the B$_{12}$ absorption is directly through the ileum by the basic diffusion process. It is this one percent which is probably the basis of the extremely high B$_{12}$ tablets we see in the health food stores.

4. An additional mechanism for maintaining a high B$_{12}$ level in the system is that high quantities are secreted by the liver into the bile. Dr. Herbert, a national expert on B$_{12}$, estimates that anywhere between 1 to 10 micrograms of B$_{12}$ are secreted into the bile, and therefore into the small intestine, each day. Normally we absorb much of the human-active B$_{12}$ back into our system through the ileum. In this process unwanted analogues are excreted. Dr. Herbert feels that vegetarians may be getting more B$_{12}$ from the reabsorption of the bile B$_{12}$ than from the foods they eat. Since humans need less than 0.5 micrograms per day, this bile secretion is indeed significant.

5. Louis Sullivan, a researcher at Harvard, showed that only 0.1 microgram of B$_{12}$ is needed to get a physiological response in B$_{12}$-deficient people. Dr.

Picture of B$_{12}$ physiology

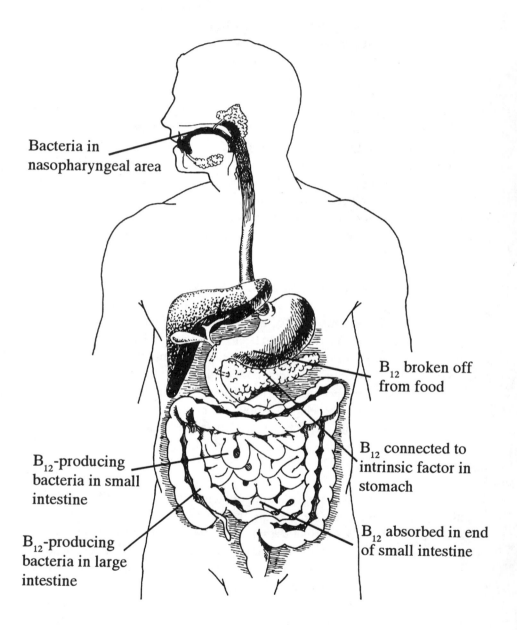

Bacteria in
nasopharyngeal area

B$_{12}$ broken off
from food

B$_{12}$-producing
bacteria in small
intestine

B$_{12}$ connected to
intrinsic factor in
stomach

B$_{12}$-producing
bacteria in large
intestine

B$_{12}$ absorbed in end
of small intestine

Fig. 16

Herbert estimates that between 0.2 to 0.25 micrograms per day is probably adequate for any individual. Dr. Herbert feels there is no objective published data that show any larger amounts of B$_{12}$ have any additional value for greater health or longevity. Other leading experts feel that 0.5 microgram per day is sufficient. Dr. Baker reports that he found the daily B$_{12}$ intake of healthy South Indian vegetarian villagers, who had no signs of B$_{12}$ deficiency, fell in the range of 0.3 to 0.5 micrograms per day. This estimate did not factor in B$_{12}$ loss for cooking their food. This range of .25-.5 micrograms per day as the minimum needed for adequate B$_{12}$ is approximately 250 to 500 times less than the 50 to 100 microgram tablets offered in health food stores for daily doses. It is estimated that about 1-3% of these B$_{12}$ tablet megadoses will cross the intestinal barrier directly.

Vegetarians have also been shown to have better absorption rates than meat eaters. Meat eaters, who might ingest 10 micrograms per day, are estimated to absorb 16%, while vegans, who may be ingesting 1 microgram per day from their food, are estimated to absorb up to 70%. This is another example of how the adaptive physiology of the human organism changes as a function of the quality of the diet. Dr. Thrash suggests that those on low-fat and low-protein vegetarian diets with good health habits may need only 0.05 micrograms of B$_{12}$ per day, and that nonsmoking vegans may not need any external source of B$_{12}$ in their diets or through supplements because their own friendly bacteria living in the nasopharynx, teeth, gums, and small intestine would produce enough B$_{12}$.

6. Vitamin B$_{12}$ is heat sensitive but not entirely destroyed by cooking. Research shows that between 23.7% to 96.4% of B$_{12}$ is destroyed by boiling or baking, depending on the food type and the length of heat processing. Boiling milk for two to five minutes decreases the active B$_{12}$ amount by 30%. Another study of longer boiling time showed a 50% loss. Sterilization of milk in sealed containers for 13 minutes caused a 77% loss. Milk pasteurization has been reported to have as low a loss as 10%. In condensed milk, the B$_{12}$ loss is between 40-90%.

7. B$_{12}$, when isolated as a single factor, is highly mutable. When it is put in a multi-vitamin, for example, B$_{12}$ often mutates into an analogue state and is no longer utilizable for body consumption. Because B$_{12}$ breaks down to analogues when in a multi-vitamin, it is advisable that if one is to take a B$_{12}$ supplement, it should be taken as a single, separate supplement rather than in a multivitamin.

Why Vegetarians do not Become B_{12}-Deficient

Now that we understand some of the B_{12} physiology, the reasons why vegetarians, and particularly vegans, do not normally develop B_{12} deficiencies give some insight into the subtleties of the B_{12} question. There is enough B_{12} in dairy products alone to supply adequate B_{12} for lactovegetarians, so they are considered less at risk for B_{12} deficiency.

One of the major sources of B_{12} for vegans is their own bacteria. Bacteria growing in the nasopharyngeal areas, as well as the teeth and gums, supplies .5 micrograms of B_{12} a day, which is enough to supply one's daily needs by itself. There is also some absorption from the bacterial production in the small intestines, as well as reabsorption from bile. Additional research has found that there is actually more B_{12} produced by the bacteria in the small intestine of a vegetarian than in that of a meat eater. This fits perfectly with the aforesaid principle that different dietary and lifestyle patterns produce different physiologies which reveal different normal baseline readings. A study of South Indian immigrants who had no B_{12} deficiencies in India, but who developed some deficiencies when they migrated away from India, sheds some additional insight into the importance of small intestinal bacteria. Researchers found that the bacteria in the stomach of the South Indians while in India had higher amounts of B_{12}-producing bacteria than that of Britishers. It was hypothesized that the move to England changed the types of bacteria colonizing the small intestine. This new and less dense strain of bacteria did not produce sufficient B_{12} to meet the B_{12} needs of the emigrating South Indians. Some studies of the well water of these same South Indians also showed that in India there was considerably more B_{12}-producing bacteria in the water, so more of their B_{12} needs were met by the B_{12} in the well water.

The B_{12} bacteria growing in water and found on vegetables that we eat are another way vegetarians get B_{12}. In an unusual study, it was found that a vegetarian community grew their food using fertilizing methods that have been used in the Orient for thousands of years, namely, using fertilizer that has composted human feces mixed in. It was found that the foods had an ample quantity of B_{12} because of this. The point is, that the B_{12} is not in the food, but on the food. It is produced by the local bacteria, and those bacteria are commonly abundant in our environment and on our food. B_{12} intake can come from multiple sources, as has been mentioned, other than merely from food.

B_{12} is found more often in root vegetables because of their contact with the soil bacteria. This means that if we are too scrupulous in washing off our food we may actually be washing away part of our B_{12} intake. Researchers have found high concentrations of B_{12} in and on mung beans, bean sprouts, comfrey leaves, fermented soybeans, peas, peanuts, lettuce, alfalfa, rice polishings, turnip greens, legume root nodules, and whole wheat. Each harvest seems to have

HUMAN ACTIVE B$_{12}$ IN SEA VEGETABLES

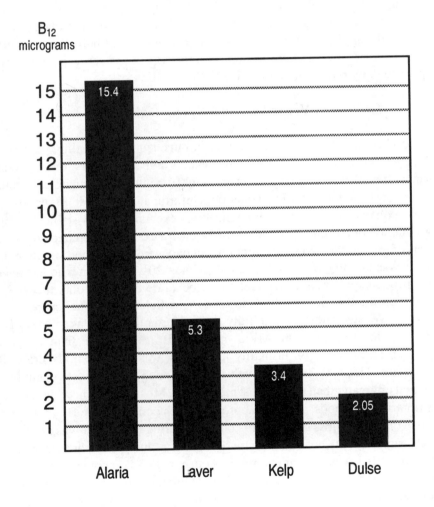

Fig. 17

variable amounts of B_{12} so that sometimes the same food may not have any B_{12} on it.

Recent research financed by the Maine Coast Sea Vegetables company at my suggestion has found that kelp, alaria (like wakambe), dulse, and laver (like nori) all have high amounts of human utilizable B_{12}. Their sea vegetables were sent to an independent lab that tests for human active B_{12}. Alaria had 15.4 micrograms ug of B_{12} per 100 grams. Laver had 5.3 ug of B_{12} per 100 grams. Kelp had 3.4 ug of B_{12} per 100 grams. Dulse had 2.05 ug of human active B_{12} per 100 grams. What this means is that one half ounce of alaria, which is a large single portion, will supply ten times the daily amount needed. One half ounce of dulse, which has the lowest amount of human active B_{12} of the sea vegetables, will supply the daily requirement (see fig. 17).

A Vegan Diet Supplies Enough B_{12}

Blood and tissue levels of B_{12} are lower but adequate in healthy vegans. In lactovegetarians and flesh eaters the B_{12} level is higher. There is some speculation that after 20 years on a vegan diet one might run into B_{12} deficiencies because of a very slow and gradual B_{12} depletion. Unfortunately, almost no research is available on vegans of over 20 years who have never taken any B_{12} tablets or food supplements containing B_{12}. Sander's research, for example, included only three vegans of greater than 20 years duration, but two were taking food supplements and one was taking a B_{12} tablet. The longer-than-20-year vegan who has never taken a food supplement of B_{12} tablet may be a rare find. It is only theoretical speculation whether they might, in fact, be B_{12}-deficient. The practical reality is that many vegans, either thoughtfully or inadvertently, have taken some B_{12}-containing food supplement. My own serum B_{12}, after more than 20 years vegetarian and 8 years on primarily live foods, was a surprisingly high 500 micrograms. This 500 microgram value is about double what most vegans have and equal or greater than that of most meat eaters. Most vegans, however, do not eat primarily live foods, a dietary approach which conserves the B_{12} in the food because there is no loss of B_{12} from cooking. During this time I was not taking any B_{12} supplements but I was regularly taking a blue-green algae from Lake Klamath, called Alphanizomenon Flos-Aquae, which I discovered through an independent laboratory analysis to be high in human active B_{12}. The laboratory report showed that one gram of the blue-green algae powder contained .279 micrograms of active B_{12}. This is equal to approximately the daily dose needed of active B_{12}. Although I did not take the Algae from Klamath Lake for this reason, it has obviously been a perfect vegetarian source of B_{12} for me. This high human active B_{12} may not be the same as green or other blue-green algaes which have been noted to have high concentrations of the inactive B_{12} analogs.

I have also observed in my clinical practice that there is a certain percentage of both meat eaters and vegetarians who seem to need B$_{12}$ supplements. One patient who was a meat eater came to me with a history of becoming ill after hepatitis, and for 20 years he needed B$_{12}$ shots on alternate days in order not to feel sick or become constipated. As I worked with him to move his diet in the direction of vegetarianism, his overall health got stronger and he then only needed to get a B$_{12}$ shot once every 2 to 6 months. I have observed other patients who, under mental or physical stress, become B$_{12}$ depleted and are helped considerably with a B$_{12}$ shot. In my earlier work as an orthomolecular psychiatrist (use of vitamins and minerals to improve mental imbalances), I observed certain patients with psychosis or borderline mental states whose minds became normal after a B$_{12}$ shot and who were able to be maintained on regular B$_{12}$ shots. There is a lot we do not understand about B$_{12}$ and human function. Even the editorial of the June 1988 edition of the *New England Journal of Medicine* by William Beck, a prominent B$_{12}$ researcher at the Massachusetts General Hospital, has suggested that newer research may ultimately justify previously judged "indiscriminate" use of B$_{12}$ injections. This comment was mostly for certain subpopulations of people who are not primarily vegetarians and yet still need B$_{12}$ because of certain pathological conditions. Dr. John Domissee, a prominent orthomolecular psychiatrist from Virginia, uses B$_{12}$ for post-traumatic stress disorders with great success. So, whether vegetarian or not, there are groups of people who need B$_{12}$ supplementation.

Causes of B$_{12}$ Deficiency

The main causes for a B$_{12}$ deficiency are either poor absorption, not enough B$_{12}$ intake, or physical or mental stress. The following situations are those which may cause either. It is my experience that these causes are far more responsible for B$_{12}$ deficiencies than general type of diet.

1. A disruption of the normal B$_{12}$ mechanism of absorption may be caused by such things as: low hydrochloric acid in the stomach, insufficient pancreatic digestive secretions, inadequate intrinsic factor production in the body, and disrupted small intestine function. Some of these things happen with a lowered quality of health and vitality, such as in older people who are not making efforts to maximize their vitality with good health habits. Some of the chief causes of poor absorption are: intestinal parasites, such as fishtapeworm; malaria; liver disease; chronic pancreatic disease; chronic infections, such as systemic mucocutaneous candidiasis; cancer; specific diseases of the gastrointestinal tract, such as regional ileitis, chronic atrophic gastritis, tropical sprue, and celiac disease; and poor digestion in general. Putrefaction in the small intestine from a high protein diet or contaminated

meat, chicken, or fish may stimulate the overgrowth of pathogenic bacteria that may also block the B_{12} uptake.

2. Surgery which has compromised intrinsic factor secretions of the small intestine or which has removed the B_{12}-absorbing segments of the small intestine.

3. Excess fat or protein may increase B_{12} needs.

4. Cooking our foods rather than eating them live depletes available active B_{12}.

5. Drug intake, such as alcohol, tobacco, coffee, para-amino salicylic acid, colchicine, birth control pills, and antibiotics increase the body needs for B_{12}.

6. Megadoses of vitamin C seem to lower serum B_{12} levels. Studies showing people who take two or more grams per day create a depletion in the B_{12}. Some have estimated that a high vitamin C intake increases the B_{12} needs tenfold. Others feel that anyone taking more than 500 mg of vitamin C per day for a long time should check their B_{12} status.

7. Foods with a high amount of B_{12} analogues, such as multiple vitamins or spirulina, might cause a depletion because the analogs and active B_{12} compete for B_{12} receptor sites. I believe further research is needed to confirm this.

8. Low B_6 and iron may also cause B_{12} depletion.

9. Raw soy products increase the excretion of B_{12}.

10. Thyroid disease has also been implicated in B_{12} depletion.

11. One of the most important causes of B_{12} depletion is pregnancy and lactation. Pregnancy causes an increased requirement of B_{12} due to the fetal drain on the maternal stores. The fetus requires about 50 micrograms of B_{12} per day. Under normal conditions, including that of healthy vegan mothers, there is enough stored B_{12} to meet the need of both the mother and the fetus. One Indian researcher concluded that vegetarians have lived for ages giving birth to healthy children and having healthy mothers who have never eaten flesh foods. This researcher felt there was no evidence to suggest that a vegetarian population consuming adequate lactovegetarian food is at any more risk than nonvegetarian mothers and babies.

While this may be true, there is one relatively small study of 17 macrobiotic babies and mothers reported in the *American Journal of Clinical Nutrition* which is of concern to me. It indicated that 56% of the macrobiotic mothers had a lower B$_{12}$ than compared to the study's nonvegetarian control group. Their infants also had a lower B$_{12}$ level. According to what we know, this lower serum B$_{12}$ would be expected. It is significant that none of the mothers showed any clinical signs of a B$_{12}$ deficiency. My concern was that at least one of the 17 macrobiotic babies had mild symptoms suggestive of a B$_{12}$ deficiency which went away when the mother was given B$_{12}$ supplementation in the form of food sources which contained active B$_{12}$. One out of 17 in such a small study is not a highly significant finding or even suggestive that a macrobiotic diet is B$_{12}$-deficient in the actual B$_{12}$ taken into the body. One possibility for these findings is that there is something detrimental in the macrobiotic diet that leads to B$_{12}$ deficiencies from poor assimilation or poor health that it creates.

There are other individual reports, as well as a Dutch study of macrobiotic mothers and infants reported in the East-West Journal May 1988 issue, showing infants of mothers on a macrobiotic diet who have developed B$_{12}$ deficiencies with some of their macrobiotic children actually developing blood changes and physical symptoms that were reversed with B$_{12}$ supplementation. This tendency may also be true for mothers and infants on fruitarian diets. Again, a possible explanation for these results is that the health of these mothers and infants was compromised in a way that lead to poor B$_{12}$ assimilation or retention.

I have also observed in my practice that there is a variety of women who have come to me, who have been both vegetarian and meat eaters, who have become B$_{12}$ deficient during pregnancy and lactation. **My impression is that B$_{12}$ deficiency with symptoms, not simply a lower serum B$_{12}$ as compared to nonvegetarians, is more because of poor health resulting in poor assimilation of B$_{12}$ or accelerated loss of B$_{12}$ from the system rather than not enough B$_{12}$ in the diet. It is possible that this may happen more easily on a macrobiotic or fruitarian diet than for other types of vegetarian diets.** My recommendations for preventing B$_{12}$ deficiencies stemming from certain diets and pregnancy are: follow Dr. Paavo Airola's suggestion of three tablespoons of brewers yeast or yeast that has been grown on a B$_{12}$-supplemented medium; sea vegetables; and one gram (approximately four capsules or one half teaspoon) of Algae from Klamath Lake. This approach has been most helpful in preventing this problem, as well as meeting the increased need for protein during this time. I have often found that one B$_{12}$ injection for a chronically depleted, postpartum woman has brought tremendous relief almost immediately. Oral B$_{12}$ supplementation often works, but not as well. Because of the general compromised health level of our total population, both vegetarians and flesh food-eating mothers would do well to pay careful attention to their B$_{12}$ levels during pregnancy and lactation.

Signs of B$_{12}$ Deficiency

A B$_{12}$ deficiency may first be suggested by symptoms of general fatigue and tiredness. Symptoms may manifest first through the blood system with anemia-caused fatigue and other blood cell changes. B$_{12}$ is important in DNA synthesis which affects the ability of all cells to reproduce and function properly. Over time, all the cells may be affected. The nerve cells are one of the primary targets. Onset of symptoms of nerve degeneration is suggested by loss of feeling in one's fingers and toes and loss of feeling in the spine. Other symptoms may be a progressively poor sense of balance, clumsiness, loss of the sense of joint position orientation, cutaneous pain upon light touching, and decreased reflexes.

Another set of symptoms that might first manifest are mental in origin. Increased irritability is often the first symptom. There may also be memory loss, inability to concentrate, depression, and other subtle symptoms which may mirror senile dementia. There may be personality changes or even hallucinations. These neuropsychiatric changes in certain people, according to Lindenbaum's recent studies at Columbia Presbyterian Medical Center, may occur without accompanying changes in the blood picture in about 30% of people. Deficiency symptoms in infants manifest as lethargy, loss of appetite, speech impairment, and other signs of slow physical and mental development.

The basic test for B$_{12}$ is a serum B$_{12}$ which tests for active B$_{12}$ in the blood. We normally have about 40% of the B$_{12}$ in the blood as analogues. The O malhamensis bacteria (bacteria that will only grow on human active B$_{12}$) test, which shows only the active B$_{12}$, is probably the most accurate. A generally safe range is between 150-200 micrograms per cc. In one recent study on students put on a vegan diet without B$_{12}$ supplements, it was noted that within one to two years most of the students' serum B$_{12}$ dropped and then leveled off slightly above 200 micrograms/cc. A basic blood test for B$_{12}$ deficiency is the one for anemia associated with enlarged red blood cells. There are some new tests which measure homocysteine and methymalonic acid in the urine (the secretion of these two metabolites are increased when the B$_{12}$ levels are lowered). This test is particularly good for screening for subtle neurological changes when the blood lab tests are normal. It is good for children and infants as well.

Because of the relativity of the serum B$_{12}$ levels and the urine metabolite levels, a B$_{12}$ deficiency should be diagnosed by evidence of clinical symptoms plus these tests being low. A low B$_{12}$ level can be used as encouragement to take more B$_{12}$-containing foods, such as yeast, sea vegetables, or the Algae from Klamath Lake. A good time to do a screening for B$_{12}$ is about two years after becoming vegetarian to see where one's B$_{12}$ has leveled off. Afterwards, one should check every three to five years since it takes that long to run out of B$_{12}$ if there is a malabsorption problem. My feeling is that any vegetarian whose health has been compromised in some manner and who chooses not to take any high

B$_{12}$-containing foods, would be wise to screen once a year for a possible low B$_{12}$ level. Although there is little need for a healthy vegan to be concerned, everyone who has gone 20 years as a vegan would be wise to check their B$_{12}$ levels. The results would be important data to share.

Summary of B$_{12}$ Discussion

Healthy vegetarians (lactovegetarians and vegans), as a matter of practical reality, do not have to worry about B$_{12}$ deficiency problems and do not have to take any B$_{12}$ supplementation, except for pregnancy, where yeast, sea vegetables, and/or Algae from Klamath Lake is advisable as a preventative measure. Synthetic B$_{12}$ supplementation or flesh foods are not really needed. For people eating 80% or more live food, even less whole food supplementation is needed. On the other hand, vegans should be aware that although the B$_{12}$ is sufficient when they are healthy, they do seem to have lower B$_{12}$ serum levels than those on a flesh-centered diet. Because of this they run a higher risk of developing a B$_{12}$ deficiency under a variety of stressors, as mentioned above. The slight risk of a B$_{12}$ deficiency for a vegetarian under stress may be well worth it as compared to the major risks to health taken by those on a flesh food diet in terms of heart diseases, cancer, decreased endurance, and the general inferior health of a flesh-centered diet as compared to a vegetarian diet. By regularly including high B$_{12}$ foods, even this risk is minimized.

The healthiest and best prevention for lactovegetarians and vegans against B$_{12}$ deficiency is to honor Mother Nature and our bodies with optimal health habits and a live food diet in which no B$_{12}$ is destroyed by cooking. I was not able to find any studies of B$_{12}$ levels in live food vegans, but my observations of the few raw food vegans who have been on such a diet for more than 20 years without any supplementation of B$_{12}$ is that they are the healthiest group of people I have ever seen in our western culture. The health and vitality of some of these people in their 70s and 80s is heart-warmingly astounding.

If you regularly use alcohol, coffee, birth control pills, antibiotics, more than 500 mg of vitamin C a day, aspirin, or have chronic digestive or colon problems, you are in danger of becoming B$_{12}$ deficient, especially if you are a vegetarian who cooks your food.

Cooking food destroys 30-90% of the B$_{12}$—protect yourself by giving up these habits and/or taking brewers yeast, bee pollen, sea vegetables, or algae from Lake Klamath.

A healthy vegetarian with a healthy lifestyle does not need to worry about B$_{12}$ deficiency, especially if 80% of the food eaten is uncooked.

Preview of Chapter 13
Doubts About a Vegetarian Diet

In this chapter we directly show, with the use of population studies and other forms of discussion, that many of the ideas held in the West and in Traditional Chinese Medicine (T.C.M.) about the "dangers" of a vegetarian diet are primarily myths. Although there may appear to be some shade of truth about some of these ideas in the short run, when the whole process of the skillful transition to vegetarianism is considered over time, these shades of truth become significantly less accurate. Are your ready to learn more information about the safety of a vegetarian diet?

I. Cultural bias of T.C.M. against vegetarianism

   A. Myth of spleen yang definition

   B. Vegetarian diet superior to meat-centered in prevention of chronic disease, creation of health, vitality, endurance

II. Why vegetarians have less anemia

III. Why vegetarians in Alaska are not cold

IV. Doctors' issues with vegetarianism

V. Vegetarian women have normal menses

Chapter 13

Doubts About a Vegetarian Diet

After considering some of the health benefits, it is time to address some of the cultural doubts arising about vegetarianism. I have already answered some of the usual questions that arise in our Western culture; now it is time to include some of the questions raised by the system of medicine known as Traditional Chinese Medicine (T.C.M.) because more and more people in the West are using this system. T.C.M. is a time-honored medical system that has a unique way of conceptualizing health and disease. The main approaches used in T.C.M. are acupuncture, herbs, and dietary advice. This system has its primary roots in China, which is still the major advocate of this system, however, variations of T.C.M. have been created in Japan and Korea and interest is now growing in the West. Within the ancient system of T.C.M. there is a widespread belief that a vegetarian diet, and especially a live food diet, will create a "spleen yang deficiency." A spleen yang deficiency is usually associated with anemia, less endurance, decreased digestive power, excess water, excess phlegm (mucous), edema, internal coldness, a weakened immune system, paleness, cyclic imbalances (including the cessation or imbalance of the menstrual cycle), and general poor health. These ideas need to be critically addressed.

Not all T.C.M. practitioners believe these symptoms automatically happen on a vegetarian diet. For example, one of the world's most respected leaders in classical acupuncture, Englishman Jack Worsley, N.D., C.A., and director of the Worsley Institute of Classical Acupuncture, does not hold this unqualified negative attitude on the merits of vegetarian diets. Other Western-trained acupuncturists are also moving in this direction of accepting the health benefits of vegetarianism as well. Like Westerners who are trained in Ayurvedic medicine who do not share certain Indian cultural beliefs about vata and live foods, these Western acupuncturists are not blindly holding onto the ancient Chinese cultural beliefs about vegetarianism. With some noteworthy exceptions, such as the vegetarian Shaolin priests, throughout history and to this day the Chinese culture has attached a higher social status to including flesh in the diet. Being a pure vegetarian in China is, to some degree, associated with poverty and lack of social standing. This bias is reflected in the Chinese medical establishment, which in turn influences medically endorsed dietary advice. Fortunately, most modern research shows that these myths are not substantiated either epidemiologically nor on the individual dynamic level.

In all fairness, I must point out that although China does not embrace vegetarianism as its main dietary system, it is not as heavy a meat-eating country as the U.S. According to the China Health Project, a major study I mentioned in the previous chapter, that was initiated in 1983 by scientists from the Chinese

Academies of Preventative Medicine, Cornell University, and University of Oxford, only 7% of the protein in the Chinese diet comes from animal sources as compared to 70% in the American diet. In the Chinese dietary pattern, eating a whole steak as the main part of a meal is considered to be imbalanced and excessive. In China, a flesh eater may have only three to four ounces of meat per day, whereas a typical heavy flesh eater in the U.S. consumes much more. The prestigious researchers of the China Health Project felt that the Chinese eating patterns were considerably healthier because so much less flesh food was eaten. In essence, the Chinese traditional diet is closer in content to a Western vegetarian diet than the typical Western, meat-centered diet.

With almost every bias, however, there is also some shade of truth that is expanded upon, and in this case, exaggerated into, somewhat of a myth regarding the dangers of a vegetarian diet. It is inevitable and unavoidable that with any kind of diet, vegetarian or otherwise, there will always be some individuals who will become imbalanced due to their own health problems and psychophysiological constitutions they bring to the situation. These exceptions may become yang deficient and/or imbalanced on a poorly chosen vegetarian diet if they do not have appropriate guidance in the type of vegetarian diet they need. It may also be possible that a flesh food diet may more quickly improve a person who is yang deficient. Although it may work quicker than a vegetarian diet, it does not mean that it is healthier in the long term than a vegetarian diet.

Another category, which I call the transition phase to vegetarianism, can also temporarily support the myths. As the body adjusts to vegetarianism and/or live foods, it is common that there may be some internal and external sensitivity to coldness for a while. When the transition is carefully, patiently, and intelligently made, one eventually passes through this coldness and begins to feel warmer. For example, during fasting, one may feel cold and weak as the detoxification process unfolds. If one happened to be seen by a T.C.M. doctor in the middle of this detoxification phase, one might receive a yang deficient diagnosis and be advised to eat meat for strength and heat. But what is actually happening is that the vital force is healing and strengthening at a deeper inner level so that by the end of the fast the person emerges stronger and more vital than when he or she began. In other words, looking at the total process gives a radically different understanding than simply looking at the apparent, observable symptoms at one point in the process. I believe this misunderstanding of the significance of the transition process is how some of the bias and confusion has manifested into a belief system.

In intelligently handling the detoxification stage of the transition to vegetarianism and dealing with the "internal process" shifting of the body's physiology, the true remedy is not flesh food, but the highest quality vegetarian foods, herbs, and enzymes that enhance and balance the transition process so the person glides to a higher level of health. Although flesh foods may temporarily balance someone, by patiently travelling through the vegetarian transition phase, one becomes grounded on a deeper level of health.

In fact, the epidemiological statistics show that in the long run flesh foods speed the aging process and lower vitality so that one becomes permanently grounded (six feet underground?) sooner. If we look at health patterns in different nations and cultures with a high incidence of longevity, more people consistently over 100 years old are vegetarians or primarily vegetarians or those who may eat meat on a monthly frequency. As previously mentioned, only 5 of 154 Bulgarians over 100 were not vegetarians. The research I've already cited shows that vegetarians have between two to three times the endurance and, at least in one study, recover from physical activity at least two times faster.

The general health data indicate that vegetarians have a lower incidence of chronic disease and cancer in all categories and superior health, vitality, and endurance. Because of this, one can deduce that their immune systems would also be stronger. Live food vegetarians, in addition, do not suffer from the chronic overstimulation of the immune system every time they eat caused by the effects of cooked food. Although I do not know of any studies comparing the immune system strengths of live food vegetarians to flesh food eaters, theoretically, the immune system of a live food eater should be stronger. I have observed in my clinical practice that live food vegetarians seem to have the most resistance to disease. This stronger immune system is contrary to what would be associated with a spleen yang deficient pattern as theoretically predicted by the T.C.M. system.

The Chinese are not alone in their cultural myths. If we were to believe the culturally biased propaganda of the beef industry, a juicy steak dripping with blood is supposedly loaded with the highest quality iron that one cannot get anywhere else. Nowadays it is easy to be scared into believing the mythology that vegetarians will become anemic and therefore spleen yang deficient. The research, however, shows this is just another cultural myth disseminated through the flesh-centered Chinese or American medical establishments. One of the most startling historical facts which repudiate this myth were the British statistics during World War II. When the meat supply was seriously curtailed due to scarcity and the diversion of meat to the fighting soldiers, the population in England had significantly less flesh foods in the diet. **The rate of anemia significantly decreased in the total civilian population during the time of the least flesh food consumption.**

Why do vegetarians have less anemia? The answer, I believe, lies in the leafy greens, which often have a higher concentration of iron than flesh foods. For example, according to the *U.S.D.A. Handbook no. 456*, gram for gram, kale has fourteen times more iron than red meat. Spinach, Popeye's comic strip power food, has approximately 11 times the iron as ground beef. Strawberries, cabbage, bell peppers, and even cucumbers have more iron per weight than ground beef or sirloin steak. Researchers have also found that vitamin C, which is high in fruits and vegetables, significantly enhances the body's ability to assimilate iron.

In the *American Journal of Clinical Nutrition,* 1984, research by Hallberg and Rossander showed that nonheme iron (iron found in vegetarian food as compared to the heme iron of flesh food) was absorbed four times greater if there were enough accompanying fruit and vegetables to provide 65 mg of vitamin C. There is at least that much vitamin C in one half green pepper. Vegetables, such as kale, spinach, broccoli, and mustard greens, are high in both vitamin C and iron. Beans and peas are also high in iron. Cooking in iron pots is another indirect source of iron. According to White, in *Let's Talk About Food,* the iron in food can be increased by 100 to 400% by being prepared in iron pots. The clinical evidence, as reported in such science journals as the *Journal of Human Nutrition, American Journal of Clinical Nutrition,* and *Journal of the American Dietetic Association,* clearly shows that in vegetarians, iron assimilation is as high as, or higher than, that of flesh food eaters. Anderson, Gibson, and Sabry, in the *American Journal of Clinical Nutrition,* report that the hemoglobin and iron levels in vegetarian women who are regularly menstruating were higher than that of women of comparable ages in the general population. The iron in the vegetarian diets of these women was also higher than in the diets of the general population.

Research cited by Rudolf Ballentine, M.D., in his book *Transition to Vegetarianism,* indicates that moderate amounts of oxalates and fiber found in a vegetarian diet do not block iron uptake. This may also be true for phytates as well. This is significant because of myths that fiber and oxalates may block uptake of iron. Dr. Ballentine points out there is some speculation by scientists that long-term vegetarians assimilate the iron from vegetables more efficiently, and perhaps differently, than meat eaters.

Two major foods which decrease iron uptake is the intake of excessive dairy products and black tea with meals. It is common that in the transition to vegetarianism people increase their dairy product consumption as a protein substitute in order to assuage their illusory fear stemming from the "inadequate protein myth." The problem is that dairy foods are very low in iron. To equal the amount of iron in a bowl of spinach, one would have to drink approximately fifty gallons of milk. In addition, dairy products are thought to have inhibitors to iron absorption which have not yet been specifically identified. Narins, in *Biochemistry of Non-heme Iron,* points out that breast fed babies have a higher rate of iron absorption than babies given cow's milk, even if their formulas are enriched with iron. This is a significant consideration because the populations that are at risk for iron deficiency are pregnant women and children. The fetus depends on iron for a normal development and in infants, iron is also specifically needed for mental development.

Eating a lot of milk products, such as milk, cheese, yogurt, butter, and ice cream, contributes to an iron deficiency. A high dairy product intake not only blocks iron uptake, but because it is filling, it diminishes intake of high iron foods such as fruits, grains, and vegetables. The few new vegetarians who may become iron deficient because of a high dairy intake, may psychologically crave what they remember on a subliminal level as the prime source of iron and find themselves craving meat. As meat is also a good source of iron, they feel better. In one's transition to vegetarianism, to avoid an iron deficiency, it is better to eat a minimal amount of dairy and lots of fresh fruits, vegetables, and grains.

The tannic acid in black teas is also a common cause of blocking iron uptake. If one insists on drinking black teas in one's diet, it is best to drink the tea at least one hour before meals. Tannic acid is also found in the skins of almonds. If one eats a lot of almonds, then it is a good idea to take off the almond skins as explained in the food preparation section.

A note of caution for those who are iron deficient. The best way to increase iron is to eat high iron foods such as kale and spinach. Iron supplementation, for a short time will not cause an imbalance, but research reported in the *American Journal of Clinical Nutrition* in 1986 shows that long-term use of iron supplementation can result in a decreased copper, zinc, and selenium absorption.

Does Vegetarianism Make You "Cold?"

What T.C.M practitioners describe as "internal cold" and "dampness," two symptoms of yang deficiency, is worth considering, especially if one is a kapha type. In the Ayurvedic system, people with predominantly kapha constitutions tend toward water imbalances and internal cold. They also have problems with excess mucous production when the weather is cold and damp. Excess mucous in itself can contribute to coldness. My clinical experience shows kapha types have considerably less mucous on a live food vegetarian diet. My findings parallel the findings of Arnold Erhet's mucousless diet approach. Erhet found that when he put himself and thousands of his followers on a diet which eliminated highly mucous foods, such as flesh food, dairy, and cooked grains, they had less mucous and phlegm. According to Erhet, my clinical experience with patients, and my own personal experience (my predominate constitutional type is kapha), a live food vegetarian diet is the best for decreasing mucous in the body. This is distinctly opposite to what is hypothesized by T.C.M. practitioners.

There is a way to create a water excess with a vegetarian, and particularly a live food, diet. It is by increasing fruit and vegetable intake and not decreasing intake of other fluids. Fruits and vegetables contain more water than flesh foods and grains. Fruits consist of approximately 80% highly structured water, the most biologically active water available. There is no better water that one can take into the body. The more fruits and vegetables one eats, the less one needs to drink water or other liquids. In this way the fluid balance can be maintained at a healthy level. Making the adjustment of drinking less fluid to avoid a fluid excess and "dampness" in the system as one increases fruit and vegetables in the diet is primarily important for those with kapha constitutions. In general, most people do not get enough fluid, so the increased intake of fruits and vegetables will usually be beneficial to health. By being aware of this dynamic interplay between water intake, biological water from fruit and vegetables, and one's constitution, one can intelligently work with the diet to become more in tune with optimal fluid needs.

"Coldness"

Initially, one may feel a little colder on a live food vegetarian diet. If one stops one's observation and efforts at this beginning transition stage, one will jump to the conclusion there is a spleen yang deficient condition developing because of the experience of coldness. If one continues to make scientific observations on the process, one will discover that after several months, and even a year or so with some individuals, one actually becomes warmer. As the body becomes healthier, the arteries become less clogged and circulation improves. With better circulation, vitality, and health, the body then begins, in the long term, to become warmer on a vegetarian and live food diet, even in Alaska. In the meantime, until one completely adjusts, dressing a little warmer, exercising, and using heating herbs and foods will make this transition easier.

This increased warmness has certainly been my own experience. My body is more tolerant of cold now than when I was on a flesh-centered diet or when I initially became a vegetarian. Earlier, I mentioned a preliminary retrospective survey that I conducted with vegetarians and live fooders in chilly Anchorage, Alaska. It was carried out at my suggestion by the owners of Enzyme Express, a wonderful live food restaurant in Anchorage. We found that one hundred percent of the vegetarian customers who filled out the questionnaire had no difficulty with the cold Alaskan weather. More than two thirds of these people ate 50% or more of their exclusively vegetarian food live. Approximately one third of the total surveyed ate 75% of their food live. All had reported increased health and vitality on this diet even in the Alaskan climate. This is consistent with the finding in *Diet for A New America* which showed that "over 95% of former meat eaters report that a switch to a vegetarian diet increases their energy, vitality, and overall feeling of well-being...." About half of these people in the Alaskan study used warming herbs and one third used exercise to help keep them warm during the winter. Most were long-term vegetarians, although 10% had made the transition to vegetarianism in the last six months.

In the transition to a vegetarian or live food diet, the moderate use of heating herbs, such as ginseng, cayenne, ginger, curry, and black pepper, helps to supply a drying and heating energy. The point is even an initial transitory coldness can be compensated for by the use of heating herbs and food as part of the diet. Although I initially used ginseng to increase yang heat, I stopped using it after one year because it made my body too hot. This was obviously a sign that the transition to increased internal heat had been made.

Another powerful approach to increasing body heat is to exercise vigorously on a daily basis. This distinctly increases body yang energy and dries the body of excess fluid. This is consistent with Ayurvedic teachings which stress the importance for kapha people to exercise regularly. With intelligent application of the use of heating herbs, foods, and exercise, the initial coldness that one may encounter transitioning to vegetarianism, particularly if one is a kapha or vata type, can be intelligently compensated for and balanced. The best use of these herbs and exercise is the time of maximum kapha imbalance toward excess mucous and coldness between 6 am and 10 am, or 6 pm and 10 pm. If one is a vata, the use of herbs and exercise is best between 2 am and 6 am, and 2 pm and 6 pm.

Be Aware of a Transition Detox

A vegetarian diet, and particularly a live food diet, is a powerful detoxifying diet. Too short a transition time from a flesh-centered diet to a vegetarian diet may precipitate a detoxification reaction or healing crises. For those who are hesitant to become vegetarians or are biased against a vegetarian diet as a way of life, the malaise often associated with detoxification reactions is sometimes pointed to as evidence that a vegetarian diet is not working or isn't good for a person. This way of thinking misses the point because the temporary weakness, nausea, and malodorous smells are actually signs that the diet is healing the body. If one makes a careful, patient transition, there is usually little problem with the transition to vegetarianism. If one begins to detoxify in a way that is uncomfortable, then one can always slow the transition process to a detoxification rate that one can more easily tolerate. Most often, the detoxification process, if it occurs at all, usually lasts a few days to several weeks, although it sometimes lasts longer.

Do Vegetarian Women Stop Having Menses?

Another mythology is that the menstrual cycle of vegetarian women will stop. The menstrual period of females will tend to stop, whether vegetarian or not, when a critical minimum percentage of body fat, which contains a certain amount of estrogen, becomes too low. This cessation of menstruation has been observed in both vegetarian and nonvegetarian female athletes. While it is true that vegetarians have less fat in their diet than the 40% fat of the typical American diet, this lower percentage of fat is associated with improved health. What I do observe is that most women who become vegetarians have a more moderate menstrual flow and become more regular.

The one exception to this is women on a fruitarian diet. After about eight months to one year on an exclusive fruit diet, many of these women have been noted to cease their periods entirely. My observation, in helping some of these women recover from the effects of a fruitarian diet, is that as soon as they return to a balanced vegetarian diet and reach the needed minimum body fat, their menstruation resumes. With a few rare exceptions, most people are not ready for a fruitarian diet. I do not generally recommend a fruitarian diet unless a person is prepared physically and spiritually and has been on live foods for an extended period of time. It is definitely not recommended when one is pregnant or is breast-feeding.

Because of the greater SOEF energy contained in a vegetarian (and particularly live foods) diet, one may experience the diet as too powerful when one has been years on a flesh and cooked food diet. The transition from cooked vegetarian foods to living foods may produce the same sort of experience. For example, when many of the people who live in India or have stayed there a long time come to America and try to eat salads, instead of the highly cooked vegetarian food to which they are accustomed, initially they often have digestive troubles. This does not mean that a live food diet weakens digestion. It is a sign that the body did not have adequate time to strengthen itself to handle the purer higher energy food. It may take several months or even years to acclimate oneself. This is why it is so important to carefully monitor the transition. In time, the digestive fire grows strong enough to handle the live or vegetarian foods. This transition process can be helped with chewing the food well and the use of ginger, cayenne, and/or using live plant digestive enzymes. If the digestive process becomes slow because one is too alkaline, then rebalancing the body toward a neutral pH by eating more acid-producing foods is worth trying. The transition to a higher energy vegetarian and live food diet can be successfully managed if one pays attention and is patient.

The research, as well as my own clinical experience, strongly indicates a vegetarian does not have to worry about iron deficiencies or developing a spleen yang deficiency. This is particularly true if one develops a vegetarian diet individualized to one's psychophysiological constitution and based on a regimen of organic, whole vegetables, grains, fruits, beans, nuts, seeds, and legumes. If one eats a vegetarian diet high in junk and other processed foods, sweets, coffee, black teas, and dairy, it is possible to run into all sorts of health problems. This is compounded if the diet is primarily cooked rather than live. A primarily live diet enhances mineral, vitamin, and protein absorption.

I hope that I have sufficiently shown **that a well-balanced, vegetarian diet does not lead to anemia, less endurance, less vitality, poor health, decreased digestive power, excessive inner "dampness," weakened immune system, cessation or imbalance of the menstrual cycle, or long-term, internal coldness. In short, one does not have to worry about becoming spleen yang deficient if one becomes a vegetarian.**

The first direct teaching in the Bible to be vegetarian comes from Genesis 1:29:

"And God said, Behold, I have given you every herb bearing seed, which is upon the face of all the earth, and every tree, in which is the fruit of a tree yielding seed; to you it shall be for meat."

Nowhere in the Bible can you find a place where God commanded that we kill and eat any of his living creatures who walk upon the face of the Earth.

VISION

BLACKBOARD FOOD FOR THOUGHT

Preview of Chapter 14
Judaism and Old Testament Teachings on Vegetarianism

This chapter clearly makes the point that the first dietary law and the diet prescribed for spiritual life in the Torah (Five Books of Moses) or Old Testament is vegetarian. It quotes Torah scholars and rabbis who support the idea that the eating of flesh foods was a temporary concession because the people were not ready to return to a vegetarian diet. There is not a positive commandment in the Torah which tells people to eat flesh food. We discuss five moral precepts that a vegetarian diet fulfills. Four of the past Chief Rabbis of the pre-State and State of Israel have been vegetarian. Israel has the highest percentage of vegetarians outside of India. Are you ready to look at your religious and cultural dietary habits in the light of this understanding of the Five Books of Moses and make the dietary changes that will bring you into alignment with them?

I.   Old Testament and prophets supportive of vegetarianism

    A. Vegetarianism the first dietary law

    B. Thou shalt not kill commandment

    C. Vegetarianism is the dietary blueprint for spiritual love

    D. Changes that occurred when flesh eating was consented to in Judaism

    E. Vegetarianism as the diet compatible with the Messianic Epoch

II. Vegetarianism fulfills five moral precepts of the Torah

    A. Compassion and noncruelty to animals

    B. Peace

    C. Preservation of personal health

    D. Feeding the hungry

    E. Preservation of the earth

III. Vegetarianism as the spiritual nutritional blueprint preparing for the Golden Age of Peace

Chapter 14

Judaism and Old Testament Teachings on Vegetarianism

The first teaching about vegetarianism in the Torah or Old Testament and also the first dietary law of Judaism is:

> "Behold, I have given you every herb-yielding seed which is upon the face of all the earth, and every tree, in which is the fruit of a tree yielding seed—to you it shall be for food." (Gen. 1:29)

It does not take much imagination to assume from this original commandment that God's intention was for humans to be vegetarians. The Talmud, the highly respected commentary on the Jewish laws made by its sages, also agrees that vegetarianism was the primary spiritual directive. It is no accident that after the giving of this dietary law, that in Genesis 1:31 it says God saw all that he had made and "behold, it was very good." In other words, vegetarianism is part of God's plan as it is described in the Torah. Other early verses in Genesis also support the idea of a vegetarian diet.

> "And the Lord God commanded the man saying: of every tree of the garden, thou mayest freely eat...."(Genesis 2:16)

> "...and thou shalt eat the herbs of the field." (Genesis 3:18)

In Exodus 20:13, it says **"Thou shalt not kill."** This sixth commandment is basic in terms of its compassion and love for all of creation. The exact Hebrew translation reads "lo tirtzach." This word refers to any sort of killing, and not just of humans. The practice of this commandment not only keeps the fundamental order in the world of nature, but supports the basic principle of compassion and love of all of God's creation that is taught in the Old Testament. It clearly supports the essential observance of vegetarianism.

Vegetarianism is the basic and unitary commandment on diet. It is a blueprint, in essence, of the basic diet needed to support a spiritual life in harmony with all of creation. It gives us a context to understand Genesis 9:3, the first of several concessions to people's lust for flesh:

> "Every moving thing that lives shall be food for you; as the green herb have I given you all."

213

Vegetarian Rav Abraham Isaac Hacohen Kook, the well-respected, Jewish spiritual leader and Torah scholar in the early part of our 20th century, and the first Chief Rabbi of the pre-state of Israel, felt that the permission to eat meat was only a temporary concession to the people. He felt that it was not conceivable that God would design a perfect plan of harmony for humanity and the earth and find that it was imperfect a few thousand years later. Rabbi Kook felt that Genesis 9:3 was a temporary concession because people had sunk to such a low level of spiritual awareness that they needed to feel superior to the animals and concentrate first on improving their relationship with each other. He felt that humanity's lust for meat was so strong that if they were denied they might even revert to eating human flesh. In his understanding, the permission to slaughter animals was a way to control the blood lust. He interpreted the permission to eat meat as a stopgap measure until a more enlightened era would be achieved and we would all return to vegetarianism.

Another change that came with the permission to eat meat was that animals and people stopped acting in a peaceful harmony. It was an acknowledgment of a significant shift in the relationship of the human organism to the world ecology.

Kosher laws were seen as a way to make meat eating tolerable, yet not particularly convenient. A renown Torah scholar, Rambam said,

> "Be holy by abstaining from those things which are permitted
> to you. For those who drink wine and eat meat all the time are
> considered 'scoundrels with a Torah license'."

The reluctance to give this permission to eat meat is evidenced by the prohibition against eating blood.

> "Only flesh with the life thereof, which is the blood thereof,
> shall ye not eat." (Genesis 9:4)

To have to remove the blood in order to be Kosher is a way of making flesh eating more difficult and a reminder of the compromise in permitting meat eating. Even while allowing the eating of meat, and not the eating of blood, the Torah gives a suggestion for respecting the life of the animal. There is also a "catch 22" quality to this Kosher law because the physiological reality of the Kosher commandment not to have the blood of the animal is not possible to fulfill. Although one can drain blood from the arteries and veins, it is not physiologically possible to drain it from the capillaries. From a scientific point of view, the only way to fully be Kosher is to be vegetarian. In Genesis 9:5 it says:

> " And surely, your blood of your lives will I require..."

Directly related to the temporary concession to the carnal desires of humanity, we see an immediate result in a decrease of life span. Humanity is forced to pay a price for its blood lust. Within one generation of the Genesis 9:3 statement to Noah, the life span decreased to approximately one third of its previous length, from approximately 900 years to 300 years, and then eventually to 70 years. Our current medical research has documented that a flesh-centered diet has a detrimental effect on health. This is the physiological modern day fulfillment of "your blood of your lives will I require."

During Exodus, it appears that God tried to make the Jews return to vegetarianism by just giving them the manna in the desert. Again, however, the flesh lust of the people made them rebel from the diet. They demanded flesh food from God.

> "And the mixed multitude that was among them fell a lusting;
> and the children of Israel also weeped on their part, and said,
> "Would that we were given flesh to eat." (Numbers 11:4)

Although Moses was frustrated with the lust of the people, God granted their request by providing them with quails blown in by the wind. But God's anger at their rebellion and their flesh-eating desires brought a plague to the people who ate the quail.

> "While the flesh was yet between their teeth, ere it was chewed,
> the anger of the Lord was kindled against the people, and the
> Lord smote the people with a very great plague." (Numbers
> 11:33) "Many died and the place where this took place was
> called the 'Graves of Lust;' there they buried the people that
> lusted." (Numbers 11:34)

It is hard to interpret this concession of eating the quail as supportive of a flesh-centered diet. It is far easier to interpret this incident as evidence of God's direction that the people be vegetarian and the consequence of meat eating would be poor health and a shortened life span.

The Torah consistently describes vegetarian foods in a positive light and as a reward. The Divine bounty of the Song of Songs is described in terms of fruits, vegetables, and other vegetarian cuisine. There is a blessing before eating vegetarian food such as the fruit of the vine and the bread of the earth, but there is no specific blessing for eating flesh food.

One of the more subtle issues in the Torah is the question of animal sacrifice. The Essenes, the least known of the three divisions of Judaism at that time, who were reported to be live food vegetarians, felt that animal sacrifice was not an original part of the Torah, and therefore were against animal sacrifice. Others, such as the highly revered Jewish scholar, physician, and Rabbi, Moses Maimondes, felt that animal sacrifice was given as a compromise because it was the general practice among all the nations to practice animal sacrifice at the time the Torah was given. He reasoned that it was enough that the Torah took away idolatry and established a faith in one God. To take away both the form of offering as well as idols would have been too big a step for these people. However, there is no reference in the Ten Commandments to having to perform animal sacrifice. Also, when animal sacrifice is first mentioned in Leviticus 1:2, it is mentioned in the context of *if you bring* an offering. The prophets at times spoke against the obligation to sacrifice in favor of direct devotion of the heart to God as the real sacrifice.

> "I have not burdened thee with a meal offering, nor wearied thee with frankincense...." (Isaiah 43:23)

> "To what purpose is the multitude of your sacrifices unto Me? sayeth the Lord. I am full of burnt offerings of rams, and the fat of fed beasts; and I delight not in the blood of the bullocks, or of lambs, or of he-goats...bring no more vain oblations...and when ye spread forth your hands, I will hide mine eyes from you; yea when ye make many prayers, I will not hear; your hands are full of blood." (Isaiah 1:11-16)

> "For I spoke not unto your fathers, nor commanded them in the day that I brought them our of the land of Egypt, concerning burnt offerings or sacrifices; but this thing I commanded them, saying, "Obey my voice, and I will be your God, and ye shall be my people...." (Jeremiah 7:22-23)

Based on the following prophecy of Isaiah, it is not unreasonable to assume that in the Messianic Epoch to which he is referring, we all will return to the first dietary law, which appears to be the original prescription of a diet for spiritual life in the Torah, and become vegetarian again.

> "And the wolf shall dwell with the lamb,
> And the leopard shall lie down with the kid;
> And the calf and the young lion and the fatling together;
> And a little child shall lead them...
> Their young ones shall lie down together,
> And the lion shall eat straw like the ox...
> They shall not hurt nor destroy in all My holy mountain."
> (Isaiah 11:69)

Although there is not enough information to absolutely prove that some of the prophets, such as Isaiah, Jeremiah, Amos, Hosea, Daniel, and Ezekiel, were vegetarian, there are certainly quotes from their teachings that suggested they taught against the killing of animals and animal sacrifice. These quotes also suggest they taught a vegetarian lifestyle, as they do not say that people should raise animals to slaughter and eat their flesh. As these were true prophets, one can only assume they lived their teachings. Examples of these teachings are:

> "...and the fruit thereof shall be for meat, and the leaf thereof for medicine." (Ezekiel 47:12)

> "He who kills an ox is like him who slays a man." (Isaiah 66:3)

> "Please test your servants for ten days, giving us legumes to eat and water to drink. Then compare our appearance with that of the youths who eat of the king's food." (Daniel 1:12-13)

> "For I desire goodness, not sacrifice; obedience to God, rather than burnt offerings." (Hosea 6:6)

> "When they present sacrifices to Me, it is but flesh for them to eat: The Lord has not accepted them..." (Hosea 8:13)

> "I will restore My people Israel. They shall rebuild ruined cities and inhabit them; they shall plant vineyards and drink their wine; they shall till gardens and eat their fruits." (Amos 9:14)

> "Thus said the Lord of Hosts, the God of Israel, to the whole community which I exiled from Jerusalem to Babylon: Build houses and live in them, plant gardens and eat their fruit." (Jeremiah 29: 4-5)

Vegetarianism naturally fulfills five of the moral precepts of the Torah:

1. Compassion and noncruelty to animals.
2. Preserving the earth.
3. Feeding the hungry.
4. Preservation of personal health.
5. Seeking peace.

Because of these teachings, it is no coincidence that there has been three vegetarian chief rabbis in 25 years of the state of Israel's existence, as well as Rabbi Kook of the pre-Israel era. Four percent of the population in Israel is vegetarian, which, outside of India, with 83% of its 680 million people who are vegetarian, is the largest percentage of vegetarians in the world. Other prominent Jewish thinkers who are or were vegetarian are: Martin Buber, one of the greatest existential philosophers; Isaac Bashevis Singer, winner of the 1978 Nobel Prize for Literature; Shmuel Yoseph Agnon, Nobel Prize recipient; Rabbi David Rosen, the former Chief Rabbi of Ireland; and Sher Yashuv Cohen, the Chief Rabbi of Haifia.

In the Talmud, Rabbi Yishmael said,

> "From the day that the holy Temple was destroyed it would have been right to have imposed upon ourselves the law prohibiting the eating of flesh. But the rabbis have laid down a wise and logical ruling that the authorities must not impose any decree unless the majority of the members of the community are able to abide by it. Otherwise the law and those who administer it get into disrepute."

Perhaps this is the crux of the issue for why meat eating has been allowed by many of the major religions, such as Judaism, Christianity, and even Buddhism. Out of compassion for the limitations of their followers, the essential compassion found in all religions for all life needed to wait until people were ready. I wonder if we have been waiting too long.

Compassion and Noncruelty to Animals and World Peace

The connection between compassion toward, and noncruelty to, animals with world peace is directly linked morally and spiritually. Killing an animal for food is still a violent act. There is no compassion in it for the animal. There is also a connection between justifying slaughtering animals for food or profit and taking the next step in the violent process, which is the killing of one's fellow human beings for some sort of "good" reason.

"He who kills an ox is as if he slew a person." (Isaiah 6:3)

George Bernard Shaw once said in his poem, *Song of Peace:*

> "Like carrion crows, we live and feed on meat
> Regardless of the suffering and pain

Animals today, such as cows, chicken, turkeys and pigs, are perceived in the same way as plants in that they are fed and watered and considered a "cash crop!"

Is that a humane way to treat God's creatures?

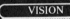

BLACKBOARD FACTS

We cause by doing so. If thus we treat
defenseless animals for sport of gain,
How can we hope to attain the
Peace we say we are so anxious for?
We pray for it, o'er hecatombs of slain,
To God, while outraging the moral law,
Thus cruelty begets its offspring—War."

Today, the cruelty extends beyond the mass killing of animals to a systematic, antilife, antihumane treatment of animals from the time they are born until they are harvested as if they were a cash crop. They are systematically deprived of their natural habitat and life cycle for the expediency of the meat industry. Individual killing of animals for food is the first step of cruelty (hunting, fishing). The profit-motivated industrialization of nature's living animals, as if they are inanimate and without any rights, feelings, or soul, is an example of the next step of the expansion of cruelty.

People in the U.S. and Canada consume over 200 pounds of animal flesh per person a year. In one year, four billion cattle, calves, sheep, hogs, chicken, ducks, and turkeys are slaughtered. In a lifetime, a Canadian or U.S meat eater eats: 11 cattle, one calf, three lambs and sheep, 23 hogs, 45 turkeys, 1,100 chickens, and 826 pounds of fish. The Hebrew word for meat is "basar." As explained by the Talmudists, it is composed of the letters "bet" (shame), "sin" (corruption), and "resh" (worms).

The famous Talmudic jurist and Rabbi, Moshe ben Nachman, who lived in the 11th century, said about avoidance of cruelty and compassion for animals:

> "...for cruelty expands in a man's soul, as is well-known with respect to cattle slaughters."

This is a prophetic comment in that a current struggle exists around the destruction of the rain forests in which the cattle farmers and other forces who want to level the forests have been involved indirectly and directly in shooting people who oppose destroying the forests for the purpose of raising cattle. The most infamous of these money-, flesh-, and lust-associated killings was the assassination by cattle ranchers of Chico Mendes, a leading environmentalist working to prevent the destruction of the Amazon rain forests. This killing of Chico Mendes forms a direct link between first killing animals for personal food, to raising animals to be killed for profit, to the next level of cruelty and violence which "expands in a man's soul," which is the killing of humans to preserve profit from killing animals.

The connection between the violence of killing animals for food, and the violence of killing humans, has been established by philosophers and religious teachers for hundreds of years. Quaker leader Thomas Tyron (1634-1703) points

The average American meat eater consumes in a lifetime:

    A. Eleven beef steers

    B. One calf

    C. Three lambs

    D. Twenty-three hogs

    E. Forty-five turkeys

    F. Eight hundred and twenty-six fish

The Hebrew word for meat is BASAR (which means shame, corruption, and worms)!

When a vegetarian looks at these facts, it is bizzare!

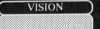

VISION

BLACKBOARD FACTS

221

out that the violence of killing animals for food stemmed from the same source of "wrath" as the killing of humans. Maimonides felt that the Torah's emphasis on compassion was to protect us from acquiring the moral habits of cruelty. The violence of killing animals for our dinner table, comes from the same rationale of justifiable violence that leads humans to kill humans. Pythagoras, the Greek mathematician and philosopher, once said:

> "As long as men massacre animals, they will kill each other. Indeed, he who sows the seeds of murder and pain cannot reap joy and love."

One of the most elegant, yet simple statements about the connection between the killing of animals and human violence and pain comes from the enlightened monk, Swami Prakasananda Saraswati. In 1987 he gave this answer to the question of the connection between vegetarianism and peace:

> "Every animal that is slaughtered for human consumption brings the pain of its death into your body. Think about it. The animal is killed with violence. That violence causes the animal to experience very intense pain as it dies. That pain remains in the meat even after you prepare and cook it. When you eat that meat, then you eat pain. That pain becomes lodged in your body, heart, and mind. That violence and pain which you consume will eat you also. It consumes you so that you must experience the same pain in your own life also."

"The earth is the Lord's and the fullness thereof." (Psalms 24:1)

This is the Old Testament teaching: that we are to help, as God's co-workers, to preserve and improve the world. It is part of the teaching of Tikkum, in which the Torah instructs that it is part of one's role in life to help heal the substance and soul of the planet. This means that we are to protect the resources of the Earth as well as the animal and human inhabitants.

A flesh-centered diet that many follow results in just the opposite. For example, according to John Robbins' book, *A Diet for A New America,* livestock uses approximately 50% of all the water in the U.S. Livestock produces twenty times the excrement as the human population of the U.S. This also increases the nitrate/nitrite water pollution in the rest of the water supplies. Extensive water use for livestock is also pushing us closer to a clean water shortage. It requires 60-100 times more water to produce a pound of beef than a pound of wheat. One estimate is that if everyone were vegetarian, there would be no need for irrigation systems in the U.S. This excessive water usage for livestock is because the land needed to grow grain for livestock takes up about 80% of the grain produced in the U.S., as well as because of the water needed for the animals. When one considers the water needed for this extra grain and for the care of the livestock, a flesh food diet creates a need for 4,500 gallons per day per meat eater as compared to 300 gallons per day needed for a vegan. A vegan saves approximately 1,500,000 gallons per year as compared to a flesh and dairy eater. Much of this information is found in a greatly expanded form in John Robbins' book, *A Diet for a New America.*

The destruction of the rain forests for grazing land and the resultant greenhouse effect is another example of the destructive results of a flesh-centered diet on our ecological system.

In Deuteronomy 20:19 it says "You must never destroy its trees...you may eat of them, but you shall not cut them down."

This statement in Deuteronomy is one of the bases of the Talmudic laws which prohibits willful destruction of natural resources or any sort of vandalism to the natural resources, even if it is by those who have a deed to the land. Estimates in the *Vegetarian Times* are that the rain forest destruction also causes the extinction of 1000 species per year. For each fast food, quarter pound hamburger, 55 square feet of rain forest are destroyed. One hundred species become extinct for every two billion fast food burgers sold. The effects of livestock land use in the U.S. accounts for about 85% of the topsoil loss of the four million acres of topsoil lost per year. A pure vegetarian diet, on the other hand, makes less than five percent of the demand on the soil in this country.

The ratio of food productivity per acre of land from livestock versus vegetarian food reveals a tremendous disparity in terms of productivity from the same amount of natural resources. For instance, one acre of land yields 20,000 pounds of potatoes versus 165 pounds of beef. An acre of grain gives five times more protein than beef. An acre of legumes gives ten times more, and an acre of leafy greens produces 25 times more, protein than one acre of beef. Grain for 100 cows will feed 2000 people. Neither land, water, atmosphere, or animal population are safe from the resource-intensive destruction that results from a meat-centered diet.

We simply cannot escape the fact that raising animals for meat and dairy has a disastrous effect on our ecological system. U.S. livestock regularly eats enough grain and soy to feed the U.S. population five times over. Over 80% of the grain grown in the U.S. is to feed livestock. This includes 80% of corn and 95% of oats. The total world livestock regularly eats about twice the calories as the human world population receives. By cycling our plant protein through the beef, the conversion to beef protein is approximately between one tenth and one twentieth of the plant protein yield. This is a 100% loss of complex carbohydrates and a 95% loss of calories when plant protein is recycled through

223

livestock. This is a rather significant waste of protein, complex carbohydrates, and calorie resources when so many people in this world suffer from malnutrition. It is an ecological shame to realize that meat eaters, according to *Diet for a New America*, use three and one half acres per year to supply their meat and dairy consumption lifestyle, whereas vegans require one quarter of an acre of land. In other words, **approximately 16 vegans can live off the same land and water supply as it takes for one meat eater.** A nondairy and nonmeat diet saves one acre of trees per year because of how little resources the diet demands. On our planet, with ever-increasing shortages of land and water, this is a tremendously significant amount of resources that are wasted, resources that we can no longer afford to be wasting.

A vegetarian diet also helps to conserve the world's fuel energy and total raw material resources. Seventy-eight calories of fossil fuel are required for each calorie of protein from feedlot-produced beef. Grains and beans require approximately .6 to 3.9 calories of fossil fuel to produce each calorie of vegetarian food. **There is about twenty times more fossil fuel energy needed to produce one calorie of beef as compared to one calorie of vegetable protein.** The energy required to produce food in the U.S. is about 16.5% of the total energy requirements of the U.S. The value of the raw materials consumed for livestock production is larger than the value of all the oil, gas, and coal produced in this country. Raw materials needed to support the livestock industry is one third of the value of all the raw materials consumed in this country. The earth resources demanded by a flesh-centered diet are enormous as compared to those required by a vegetarian diet. **A flesh-centered diet is a significant stress on the earth's ecological balance and resources. It is an unnecessary hoarding of resources.**

Feeding the Hungry

Neither humans nor animals are safe from the collective effects of a flesh food diet. Sixty million people starve to death per year on this planet. The reasons for this terrible state of affairs are also associated with many political, economic, and natural disasters, et cetera. However, the fact remains that because a flesh-centered diet creates an overextended use of water, land, energy, and other resources, it is estimated by nutritionist Dr. Jean Meyer of Harvard, that if meat eaters ate just ten percent less flesh per year, the resources saved would be enough to feed all these sixty million who starve to death.

The number one health problem in the world today is chronic malnutrition. The United Nations estimates that one half the world's population suffers from malnutrition and 700-900 million people are seriously malnourished. Twenty-five percent of the world's children suffer from a lack of food. Forty-two thousand children die per day from malnutrition. That comes to 15 million per year or 30% of all the world's deaths per year. **In the last five years, more**

Forty-two thousand children die per day from malnutrition — that's 15 million children per year who starve to death. U.S. livestock eat enough grain and soy foods to feed our population five times over!

Over 80% of corn and 95% of oats is fed to livestock!

One acre of land gives only 165 pounds of beef protein. Yet one acre of land will produce 20,000 pounds of potatoes!

While we feed our cattle to fatten them up for our flesh desires, 60 million human beings are starving to death each year.

If we only cut back our flesh food intake by 10% a year, there would be enough resources and grain to feed these 60 million people for a year.

VISION

BLACKBOARD FACTS

people died from malnutrition than from all the wars, revolutions, and murders of the last 150 years.

In the Jewish tradition, the Talmud teaches that providing sustenance to the hungry is as important as all the other commandments of the Torah combined.

> "To loose the chains of wickedness, to undo the bonds of oppression, and to let the oppressed go free....Is it not to share thy bread with the hungry? (Isaiah 58:6-7)

The Midrash—a highly respected compilation of rabbis on the five books of the Torah—says that whenever we give food to the poor it is as if one is feeding God. The feeding of the hungry extends even to one's enemies.

> "If your enemy is hungry, give him bread to eat. If your enemy is thirsty, give him water to drink. (Proverbs 25:21)

The ethic of feeding the hungry can be seen directly in Leviticus 19:9-10:

> "And when you reap the harvest of your land, thou shalt not wholly reap the corner of thy field, neither shalt thou gather the gleanings of thy harvest. And thou shalt not glean thy vineyard, neither shalt thou gather the fallen fruit of thy vineyard; thou shalt leave them for the poor and the stranger."

A flesh-centered diet creates a hoarding of the resources in a way that greatly contributes to world hunger. World hunger, however, reflects a social and political disharmony as much as it does a resource problem. But it does help to have ample resources. Vegetarianism is a major step in creating a reorganization of how our world food resources are used.

The implication of the above statistics is that one who is a vegetarian is indirectly helping to feed the hungry of this planet.

Preservation of Personal Health

The renown 12th century physician, rabbi, and sage, Maimonides, in his commentary on the Torah, makes it obvious that one must not place one's health and life in danger. This teaching includes the importance of actively living in a way that will bring good health. In Deuteronomy 4:9 it says:

> "Take heed unto thyself and take care of thy life."

It is obvious at this point that a vegetarian diet is the most healthy diet.

Summary

A vegetarian diet is the basic spiritual diet of the Torah and is consistent with many of its key teachings. Vegetarianism is compatible with, and supportive of, **any spiritual path** because it is conducive to spiritual growth of the individual. A vegetarian diet is automatically Kosher. It is the essence of sharing because it puts far less stress on the environment and allows far more of the earth's bounty to be shared with everyone. It brings peace to the world because it establishes habits of peace and a relationship of peace with all of nature. By learning compassion for all of God's creatures, we develop habits that allow us to show peace and compassion for our fellow humans. Such a diet also brings us into a harmonious balance with the ecology of the planet. In this way **a vegetarian diet is the basic nutritional blueprint not only of the Torah, but for enhancing aspects of spiritual life for all of humanity. It is part of the plan for the coming Golden Age of world peace.**

Five basic biblical moral precepts according to Jewish tradition are:

1. *Compassion and noncruelty to animals*
2. *Preserving the Earth*
3. *Preservation of personal health*
4. *Feeding the hungry*
5. *Seeking and creating peace in the world*

Following the original vegetarian diet prescribed in Genesis 1:29 automatically fulfills these teachings.

BLACKBOARD FACTS

Preview of Chapter 15
Jesus and Vegetarianism

Although it cannot be proven that Jesus did not eat flesh food, the following evidence suggests: He grew up in an Essene community which was vegetarian and against animal sacrifice; His family, and probably all His disciples, were vegetarian; and many of the early Christians were vegetarian and some claimed to have been directly instructed by Him to be vegetarian. The fact that Jesus was the master example of love and reverence for all life strongly suggests that he was vegetarian. Although it may be easier for us to believe and project that a Son of God would not have us return to God's original dietary blueprint of how to eat as revealed in Genesis 1:29 and pointed out in the previous chapter, we may have to accept that Jesus came to help us return to the original spiritual plan of God. Are we ready to give up our human projections of Jesus so that we can see him in his original light and teaching?

I.   Jesus and vegetarianism

    A. Dead Sea Scrolls

    B. *Essene Gospel of Peace*

    C. Inaccurate translations from Council of Nicea

II. The historical Jesus

    A. The Essene Jesus

    B. *Gospel of the Hebrews*

III. History of vegetarianism in early Christianity

IV. The Vegetarianism of the disciples

    A. Writings on the disciples' eating habits

V.   Many early Christian leaders were vegetarian

VI. Summary

    A. Historical evidence suggests Jesus was a vegetarian

    B. Messianic prophecy includes a vegetarian Messiah

VIII. Contemporary Christian vegetarians

    A. Ellen G. White - Seventh Day Adventist

    B. Christian vegetarian writers in early America

Chapter 15

Jesus and Vegetarianism

Whether or not Jesus was a vegetarian is a delicate subject that has no definitive answer because of variations in different historical accounts. The Dead Sea Scroll materials unearthed in 1947 indirectly suggest that Jesus was a lifelong vegetarian. This is because they indicate that the Essenes were vegetarian and historically there is evidence that Jesus was raised in an Essene community, therefore it is highly likely that He and His family were vegetarian. The *Essene Gospel of Peace Book I,* taken from the original, Aramaic, third century manuscript discovered in 1927 in the secret Vatican archives by Dr. Edmond Bordeaux Szekeley, directly and strongly suggests that Jesus was a lifelong vegetarian. It reveals His direct teachings against the eating of flesh. Nevertheless, as these documents come to the surface, there is still lack of definitive proof and confusion about mistranslations and conscious and unconscious changes made in the scriptures as we see them today. This is especially true with the claims of various changes and deletions in the Gospels and Epistles that in all probability largely occurred at the Council of Nicea in 325 A.D. According to *The Prophet of the Dead Sea Scrolls* by Upton Clary Ewing, a theologian praised by world-famous Albert Schweitzer, M.D., as the "renaissance of Leonardo da Vinci:"

> "There is hardly a single scholar among Bible exegetists who
> will not agree that there are many inconsistencies and contra-
> dictions to be found in the Gospels and the Epistles."

Perhaps this inability to make a final proof one way or the other is fortunate, as no one's faith need be flatly challenged by this chapter. There is room to ultimately believe whatever one feels comfortable to believe. This topic is not meant to challenge anyone's religious beliefs. It is meant to raise issues and information that is not readily available in order to aid and support those who are Christian vegetarians already, or those Christians contemplating the transition to vegetarianism as part of the medicine for healing themselves and this planet. The following information is for those who are confused or disempowered in their desire to be vegetarian by the commonly held interpretations, based on the currently used editions of the New Testament, that maintain Jesus was not a vegetarian.

To understand the relationship of Jesus to vegetarianism, we must probe into a realm in which much of the historical documentation has been lost, and into that which is left, which is partially confused by the subtleties in the translation from the Greek to English. The accuracy of the translations have also been affected by the limited understanding and philosophy of those who were doing the translating. For example, the word "meat," which appears 19 times in the New Testament, seems to imply that Jesus sanctioned meat eating. The most accurate understanding, however, of the word meat in the translation from Greek to English does not imply flesh food at all. The Greek word translated as "meat" is more precisely translated as "food" or "nourishment," and not animal flesh as we currently think of when we hear the term "meat." For example, Jesus did not actually say "Have ye any meat?" as in John 21:5 but "Have ye anything to eat?" And when the Gospels say that the disciples went away to buy meat (John: 8), it merely means to buy food.

Similar mistranslations have occurred with the use of the word fish. The misunderstanding of the use of this word results in a portrayal of Jesus as eating fish and encouraging the eating or killing of fish by others. In the early church, the word fish was a secret term. The Greek word for fish is I-CH-TH-U-S. It is made up of the first letters of the words: Jesus Christos Theou Uios Soter. This translates as Jesus Christ Son of God Savior. The fish is also found as a Christian symbol in the catacombs. It is also symbolic of the Piscean Age which was emerging at that time. It is entirely conceivable that the word fish, as used in the New Testament, was used primarily in this deeper mystical way. Since Jesus taught in parables and metaphors, I believe its use in the New Testament was used to communicate this deeper meaning of fish rather than the literal idea of a dead fish that was physically eaten. In this context, the feeding of the fish to the people is a metaphor for the feeding of the higher teachings of the Master to the masses. In a second century book by Irenaeus (120-202 C.E.) it is twice stated that Jesus fed the multitude of 5000 with bread alone. Others have pointed out that there is a submarine plant called the fish plant that was used as a food in that era as well as during Babylonian times. These fish plants are dried in the sun, beaten into mortar, and baked into bread-like rolls and sold in the open market. Perhaps in the translation, the plant portion of the word designated as the fish plant was omitted. It was only in the fourth century that fish was added to the bread offering in the scriptures. This suggests the second century version of the *Gospel of the Hebrews* might be more authentic. In this second century translation, it says in Lection XXIX, verses 7 and 8:

> "And when He had taken the six loaves and the seven clusters of grapes, He looked up to heaven, and blessed and broke the loaves, and the grapes also, and gave them to His disciples to set before them, and they divided them among all."

> "And they did all eat and were filled. And they took up twelve baskets full of the fragments that were left. And they that did eat of the loaves and of the fruits were about five thousand men, women, and children, and He taught them many things."

In any case, the souls of the 5,000, we can assume, were at least fed with the mystical meaning of fish.

The Historical Jesus

It is a lot easier to understand Jesus' teachings about vegetarianism when He is understood in His historical context. He and His family were associated with the Essene movement of the times. The Essenes were Jewish communities made of very evolved people who had broken away from the mainstream of Jewish thought several hundred years before the time of Jesus. They were vegetarians in accordance with the highest meaning of the Law of Moses which said that, "Thou shalt not kill." They were also against the practice of animal sacrifice. In *The Prophet of the Dead Sea Scrolls*, Ewing quotes Philo of Alexandria, a historian writing during the time of Jesus' ministry, who said:

> "They are called Esseni because of their saintliness. They do not sacrifice animals, regarding a reverent mind as the only true sacrifice."

Ewing quotes Professor Teicher in saying:

> "But we have there (in the Essene scriptures) the emphatic prohibition of eating animals. No consumption of meat means no killing of animals and both together means no sacrifice of animals."

The book, the *Dead Sea Scrolls,* by Millar Burrows, quotes from the Essene scriptures:

> "Let not a man make himself abominable with any living creature or creeping thing by eating of them."

The lives of the Essenes required a discipline and purity of mind, body, and spirit that was beyond the practice of the typical religious person of the time. The Essenes developed self-sufficient communities in the peace of the desert in order to make it easier to focus on God. It is thought that Jesus and His parents were part of the Essenes, some of whom were also called the Nazarenes. It is said that Jesus escaped to an Essene community in the desert to avoid the murderous intent of King Herod. It was in the Essene communities that He was raised and trained. Some of the Essenes, such as John the Baptist, as well as the Master Jesus Himself, went out into the public to uplift the people. As part of their teaching of compassion and love for all life, they taught vegetarianism. For example, in

The Essene Gospel of Peace Book One (p. 36), discovered in 1927 by Dr. Edmond Bordeaux Szekely, Jesus is quoted as saying:

> "God commanded your forefathers: 'Thou shalt not kill.' But their heart was hardened and they killed. Then Moses desired that at least they should not kill men, and he suffered them to kill beasts. And then the heart of your forefathers was hardened yet more, and they killed men and beasts likewise. But I do say to you: Kill neither men nor beasts, nor yet the food which goes into your mouth. For if you eat living (uncooked) food, the same will quicken you, but if you kill your food, the dead food will kill you also."

What is important here is that this teaching is a direct quote of Jesus from an original Aramaic third century manuscript found in the secret archives of the Vatican. It is not a teaching by implication. The message is consistent with Jesus' own dietary practice and of His community of birth and where He grew up, which also practiced vegetarianism. Aside from these exciting findings, most of the information concerning Jesus' explicit teachings on this subject has been lost or destroyed. One exception is the work by Epiphanius (315-403 A.D.), a Catholic bishop of Constantia in Cyprus. In his book, *Panarion* (as explained in the book, *A Critical Investigation of Epiphanius' Knowledge of the Ebionites: A Translation and Critical Discussion of "Panarion,"* by Glenn Alan Kochit), Epiphanius points out that according to the Ebionites, a group of early Judaic Christians who were vegetarians:

> "Whenever you speak to them (Ebionites) concerning flesh food, the Ebionites reply they were vegetarian because "Christ revealed it to me." (This was a direct teaching they were referring to and not a revelation.)

There is also another early book called *The Gospel of the Holy Twelve,* also known as *The Gospel of the Hebrews,* the *Essene Gospel,* the *Gospel of the Ebionites,* or just plain "the Gospel." This book has been translated from the Aramaic by the Englishman Reverend Gideon H. Ousley (1835-1906). Ousley claims that it is the translation of the original gospel and that it had been preserved first by the Essenes and then later in a Tibetan monastery after the Essenes were forced to leave their communities in 68 A.D. by the advancing Romans. The Essenes apparently hid many of their scriptures in the desert (such as the Dead Sea Scrolls) and took some with them as they dispersed. Reverend Ousley claims that this Gospel was taken to a Tibetan Buddhist monastery by Essene monks. It was in the Tibetan monastery that Reverend Ousley found it.

If this is authentic, as some scholars believe, it would be the most ancient, authentic, and complete writings about Jesus and His teachings available. Dr. Ewing felt that this might be the original gospel, but it might have been known primarily as "the gospel" and was written in western Aramaic. Jesus' teaching of vegetarianism in the *Gospel of the Hebrews* is both poetic and clear as He answers a doubting Sadduce man who had asked Jesus, "Tell me, please, why sayest thou, do not eat the flesh of animals...?" Jesus' beautiful answer to him was:

> " 'Behold this watermelon, the fruit of the earth.' Jesus then broke open the watermelon and said: 'See thou with thine own eyes the good fruit of the soil, the meat of man, and see thou the seeds within, count ye them, for one melon maketh a hundredfold and even more. If thou sow this seed, ye do eat from the true God, for no blood was spilled, nay no pain nor outcry did ye hear with thy ears or see with thine eyes. The true food of man is from the mother of the earth, for she brings forth perfect gifts unto the humble of the land. But ye seek what Satan giveth, the anguish, the death, and the blood of living souls taken by the sword. Know ye not, those who live by the sword are the ones who die by the same death? Go thine way then, and plant the seeds of the good fruit of life, and leave ye off from hurting the innocent creatures of God.' "

In a teaching to His disciples in Lection XXXII, verse 4, of the *Gospel of the Hebrews*, Jesus is completely clear about His opposition to killing and eating animals:

> "For of the fruits of the trees and the seeds of the herbs alone do I partake, and these are changed by the Spirit into my flesh and my blood. Of these alone and their like shall ye eat who believe in me, and are my disciples, for of these, in the Spirit, come to life and health and healing unto man."

In the same section, verse 9, Jesus explains the problem of the custom of flesh eating with an understanding of the past and a prophecy for the future return to vegetarianism for the whole world:

> "Verily I say unto you, in the beginning, all creatures of God did find their sustenance in the herbs and the fruits of the earth alone, till the ignorance and the selfishness of man turned many of them from the use which God had given them, to that which was contrary to their original use, but even these shall yet return to their natural food, as it is written in the prophets (Isaiah), and their words shall not fail."

In Lection XXXVIII, verses 3, 4, and 6 of *The Gospel of the Holy Twelve,* the spiritual meaning of the *awareness and practice of the oneness with all of life* is translated into His teachings of vegetarianism, and noncruelty to animals and all of life; His words are consistent with the awareness one would expect from someone of Jesus' great spiritual stature:

> 3 "God giveth the grains and the fruits of the earth for food; and for righteous man truly there is no other lawful sustenance for the body."
>
> 4 "The robber who breaketh into the house made by man is guilty, but they who break into the house made by God, even of the least of these are the greater sinners. Wherefore I say unto all who desire to be my disciples, keep your hands from bloodshed and let no flesh meat enter your mouths, for God is just and bountiful, who ordaineth that man shall live by the fruits and seeds of the earth alone."
>
> 6 "And whatsoever ye do unto the least of these my children, ye do it unto me. For I am in them and they are in me. Yea, I am in all creatures and all creatures are in me. In all their joys I rejoice, in all their afflictions I am afflicted. Wherefore I say unto you: Be ye kind one to another, and to all the creatures of God."

History of Vegetarianism in Early Christianity

From Epiphanius' book it is shown that the immediate followers of Jesus, the Judaic Christians, were vegetarians until the fifth century. This was about 100 years after the historical struggle between the three main factions of Christianity of those times: Judaic Christians, Christian Gnostics, and Catholic Christians. According to the evidence presented in the *Vegetarianism of Jesus Christ* by Charles Vaclivik, the Judaic Christians, were lead, for 30 years after Jesus left the physical realm, by His brother James. Vaclivik's historical evidence suggests the Judaic Christians were the very first Christians. They were the ones who actually walked and prayed with Jesus. After them, the Christian Gnosticism developed, and around 70 A.D. the Catholic Christians began their ascent to power. The Judaic Christians and Gnostics were vegetarian and the Catholic Christians were not. Many early Christian leaders were also vegetarians. Clement of Alexandria (A.D. 160-240) wrote,

> "It is far better to be happy than to have our bodies act as graveyards for animals."

St. John Chrysostom (A.D. 345-407) also taught the unnatural eating of flesh meat was polluting.

Many scholars feel that the original Christian documents were altered at the Council of Nicea in 325 A.D. to make them acceptable to the emperor, Constantine. Steve Rosen, in *Food for Spirit*, points out that flesh food eating was not officially permitted until the fourth century, when Emperor Constantine, through his powerful influence, made his version of Christianity the official version for everyone. Vegetarian Christians had to practice in secret or risk being put to death for heresy. Rosen writes that Constantine used to have molten lead poured down their throats if they were captured. By the fourth century, the Catholic Christians became considerably more politically powerful than the other two groups. Most of the literature of the Judaic Christians and Gnostics was essentially destroyed during the political repression of this time period. In the book, *The Vegetarianism of Jesus Christ*, it is postulated that the translations after this time may have been altered away from a vegetarian menu, as the Catholic Christians did not believe in vegetarianism and/or were not ready for it. If people are surprised that there was more than one Christian faction in the first 100 years after Jesus, it is useful to remember that we now have hundreds of different Christian churches.

Jesus and Animal Sacrifice

Epiphanius also points out that the Essenes were not only vegetarians, but also opposed animal sacrifice. It is in this context that one gets a further understanding of why Jesus chased out the money lenders from the Temple and freed the animals who were going to be sacrificed. It was the money lenders who exchanged money so that Jews coming from foreign lands could purchase animals for sacrifice. The teachings of Jesus and the Essenes stood directly against the practice of the other Jewish sects and that of the Romans, who also practiced animal sacrifice. Titus Flavius Clemens, one of the most respected of the early Christian fathers, is quoted in *Ethics of Diet* by Howard Williams as saying,

"Sacrifices were invented by men as a pretext for eating flesh."

This seems to be essentially the Essene understanding of the motivation behind sacrifices. According to Ewing, the Essene understanding of diet was based on the commandment, "Thou Shalt Not Kill" and the first dietary commandment of Genesis 1:29, quoted earlier in this chapter, which gave humanity fruits, nuts, seeds, vegetables, grains, and grasses to eat, but specifically not flesh food. The position of Jesus against animal sacrifice is, of course, consistent with His humaneness, His love for all of God's creatures, and His vegetarianism. According to the *Hastings Encyclopedia on Religion and Ethics,*

> "The Gospel according to the Apostles was used by the Ebionite (viz Nazarenes). Herein is found the 'Essene Christ.' He denounces sacrifice and the eating of flesh."

Epiphanius quotes Jesus, in His confrontation with the high priest in the Temple after He has chased out the money lenders,

> "I come to abolish sacrifices, and unless you cease sacrifices my anger will not cease from you."

The Gospel of the Hebrews also clarifies that Jesus not only taught not to eat our animal friends, but had come to end blood sacrifices. In Lection XXI, verse 8, teaching to His disciples He says:

> "I am come to end the sacrifices and feasts of blood; and if ye cease not offering and eating of flesh and blood, the wrath of God shall not cease from you; even as it came to your fathers in the wilderness, who lusted for flesh, and they ate to their content, and were filled with rottenness, and the plague consumed them."

Many feel that Jesus ate the lamb of the Passover meal and use this as indirect evidence that He did not teach or practice vegetarianism. In the *Gospel According to the Hebrews,* Lection LXXVI, section 27, which predates the present edition of the Gospels used today, Judas is quoted as inciting Caiaphas against Jesus for not eating lamb at the Passover:

> "Now Judas Iscariot had gone to the house of Caiaphas and said unto him, Behold He (Jesus) has celebrated the Passover within the gates (of Jerusalem), with the Mazza in place of the lamb. I indeed bought a lamb, but He forbade that it should be killed, and lo, the man of whom I bought it is witness."

It is important to remember that the information in the Gospels came from earlier Judaic sources and not vice versa. Changes in translations commonly occur, and this could be one of them. Again, His refusal to eat the Passover lamb is consistent with His role and high spiritual awareness as the great Essene Teacher of the time and also His actions against animal sacrifice in the Temple.

The Vegetarianism of the Disciples

Dr. Ewing points out that the highly respected Church Father Eusebius, quotes Hegesippus (about 160 A.D.) who said that James, the Disciple and brother of Jesus, who became head of the Judaic-Christians after Jesus, was a vegetarian who "drank no wine, wore no wool, nor ate any flesh." It was said that he followed this practice from birth. It is likely that all of Jesus' family, including Himself, were raised as vegetarian and lived that way as adults. It is also likely, that in the light of the overall evidence, all but one of the disciples were initially vegetarian. Ewing quotes the Clementine Hominies XXII, 6, which also suggests that most of the disciples, if not all, were vegetarian:

> "They followed the Apostles in their custom of daily lustrations. They refused to partake of flesh or wine, taking as their pattern, St. Peter, whose food was bread, olives, and herbs...."

Clement of Alexandria, in his book *The Instructor*, states:

> "Accordingly, the apostle Matthew partook of seeds, and nuts, and vegetables, without flesh."

Peter was also historically known to be vegetarian as well. He was quoted as telling Clement,

> "I live on bread alone, with olives, and seldom even with potherbs."

Peter is also cited in the Clementine Hominies XII, which dates back to the middle of the Second Century, as being vegetarian. Dr. Ewing quotes an early Christian document which quotes Peter as saying:

> "The unnatural eating of flesh is as polluting as the heathen worship of devils, with its sacrifices and impure feasts, through participation in which a man becomes a fellow eater with devils."

In a letter to Trajan, the Roman Emperor, Pliny, the historian and governor of Blithynia (an area where Peter was teaching), describes the early Christian practices:

> "They affirmed the whole of their guilt, or their error...binding themselves by a solemn oath never to commit any sin or evil and never to falsify their word, nor deny a trust, after which it was their custom to depart and to meet together to take food, but ordinary and harmless (vegetarian) food."

Dr. Ewing also quotes an early Christian document which presents Thomas as:

> "...fasting, wearing a single garment, giving what he has to others, and abstaining from the eating of flesh and the drinking of wine."

John the Baptist also was a vegetarian. *The Gospel of the Hebrews* describes the food of John the Baptist as:

> "...wild honey and cakes made with oil and honey."

The word locust, which is commonly given, is a mistranslation. The Greek word for oil cakes is 'enkris' and the Greek word for locust is 'akris.' This translation of cakes of honey and oil is in keeping with the appearance of the angel, Gabriel, to John the Baptist's mother instructing her that John should be raised on honey and butter.

Another major follower of Jesus was Paul. Paul may have been the only major early teacher who was not initially vegetarian. He appears to have become vegetarian a little later in his ministry. In Corinthians 8:13 Paul states:

> "Therefore if food makes my brother stumble, I will never eat flesh at all, that I may not make my brother stumble."

According to Dr. Ewing, the well-respected Christian Father, Flavius Clemens, the founder of the Alexandrian School of Christian Theology, wrote in 190 A.D.:

> "It is good neither to drink wine nor to eat flesh, as both St. Paul and the Pythagoreans acknowledge, for this is rather character-istic to a beast, and the fumes arising from them (flesh pots) being dense and darken the soul....For a voice will whisper to him (Paul) saying 'Destroy not the work of God for the sake of food. Whether ye eat or drink do all to the glory of God'."

Vegetarianism of Early Christians Leaders

As already pointed out, many of the early Christians, such as the Judaic Christians, the early Gnostics, the Ebionites, and the Montanists, were vegetar-ian. Early church fathers, such as Tertullian, St. John Chrysostom, Clement of Alexandria, Origen, St. Benedict, Eusebius, Pliny, Papias, Cyprian, and Pantaenus, all supported vegetarianism as part of Christianity. It is no accident that these

Christian leaders of the time were vegetarians, as they were still influenced by the direct teaching of the first Christians.

One of the great figures of Latin Christianity was Florens Tertullianis who was born in Carthage about 155 A.D. His spiritual understanding was so profound that he is referred to by the Bishop of Carthage as the "Master." In *Ethics of Diet*, Tertullianis makes the underlying point on the issue of the vegetarianism of Jesus. He is quoted as saying:

> "How unworthy do you press the example of Christ as having come eating and drinking into the service of your lusts: He who pronounced not the full, but the hungry and thirsty blessed, who professed His work to be the completion of His father's will, was wont to abstain—instructing them to labor for that food which lasts to eternal life, and enjoining in their common prayers, petition not for flesh food but for bread only."

Concluding Points

The historical evidence from the writings of the early Christian Fathers, the Jewish philosopher, Philo, the Dead Sea Scrolls, the Gospel According to the Hebrew's, the *Essene Gospel of Peace Volume I*, and evidence from the work of the Catholic historian, Epiphanius, all indicates that the Essene culture in which Jesus was raised, His family, most, if not all, of His twelve disciples, and His early Christian followers were vegetarian. The prophecy of His coming in Isaiah 7:14,15 even foretells of Him being a vegetarian:

> 14 " Therefore the Lord Himself shall give you a sign; Behold a virgin shall conceive, and bear a son, and shall call His name Immanuel (with us is God).

> 15 Butter and honey shall He eat, that He may know how to refuse the evil, and choose the good."

The historical evidence also strongly suggests that Jesus did teach vegetarianism, was a vegetarian, and therefore did not eat flesh food. This is consistent with His teachings of love of all God's creatures, His commitment not to kill any life according to the highest understanding of the Law of Moses that "Thou shalt not kill" (man or animal), the original teachings of vegetarianism in Genesis 1:29, and His stand in the Temple against the sacrifice of animals. Jesus taught that compassion should extend to all of God's creatures. Jesus taught a humane way of life and was a shining example of a fully humane human being. To be humane is to be kind, merciful, and not to kill any living creature. The slaughter of animals can in no way be considered humane.

Although there is compelling and strong evidence that Jesus was vegetarian, there is no absolute proof of this. This leaves the door open for readers who do not wish to entertain this understanding to maintain whatever belief system they want. Could, however, a living Son of God teach anything less or live any way less pure than this?

Contemporary Christian Vegetarians

More recently we have the Seventh Day Adventists whose many members are vegetarian. John Wesley, the founder of Methodism, was also vegetarian, as was Sylvester Graham, the Presbyterian minister known for the "Graham cracker." What is believed to be the first book on vegetarianism published in the U.S., *Abstinence from Flesh of Animals,* was written by William Metcalf, a pastor of the Bible Christian Church of England. Christian monks, such as the Trappist, Benedictine, and Carthusian orders; the Universal Christian Gnostic Movement; and the Rosicrucian Fellowship, practice a vegetarian diet. Many Franciscan monks follow a vegetarian diet. Some of this has changed since the 1965 Ecumenical Council which relaxed the regulations regulating flesh food eating. In September 1990 at Brown University, Bishop Desmond Tutu from South Africa elegantly stated the meaning of vegetarianism in the context of the promise of world peace and equality for all of God's children. To paraphrase him, he said that in God's garden, we are all vegetarians. Since vegetarianism was God's original plan, although shattered temporarily, it will be again!

The Seventh Day Adventists, Modern Vegetarian Christians

In June 1863, Ellen White, a devout Christian woman who had been receiving revelations since 1844, began to receive specific revelations pertaining to reforming the health practices in the Adventist movement. This vision in 1863, often referred to as the "Otsego Vision," forms the core of the Seventh Day Adventist (SDA) diet and health practices. She claimed to have received her revelations directly from God. Many of them were said to also come through angelic messengers. The most frequent of these angelic messengers was Gabriel. Her revelations became a tower of guidance for the growth of the Seventh Day Adventist movement. Vegetarianism, however, was not, and is not, an absolute precondition for joining the Seventh Day Adventist Church.

Mrs. White makes the clear connection between one's ability to lead a spiritually sensitive, moral, and physically healthy life which enables one to serve God to one's highest ability, and the importance of eating a moderate, simple, vegetarian diet. This is also a diet devoid of overindulgence in even too much "healthy" foods or stimulating, rich foods. Her teachings did not recommend stimulants like coffee and other drugs which alter spiritual awareness.

She taught that taking care of one's personal health was a Christian duty. In the 1976 edition of the *Seventh Day Adventist Encyclopedia*, it is said that the

> "SDAs believe that Christians should have a concern for health not because of any ceremonial or legalistic significance, but for the practical reason that only in a sound body can they render the most effective service to God and to others....Health is related to religion in that it enables men to have a clear mind with which to understand the will of God and a strong body with which to do the will of God."

> "SDAs believe that at the fall of man all three aspects of man's nature—the physical, the intellectual, and the spiritual—were affected; and that Jesus, who said He had come to restore that which was lost, seeks to save the whole man."

In her book, *Counsels on Diet and Foods,* section 111, Ellen White says:

> "Grains, fruits, nuts, and vegetables constitute the diet chosen for us by our Creator. These foods, prepared in as simple and natural a manner as possible, are the most healthful and nourishing. They impart a strength, a power of endurance, and a vigor of intellect, that are not afforded by a more complex and stimulating diet."

In section 112 she is even more specific:

> "God gave our first parents (Adam and Eve) the food He designed that the race should eat. It was contrary to His plan to have the life of any creature taken. There was to be no death in Eden. The fruit of the trees in the garden was the food man's wants required."

In section 115 she shared her revelation of God's original and present plan:

> "Again and again, I have been shown that God is bringing His people back to His original design, that is, not to subsist upon the flesh of dead animals. He would have us teach people a better way....If meat is discarded, if the taste is not educated in that direction, if a liking for fruits and grains is encouraged, it will soon be as God in the beginning designed it should be. No meat will be used by His people."

Her teachings made a clear connection between the diet one eats and the spiritual and moral sensitivity, clarity of mind, and strength of character needed to follow the spiritual life in an enduring way. In section 95 she says:

> "Foul blood will surely becloud the moral and intellectual powers, and arouse and strengthen the baser passions of your nature. Neither of you can afford a feverish diet; for it is at the expense of the health of the body, and the prosperity of your own souls and the souls of your children."

> "You place upon your table food which taxes the digestive organs, excites the animal passions, and weakens the moral and intellectual faculties. Rich food and flesh meats are no benefit to you...."

> "I entreat you for Christ's sake, to set your house and hearts in order. Let the truth of heavenly origin elevate and sanctify you, soul, body, and spirit. 'Abstain from fleshly lusts, which war against the soul'."

In section 92 she adds:

> "Indulgence of appetite strengthens the animal propensities, giving them the ascendancy over the mental and spiritual powers."

> "Abstain from fleshly lusts, which war against the soul, is the language of the apostle Peter."

The teaching that what and how we eat directly affects our spiritual sensitivity is a teaching consistent with the original teachings of Jesus. Although the *Essene Gospel of Peace Book One,* which essentially describes Christ's teaching of a live food, vegetarian diet as a part of the cleansing, rebirth, and harmonizing with the spiritual path, was not available to Ellen White in the 19th century, she indirectly refers to this core teaching. In section 73 she says:

> "The Redeemer of the world knew that the indulgence of appetite would bring physical debility, and so deaden the perceptive organs that the sacred and the eternal would not be discerned...."

The main point of her revelations was that it was time for all people to return to the original diet prescribed by God in Genesis 1:29. Ellen White was divinely directed to help people understand a vegetarian diet would help them physically, emotionally, mentally, and spiritually prepare for the Second Coming.

In The Gospel of the Holy Twelve, Lection XXXVIII, Verse 4, Jesus says:

"...wherefore I say unto all who desire to be my disciples, keep your hands from bloodshed and let no flesh meat enter your mouths, for God is just and bountiful, who ordaineth that man shall live by the fruits and seeds of the earth alone."

Remember:

"It is far better to be happy than to have our bodies act as grave-yards for animals."

— Clement of Alexandria (A.D. 160-240)

VISION

BLACKBOARD QUOTES

Preview of Chapter 16
Vegetarianism in the World's Religions

In appreciating the importance of a vegetarian way of life it is helpful to understand that vegetarianism is a world-wide teaching that seems to be part of many of the major world religions from the beginning of many of these teachings. It seems that in each part of the world people have independently acknowledged the importance of vegetarianism as a way to create peace, harmony, health, and spiritual growth. Are you ready to create less pain in the world and bring more peace and harmony by making the transition toward a vegetarian way of life?

    I.   Buddhism

   II.   Zoroastrianism

  III.   Jainism

  IV.   Sikhism

   V.   Islam

  VI.   Hinduism

 VII.   Principle of Ahimsa

       A.   Vegetariansim as a major way to create less pain

       B.   Dilemna of surviving without creating pain in the world

Chapter 16

Vegetarianism in the World's Religions

Universal compassion for all of God's creatures is also consistent with the highest ideals of many of the world religions, such as Zoroastrianism (Parseeism, as it is called in India), Buddhism, Hinduism, Pythagoreanism, Jainism, and Sikhism, all of which teach vegetarianism. Presently it is not universally practiced in Buddhism and Sikhism for perhaps the same reasons as in Judaism and Christianity. Buddha, however, is quoted in the Lankavatar as saying:

> "For the sake of love of purity, the bodhisattva should refrain from eating flesh....For fear of causing terror to living beings, let the bodhisattva, who is disciplining himself to attain compassion, refrain from eating flesh....It is not true that meat is proper food and permissible when the animal was not killed by himself, when he did not order others to kill it, when it was not specifically meant for him....Again, there may be some people in the future who...being under the influence of the taste of meat will string together in various ways many sophisticated arguments to defend meat eating....But meat eating in any form, in any manner, and in any place is unconditionally, and once and for all, prohibited....Meat eating I have not permitted to anyone, I do not permit, and will not permit."

In the Surangama Sutra it is written:

> "After my parinirvana (supreme enlightenment) in the final kalpa (time era) different kinds of ghosts will be encountered everywhere deceiving people and teaching them that they can eat meat and still attain enlightenment....How can a bhikshu (seeker) who hopes to become a deliverer of others, himself be living on the flesh of other sentient beings?"

This teaching in the Mahaparinirvana Sutra sums it up in terms of the importance of vegetarianism for Buddhism and perhaps all spiritual paths:

> "The eating of meat extinguishes the seed of great compassion."

The present Dali Lama has expressed a strong conviction numerous times that it is important not to harm other sentient beings (including animals). He considers it part of the Buddhist practice of harmlessness not to eat meat. Although Tibetans as a culture ate meat, Buddhists in general do not. Now that the Tibetan Buddhists are in exile, the Dali Lama feels all Tibetan followers, as well as other Buddhists, should conform to the Buddhist practice of vegetarianism. The Dali Lama himself is working in the direction of becoming a vegetarian.

In Jainism, ahimsa, the doctrine of nonviolence, is a central theme. Because of this, the Jains have maintained a strong and unbroken vegetarian lifestyle throughout its history. Some Jains are so committed to nonviolence that they wear a mask over their mouths so that they do not accidentally swallow any insects and they also sweep the path in front of them as they walk so as not to step on any living creatures.

The Zoroasterian religion goes back many thousands of years and is perhaps the first religion in recorded history that taught the principles of a balanced way of life, including vegetarianism and an ecological awareness. In this religion, the title of Zarathustra was given to great sages over time, but has been most associated with their last spiritual leader who lived around 600 B.C. He was a strong advocate of a vegetarian life style.

Sikhism, developed by Guru Nanak in the fifteenth century, is not strictly vegetarian because some of its roots are from the Islam tradition. According to *Vegetarianism in Sikhism,* by Swaran Singh Sanehi, a Sikh scholar, the Sikh teachings of Guru Nanak support the practice of vegetarianism fully. Guru Nanak was said to have considered the eating of flesh food improper, especially if one were using the practice of meditation as part of one's spiritual life. In the West, the 3HO Golden Temple Movement is one of the biggest western Sikh organizations and they are completely vegetarian. The Namdhari sect of Sikhs is also vegetarian.

Vegetarianism in Islam

Although vegetarianism is not specifically endorsed by Islam, there is also evidence of some support for it in the Islamic religion. Mohammed is quoted as saying,

"Whosoever is kind to the creatures of God is kind to himself."

The prophet's earliest biographies showed his universal compassion for all of creation. He spoke out against the mistreatment of camels and the use of birds for the targeting of marksmen. The Koran (s. 6, vs. 38) says,

"There is not an animal on the earth, nor a flying creature on two wings, but they are peoples like unto you."

Mohammed was said to prefer vegetarian foods, such as milk diluted with water. He was said to eat only pomegranates, grapes, and figs for weeks at a time. He is quoted as saying to some hunters, "Maim not the brute beasts." At another time Mohammed said,

> "There are rewards for benefiting every animal having a moist liver (all living creatures)."

Mohammed was not the sole voice sympathetic to vegetarianism in Islam. Al-Ghassali (1058-1111 A.D.), a brilliant Muslim philosopher, wrote:

> "Compassionate eating leads to compassionate living."

Although vegetarianism is not mandated in the Sufi path (of Islam), many of the Sufis (Islamic mystics) practice vegetarianism for spiritual reasons. The Sufi mystic, Hazrat Rabia Basri, would often be surrounded by animals when she meditated in the woods. One day, a disciple approached her in the woods and the animals ran away. He felt bad that the animals ran away from him. He asked her advice on the issue. She asked him what he had eaten that day. When he revealed that he had eaten some animal fat, Rabia explained that the animals run from those who eat their flesh. The Sufi's as a group, however, do not specifically advocate a vegetarian way of life. It is left for each individual to decide whether to make it part of their spiritual life or not.

The Islamic Holiness, M.R. Bawa Muhaiyaddeen, considered by many as an Islamic saint, was a vegetarian. He shares some specific teaching about vegetarianism that is universal for all. In his book, *The Tasty Economical Cookbook—Volume II,* he says:

> "A true human being must have compassion toward all lives. There are so many ways to eat good clean food, without killing or tormenting other lives, and without eating the flesh or bones of other lives....If a man eats meat, he will take on the qualities of the animals he eats. The qualities of all these animals can be imbibed by eating their flesh....And once those qualities enter, the man's anger, his hastiness, and his animal qualities will increase. The animal's blood will intermingle with his blood....These animal qualities are what causes one man to murder another, to harm and torment another."

In an unpublished discourse, Bawa Muhaiyaddeen gives a specific answer to the question of Islam and Sufi practice of vegetarianism as well as a universal answer about the practice of vegetarianism. From a spiritual perspective, a deeper level of vegetarianism is from the inside out, rather than from the outside in. He clarifies vegetarianism as the result and natural consequence of the development of spiritual consciousness:

"When a man's mind attains a state of completeness in wisdom and when he reaches a state where he will not hurt any life within himself (in one's mind), then he will not harm anything on the outside either. Inside he will not intend any harm or pain to any other life. Nor will he do anything harmful or eat any life on the outside. This is a state of wisdom, clarity, and the light of God. This is Sufism."

"Man is such a dangerous animal, and it is only when he changes his behavior that he becomes a good man, a true human being. When he changes into a good man, he will no longer have within himself the thoughts of killing or gaining victory over another life. He will not have within himself the qualities of distressing other lives, of wanting to harass or ruin other lives. If he does not kill anything on the inside, then he will not kill anything on the outside."

"Once a person has the wisdom, the potentialities, and the qualities of the true human being, once he attains that liberation, he will have reached the exalted state of God. The darkness in him will have been dispelled and he will love his neighbor as he loves himself. Once he attains the quality of loving every other life as he loves his own, he will never kill another life. Nor will he ever cause pain to another life. Because he feels that the other life is also his own flesh, he will never eat flesh."

"...such a one will not eat flesh. He will not eat another human being (within his heart) nor will he eat an animal. Some people will not eat animals (on the outside), but they will devour other human beings (within their hearts and minds)."

The same difficulty in Islam seems to exist in Judaism and Christianity. It is that initially a vegetarian way of life is too big a change for people and becomes a stumbling block for the people to hear. According to Bawa Muhaiyaddeen, initially,

"The Prophet came and told them, 'Do not kill. It is a sin. You are taking another life'."

Because the people were not able to follow this teaching, Mohammed then had to limit, but ultimately allow, the eating of flesh because the people were not of the consciousness that allowed them to go beyond their blood lust. As in Judaism, certain laws were given which limited the quantity of killing of animals by making the laws very difficult to follow. These laws are called qurban, or the slaughtering of animals after certain prayers are recited and while you look the animal in the eyes.

As with the Kosher laws, the Koran lists forbidden foods rather than the foods one must eat. These forbidden foods center around meat. It has elaborate regulations for preparation which limit the amount of animals one is able to kill and therefore make eating meat considerably more of a burden than eating a vegetarian diet. Muslim vegetarians, like Jewish vegetarians, have no real scriptural dietary restrictions. Because Allah is praised as merciful and compassionate, vegetarianism and other types of compassion toward animals is a way of following the Islamic teachings. Although Islam, like other modern religions, does not advocate vegetarianism to the masses, vegetarianism is quite compatible with its essential teachings.

Hinduism and Vegetarianism

Hinduism is one of the religions which has maintained its vegetarian perspective perhaps from the beginning of written history. There are about 550 million Hindu vegetarians. It is clearly part of the spiritual path as described in the Vedas, which are the ancient spiritual scriptures that are somewhere between six to eight thousand years old. The Vedas are the underlying thread of a wide variety of spiritual paths involved in the practice of Hinduism. Also involved in the practice of a vegetarian diet is the science of Yoga and the science of Ayurvedic medicine that itself originates from the Vedas. As pointed out earlier, Ayurveda describes three diet types. One of them, called the sattvic diet, is a diet for enhancing inner peace and spiritual development; it is a simple vegetarian diet. Ahimsa is another primary force behind vegetarianism in India. Ahimsa may be broadly defined as a dynamic compassion for all of life. Mahatma Gandhi, a vegetarian, taught that the two pillars of ahimsa are truth and compassion.

The following quotes represent the main emphasis of the Vedic teachings on vegetarianism. They emphasize compassion, respect, and nonviolence for all of God's creation:

"Having well considered the origin of flesh foods,
And the cruelty of fettering and slaying corporeal beings, let man
entirely abstain from eating flesh." (Manusmriti 5.49)

"You must not use your God-given body for killing God's creatures, whether they are human, animal, or whatever." (Yajur Veda 12.32)

"By not killing any living being, one becomes fit for salvation."
(Manusmriti 6.60)

Ahimsa

The principle of ahimsa can also be found in the Buddhic Eightfold Path, which has been a guide to living a harmless, compassionate life for thousands of years. In *Ahimsa,* by Nathaniel Altman, Buddha is quoted as saying:

"Him I call a Brahmin who is free from anger, who gladly endures reproach, and even stripes and bonds inflicted upon him without cause. Him I call a Brahmin who slays no living creatures, who does not kill, or cause to be killed, any living thing."

Often translated as nonviolence in the West, the principle of ahimsa has a broader meaning in the East. Ahimsa incorporates an active stance in the world with a dynamic compassion for all of life. Nonviolence, without the dynamic aspect, has more of a passive, restraining from violence connotation. Ahimsa is acting from a compassionate awareness and empathic identification born of a reverence for life that affects every facet of daily existence. It involves a personal responsibility to respect, and work for, the well-being of all sentient beings. Although often thought of as compassion between humans, ahimsa is compassion for all of the earth and its life forms.

One consideration that arises in the discussion of ahimsa and vegetarianism is the killing of plants. Ever since the publishing of *The Secret Life of Plants,* which scientifically documents the pain plants experience in being harvested and cut up, I have been aware that plants do experience some pain. For most of us, it is necessary for our survival to eat plants. Our very existence causes some sort of pain on the planet, but there is a relativity to it. For those who want to equate all pain as equal in order to justify their flesh-centered diet, I find it hard to compare the blood slaughter and eating of a sentient being, such as a cow, with the simple harvesting and eating of a carrot. To even the most callous observer, the experiences are magnitudes different in pain and violence.

A vegetarian also creates less pain than a nonvegetarian because they are not indirectly or directly participating in the systematic slaughtering and pain of billions of animals every year. The U.S. Department of Agriculture reports that 4.5 billion cattle, calves, sheep, lambs, hogs, chickens, ducks, and turkeys are slaughtered yearly in the U.S. A vegetarian also causes less overall death to plants than a meat eater because the animals the flesh eater raised for consumption has eaten thousands of plants before they themselves are slaughtered. There is also a significant difference between the gross exploitation of animal life because of greed and a flesh-centered diet and living simply and relatively harmlessly by living on a vegetarian diet so that others, including the planetary organism, Gaia, or Mother Earth, will simply live and survive.

It is possible that there may be no perfect state of nonviolence while we are in a physical body. Although vegetarians cause significantly less pain and global ecological destruction than flesh eaters, fruitarians cause even less pain than vegetarians because they do not destroy the life of the plant when they pick fruit off trees. Those rare few who live on just water and air cause even less pain than fruitarians. Ahimsa is a practice that strives to create less and less disorder and pain in the world as we do our best to live our lives with ever-increasing harmony, compassion, and love. Theoretically, since there is no cut-off point where we stop causing pain by our very existence, the guilt about causing pain could be endless. Perhaps we were given the grace of Genesis 1:29, God's command to be vegetarian, as a way to establish a relatively peaceful, guilt-free way of living on the planet.

Because our planet offers herself for our survival, I feel humble and grateful to the planet for the pain she endures. We would do well to take the minimum from Mother Earth and cause the least amount of pain and destruction so that the mutual survival of all life on the planet will be harmonically assured.

It's no accident vegetarianism is compatible with the teachings of:

Christianity
Judaism
Hinduism
Buddhism
Islam
Jainism
Sikhism
Zoroastrianism

Vegetarianism preserves life, health, peace, the ecology, creates a more equitable distribution of resources, helps to feed the hungry, encourages nonviolence for the animal and human members of the planet, and is a powerful aid for the spiritual transformation of the body, emotions, mind, and spirit.

VISION

BLACKBOARD FOOD FOR THOUGHT

Part III

Transition to Vegetarianism

At this point you have been empowered by the knowledge of how to individualize your diet, about acid/base balance, constitutional type, psychology of eating, process of assimilation, and had doubts and fears addressed about becoming vegetarian. You understand the impact of diet on the ecology of the planet, cruelty or compassion for animals, individual health, feeding the hungry, and peace in the world. You understand the connection between diet and spiritual life. You have had a chance to contemplate food as a love note from God and may have even tried taking the time to read some of these daily notes. If you are already vegetarian and have done all these, you might have already become a—sensitive, aware, alert, and compassionate—**conscious eater.** For others for whom this book is a bridge into this new world of health and spirit, there is one more major step in the process: how to make the transition to a vegetarian diet.

There are many ways to become a vegetarian. This section outlines the changes and steps one often takes. Questions about the transition are explored. The reader is given guidance regarding how to move from the present diet to lactovegetarian to vegan to live food, vegetarian diet. Enjoy the walk, take your time, and be gentle with yourself. Vegetarianism is about peace, and the first place to start is to be peaceful with yourself during the transition. Once you have made the major change to vegetarian, the individual diet that suits your own life style and health needs will gradually emerge. Those who move too fast do not always last.

Before moving further, it is important to condition your body, mind, and spirit. Perhaps part of you has even wanted to give up reading the rest of the book because you do not feel ready to become a conscious eater. That may just be your flesh-eating and culturally ingrained old habits fighting back as your intuition, intellect, and spirit are working to guide you to the highest level of conscious eating you can attain. Don't let your resistances control you.

Before moving foreward in this section, I suggest you focus on yourself for a few moments. See yourself as strong and healthy, free of pain or sickness, with a pure spirit and God-like mind. Now close your eyes and breathe in radiant health and exhale all negativity and sickness. Do this seven times. Now, see the new you as a— **conscious eater.** Take as long as you need to pray or meditate until such a vision of your Divine potential appears. Feel the experience of this vision in your body as you are filled with health, spiritual power, and sensitivity. Experience the emotions and thoughts associated with the new you as a **conscious eater.** How does it feel to align yourself with the Divine intention of thousands of years? How does it feel to prepare yourself for the promised Golden Age? Write down your experience and date it in the spirit-mind-body vision goal sheet at the back of the book. As this vision grows with your experience, continue to record your goals. Enjoy!

Preview of Chapter 17
The Change to Vegetarianism

For many people, changing to a vegetarian diet is a major lifestyle change. Without an understanding of the subtleties of the process it is easy to become confused and discouraged. This chapter speaks to those physical, emotional, mental, and spiritual issues. I also put vegetarianism in perspective spiritually by making the point that although a vegetarian diet helps the spiritual process, one cannot eat one's way to God. As you read this chapter try to see where you experience your own resistances. Are you ready to let go of these resistances? Are you ready to adopt a diet that will most likely make you more sensitive to the presence of God in your life?

I.   The change to vegetarianism

    A. Reasons for the transition

    B. Outstanding people who are vegetarians

II.   Physical detoxification

    A. Physical symptoms of detoxification

    B. Healing crises

    C. One becomes cleaner and more vital

III.   Psychophysiology of dietary change

    A. How we look, how we feel

    B. Anti-aging research

    C. Releasing old thoughts in process of healing

IV.   Perspectives on dietary change

V.   Four transition stages

Chapter 17

The Change to Vegetarianism

When asked about switching to vegetarianism, some people have the mind set, "Why bother, I like my charbroiled steak. All this stuff about becoming vegetarian makes me feel guilty. Why not just ignore it?" Unfortunately, in this case, ignorance is not bliss. To ignore the harmful effects of diet is nothing less than an accelerated path to physical degeneration, pain, misery, and disharmony with self and nature. This is especially true with the present state of the world. A vegetarian diet helps one attune to the worldwide evolutionary change that is occurring in the direction of peace and harmony for all of creation. The information and ideas that have been shared about vegetarianism are not meant to make anyone guilty, but to educate so that one can begin to make intelligent, informed choices for one's life, health, and happiness. Guilt comes from knowing what is most appropriate for one's well-being and choosing not to follow the dictates of one's conscience. Guilt is one's own creation stemming from resistance to change. It comes from not being able to let go of old habits and addictions that one intuitively knows do not serve one's ultimate well-being and that of the planet.

There is an intuitive "yesness" that many people have found works for them as they have applied these concepts in their transition to vegetarianism. The information I have presented is best used as guidelines, concepts, and tools to empower and enhance well-being. There is no single answer for everyone, but there are compelling reasons to make such a change in one's life. The following is a review of some of those reasons.

Reasons for Transitioning to a Vegetarian Diet

1. **A vegetarian diet, developed in a conscious, gradual, and scientific way, is an overwhelmingly superior diet for health, vitality, endurance, and general well-being.**

2. **Vegetarian food tends to create a calmer, more centered, and clearer emotional and mental state.**

3. **A vegetarian diet is a distinct aid for enhancing spiritual life and awareness. Throughout history, almost all major spiritual paths have acknowledged this awareness, including Genesis 1:29, the first dietary commandment and the first direct teaching to be vegetarian in the Bible.**

4. A vegetarian diet enhances the flow of the spiritualizing force in the body. A flesh-centered diet acts as a sludge to the purifying movement of this holy force in all the basic elements of the body, mind, and spirit.

5. A vegetarian diet brings one into ecological harmony with all of creation. In comparison with a flesh-centered diet, it is vastly superior in its ability to conserve land, water, and energy, and enhance the quality of both human and animal life. It brings us into harmony with the biological cycles of the biosphere, such as with the natural oxygen/carbon dioxide cycle of our breath and that of the plant kingdom.

6. A vegetarian diet connects one with the solar, lunar, and stellar forces of the universe. It allows one to extract energy from Mother Nature through the balancing principle of the rainbow diet.

7. A vegetarian diet minimizes the violence and exploitation of our animal friends on the planet. In this nonviolent space, it allows compassion for all life to blossom. A vegetarian diet would help bring planetary peace on every level.

8. A vegetarian diet minimizes the hoarding, wasting, and inefficient use of natural resources and energy for producing food. It minimizes the wasting of the food itself, particularly in the form of grain fed to livestock. Because of this, a vegetarian way of life would make it possible (if the social, political aspects of our society were ready) to end the 60 million deaths per year due to starvation. It would also help end the disease and misery of millions more suffering from malnutrition. The abundance of food created by the worldwide adoption of a vegetarian diet would prove that starvation on the planet is caused more by a scarcity of justice than of food.

9. A vegetarian diet is considerably less expensive than a flesh-centered diet, and would be even more so if the meat industry in the U.S. were not significantly subsidized by the government.

10. A shift to a vegetarian way of life is part of a major planetary shift in consciousness. It is the dietary blueprint for the Golden Age we are entering.

A number of outstanding individuals throughout history have undoubtedly understood these principles in their choice of being a vegetarian. The following individuals chose to be vegetarian for many of the above reasons: Jesus, Buddha,

Krishna, Rama, Zarathrustra, John the Baptist, John the Divine, Matthew, Pythagoras, Plato, Virgil, Horace, Rabia Basra, Henry David Thoreau, Ralph Waldo Emerson, Benjamin Franklin, Richard Wagner, Voltaire, Sir Isaac Newton, Leonardo da Vinci, William Shakespeare, Charles Darwin, H.G. Wells, George Bernard Shaw, Mahatma Gandhi, Leo Tolstoy, Albert Schweitzer, and Albert Einstein, among others.

The process of becoming a vegetarian is one of self-discovery and self-transformation. Because food is more primary than sex, whatever changes we do make have a deep impact on us on an emotional, mental, and spiritual level. With each change of habit, a little more consciousness is liberated. Part of the self-discovery process is that as we change, old thoughtforms must be brought up, examined and ultimately discarded.

A rapid shift to a vegetarian diet also may create a physical detoxification. Because of these reasons, **the number one rule for making the transition to vegetarianism is to move slowly and gently.** If we are to be at peace with ourselves, each step in the process must be one which feels harmonious. Most people can deal with change if it is gradual. If the change comes too quickly, it then becomes a shock to the system. Usually, the complete transition may take several years. I've seen it happen in a few weeks or in as much as ten years. In the overall picture, how long the process takes doesn't matter. What matters is that one has chosen to move along the evolutionary continuum toward health, harmony, and peace. At each step of the way one creates more peace and does less damage to others and oneself. Even taking the life of plants for food has some violence, so it is important to humbly remember that whatever one does on the physical plane will never be perfectly in harmony, but it will be increasingly harmonious. By moving slowly, one avoids the pitfall of overreacting on a physical, emotional, and psychological level to the attitudinal changes that are made in the transition to vegetarianism. In this way, one avoids becoming discouraged. In order to work with these changes in a beneficial way, it is important for one to develop some understanding of how they unfold.

Physical Detoxification

Because of the toxicity of the inner environment of our bodies and the outer environments we live in, it is safe to say that all of us have some stored toxins in our system. As one shifts to a healthier diet and away from a flesh-centered one, the stored toxins in the system begin to come out of the tissues. The process of detoxification can be understood by the physical phenomenon known as diffusion. The chemistry of the diffusion process says that elements move from areas of higher concentration to those of lower concentration. With a more toxic diet, such as a flesh-centered one, nutrients, as well as accompanying toxins found in these foods, flow into the blood and lymph from the intestinal tract. If

257

their concentration is higher than the toxins in the cells, as is often the case with a flesh-centered diet, these toxins diffuse their way into the cells, where they are then stored. When the toxicity level of our diet is decreased by switching to a vegetarian diet, the difference of the concentration of toxins between the intracellular fluid and extracellular fluid changes. The cells become more concentrated with toxins than the extracellular fluid because less toxins are put into the extracellular fluid by a vegetarian diet. Because of the law of diffusion, which says that elements flow from areas of higher concentrations to areas of lower concentrations, the toxins which are now more concentrated in the cells begin to flow back into the extracellular fluid. Toxins are diffused into the blood stream and then later go to the liver, kidneys, gastrointestinal tract, and skin systems, whose jobs are to eliminate these toxins from the system. If the organs of elimination become overworked, then they may go into malfunction. This is called a healing crisis. Typical detox and healing crisis symptoms are bad breath, pimples on the body, nausea, headache, liver pain, odoriferous stool and urine, and general malaise. Sometimes the blood, organs, and glands become so overloaded with toxins that one actually gets sick. Sometimes the toxins come out in the form of a past disease which our organism is releasing from the system. The health pioneer J. H. Tilden, M.D., actually defines disease as a toxemia crisis. Although there may be other primary causes for disease, such as deficiency and genetic causes, the root of many diseases come from the toxins produced by the excesses so prevalent in western society.

Healing crises usually occur when the body vitality reaches a point where it is healthy enough to throw off the toxins. A crisis may last for a few days or even weeks. In my clinical experience, one is unlikely to have a major healing crisis if one detoxifies slowly over a few years rather than going onto a diet that is so clean and pure that the detoxification process is greatly accelerated. Speeding up the recovery from a healing crisis is facilitated by daily enemas, plenty of rest, taking in alkalinizing fluids, such as fruit and vegetable juices which neutralize acid toxins, and maintaining a positive attitude. Seven to ten day "relative" fasts can also speed up this overall detoxification process. I define a "relative fast" as follows: if one is on a flesh-food diet, one would undertake several "meat" fasts by eating an ovo-lactovegetarian diet. If one is a lactovegetarian, eating a dairy-free diet for awhile or doing several juice fasts may help one shift to a cleaner diet.

In my clinical experience with juice fasting, although people may get transitory healing crises for several days, the fasts provide a controlled and safe situation where one can "reset one's dietary dial" to a healthier diet. After a few times of positive experiences of fasting on a purer diet, one has enough positive feedback so that the transition to the next step goes much more smoothly. After each stage of the transition, people seem to rise to a new level of well-being, energy, love, and light. More energy becomes available to experience one's aliveness in service of the spiritual awareness that is so important for our sensitivity and openness.

Although the discussion thus far has focused on the accumulation of toxins from dietary origin, any habit of body or mind which decreases our vital energy results in the accumulation of toxins in the body. Along with a healthy diet, one needs to develop a new lifestyle that also further enhances one's total well-being. The better one feels, the easier it is to find time to exercise, meditate, rest, drink good water, sun oneself, deep breathe, spend time with one's significant others, and experience the joy of the communion with the Divine. All these factors increase the vital force, which then helps one detoxify more easily and at progressively deeper levels.

It is also useful to understand that acid toxin production is a normal part of our metabolism. Exercise produces lactic acid build-up. Protein digestion produces sulfuric and phosphoric acid. Cell metabolism produces carbonic acid. A vital body can easily discharge these toxins, as well as many environmental toxins to which one might be exposed. The idea is not to obsessively spend time running from toxins, but to develop such a vital body force and such good health habits that one is able to handle the different environmental toxic stresses to which one is exposed. This does not mean one ignores common sense avoidance of toxic environmental situations.

In this detoxification process, one becomes cleaner and more vital over time. If people move too fast, however, they may become so pure that they actually become too sensitive to the environment or so filled with vital energy that they may become ungrounded in their lives. This is where the art of spiritual nutrition becomes important. It guides one to go beyond rigid concepts based on the mythical ideal. **The core idea of the art of spiritual nutrition is to find a diet that best establishes balance, function, and harmony in one's life.** This artful, intelligent, appropriate diet choice both supports one's daily function in the world and enhances one's communion with the divine.

The Psychophysiology of Dietary Change

Dietary change of any sort forces us to face patterns, habits, conscious and unconscious psychological attachments, our own ego defense systems, and also an acceptance of our new body image. It is an opportunity, through the self-knowledge that comes from dietary change, to expand our awareness and clarity about who we are. It is a healing step that can potentially be a catalyst that brings us into a new level of personal health. Along with psychological changes usually comes a change in our body image, sensitivity, and physical body structure.

Not all of this comes effortlessly or is necessarily easy to accept. Once when I was interviewed by a Canadian national T.V. network, the quite portly T.V. interviewer looked at a photograph of me twenty-five years ago when I was a

188-pound, bull-necked, all-New England, football middle linebacker and guard, one of eight national scholar athletes picked by the National College Football Hall of Fame, and the co-captain of an undefeated college football team. He then said to me "You looked so strong and healthy then and now you look so 'thin' and 'puny' compared to your football days." Well, I can't say I enjoyed being called puny on a national T.V. interview. It was a direct challenge to my new body image, but he got directly to the point of controversy: real health as compared to "looking healthy." "Looking healthy" is a subjective cultural concept that is not grounded in the science of health and longevity. Not too many years ago there were many young, steroid-raised athletes who looked very strong and buff on the outside, but who were tragically pointed toward serious health problems such as cancer and liver disease. Nevertheless, creating a new body image that does not fit with cultural stereotypes of health is not easy.

When I returned from India after a one year stretch of studying and working in a medical clinic, the contrast between the "normal" Indian body and the "normal" American was quite dramatic in the reverse. Almost everyone in America looked overweight to me. Is there an objective standard that can help us get some clarity?

As one observes various cultures around the world, those with the best quality of health and longevity are those who eat one third to one half the protein and total calories that Americans do. These people would be judged "thin" and "puny" by our subjective cultural standards. Even by our objective, generally accepted standards, according to the Metropolitan Life Insurance Ideal Weight tables, there are many people who are overweight in the United States. Most of the cultures known for health and longevity, who may appear thin to us, are actually the appropriate weight associated with health and longevity.

Stewart M. Berger, M.D., in his book, *Forever Young,* has a weight scale for optimal longevity that shows I am at the optimal weight for a youthful longevity. I pointed out to the Canadian interviewer that my weight as a football player was thirty-two pounds greater than the maximum for my weight to height range according to the Metropolitan Life Ideal Weight scales. I also pointed out that my flesh-eating, extra thirty-two pounds was all muscle designed to tackle or block opposing players. Since I was no longer playing football, this extra 32 pounds of muscle was no longer needed. In fact, I explained that with my new body, I felt considerably more healthy than I did in my football player body. This new body that is built primarily on living food is considerably more flexible, pain-free, physiologically more balanced, more vital, and more full of light than in my college years.

Although during high school and college my health would have been considered "good," I still got the average amount of colds and flus, had energy fluctuations, and had less mental endurance than I do now. My health and vitality back then isn't close to the quality of my almost disease-free health now. Since beginning a 95% live food diet in 1983, I've experienced an ever-increasing vitality and digestive power, strong immune and endocrine systems, and increased life force.

Being at one's ideal weight does not mean one loses relative strength or endurance, even if it doesn't fit with the stuffed body image of "healthy." On my forty-seventh birthday I was still able to do ninety-nine consecutive push-ups and one hundred sit-ups without breaking into a sweat.

In addition to observing the lifestyle patterns of cultures which enjoy greater health and longevity, some of the research by Roy Walford, M.D., one of America's leading anti-aging researchers, is highly noteworthy. Dr. Walford, in his book, *How to Double Your Vital Years,* shows with hard scientific research data from animal studies that by eating a high-nutrient, low-calorie diet (what he calls a high/low diet), animals are found to have increased their longevity by 50%. This is equivalent to humans living to be 150 to 160 years of age. This high/low diet is designed to find the point of maximum metabolic efficiency, maximum health, and maximum life span. His recommended calorie intake for maximum health and longevity is approximately 1500 calories per day. He cites research that he feels is beyond any reasonable doubt that shows that a high/low diet significantly extends life span, retards the rate of aging, and retards the onset of the major, chronic, degenerative diseases. He reports that the maximum life span in some mice in his minimal eating experiments was three to four times greater. Dietary restrictions, imposed even at late stages in the animal's life, greatly extended life span. Walford says that he is:

> "...convinced with a high order of probability that the same kind of diet will produce the same sort of results in humans."

Walford feels his approach would cut disease susceptibility in half. Humans, like the research animals, would reap health and longevity benefits by starting this low-calorie, high-nutrient diet even in middle age or later. Walford himself is following the principles he expounds upon in his research in his own life. Dr. Walford points out that 25% of women, and 12% of men, in the United States are obese. Obesity is defined as weighing more than 20% or more above the body weight ascribed by experts to a person's height and relative bone structure. It is indeed time we begin to reconsider a new cultural definition of health along with a corresponding change in what a healthy body is supposed to look like.

What happens almost universally when one stops eating flesh foods is that one drops excess weight. The loss of superfluous, unneeded weight continues when one stops eating dairy products. One's true, ideal weight is often easily discovered after one adopts a live food diet. A body built on high quality, natural, whole, organic, nature-developed foods is also of higher quality than body

261

weight that was built on poorer quality commercial foods, or the new, "improved" fast foods the industry is coming out with.

Walford suggests that most of us would do well to eat less. By cutting down to 1500 calories, over a few years one soon learns that whatever is eaten at 1500 calories per day better be especially good and healthy. A vegetarian, live food diet allows one to eat the least amount of food and receive the most nutritional and energetic impact. As in my case, without counting calories, a live food diet naturally has the ability to bring one to one's optimum weight.

It also takes time to get used to one's new body. The process is easier when one has people around who are not infecting one with irrational fears born of cultural biases about the "dangers of vegetarianism." To balance this popularist view, which is primarily based on ignorance, it is good to have objective, supportive data from cross-cultural studies, modern actuarial and scientific research, and convincing animal research.

Another part of this transition in the process of healing is the release of old, contracting thoughtforms. In my work with patients, students, and myself involving meditation, the Zero Point Process, prayer, spiritual awakenings, energetic healing, hands on healing, and dietary change, I have noticed there seems to be a common pathway by which what I call "mental toxins" are released. All of these processes enhance the spiritual energy that comes into the system and the amount of energy the system is able to handle. The more our bodies move toward health, the higher our vibration and vital force becomes. Many people believe that even though the mechanism is too difficult to scientifically establish at the present level of research technology, negative thoughtforms are stored in the subtle system of the body at lower vibrational rates. When the body begins to operate at a higher vibrational rate, these lower vibrational rate thoughtforms are forced out. They may come out in dreams, meditations, contemplations or just during the day. Dietary changes seem to be the most mild form of releasing negativities. Of all the forms of diet, the live food diet brings out the most rapid release of old, limiting thoughtforms.

Although relatively mild, for people who are not expecting it, this release of previously suppressed materials is one of the reasons a live food diet may be initially difficult for people to sustain. This is why I recommend live foods as part of a continuum rather than having people jump right into it. By gently passing through the various stages of a vegetarian diet, our minds and psyches are able to become more peacefully accustomed to the increased life force and accelerated release of negative thoughts that is associated with the healing and purification process. The body needs time to readjust on both the physical metabolic and mental levels of experience.

Perspectives on Dietary Change

Changing one's dietary pattern is not a search for a perfect diet because the only thing which is perfect is beyond the body-mind complex. The only thing that is perfect is the Truth of God, in all, as All. We are already imbedded in this perfection except that most of us are not aware of this reality. A healthy diet is an aid in clearing our consciousness and body so that we can be more receptive to the experience of this absolute level of truth. However, it must be remembered that despite all the emphasis and importance I have placed on right diet, **one cannot eat one's way to God**. Diet is not the key to spiritual life, but it is a positive helping factor that assists in opening the door to communion with the Divine.

Besides enhancing our communion with the Divine, an appropriate diet can help us reach stages of health in which we can fully enjoy life and live more youthfully, longer. Diet is not religion or an obsessive form of searching for God. Diet is simply one part of a balanced, harmonious life which is in attunement with universal laws. As has been mentioned, an appropriate diet can also help bring one into harmony with the social, ecological, and political issues of the planet. Interestingly enough, although coming from a different perspective, this intuitive, individualized dietary approach of conscious eating yields about the same results in terms of total daily calories and body weight as Walford's scientifically approached, calorie-counting diet. With the harmony of whole-ness approach, however, you never have to look at a calorie counter.

This conscious eating approach is the reflection of, and contributor to, our state of internal balance and external harmony with ourselves, our society and our planet. It is part of the unfolding process of being in harmony with the primary natural laws of the universe. A healthy diet is most appropriately developed, not as a mechanical process separate from our life, but in a full spiritual context of right livelihood, good company, loving our neighbors as our true selves, meditation and/or prayer, and starting each thought, word, and action with love. It is through this perspective that we are best able to develop an individualized diet that best reflects the highest state of awareness and is completely appropriate to maximal function in the world.

Transitioning

In the western, industrialized, mechanized, left-brained lifestyle of today's world, our relationship with nature has become confused, exploitive, and very fragile. How else could the FDA have approved such an obvious health-destroying process as the irradiation of fresh fruits, vegetables, wheat, spices, herbs, pork, and poultry products as a way of preserving them? This decision of the FDA reflects the extent to which many of us have broken our ties to nature.

What seems normal is abnormal and vice versa. According to an article in the *East West Journal* by Becky Gillette and Kate Dumont on Roy Walford's research, fully two thirds of Americans die from diseases caused by a poor diet. Approximately 1.5 million people died of diet-related disease in 1987. One has the choice to avoid these diet-related diseases by adopting the type of diet that both cures and prevents the chronic degenerative diseases from which so many suffer.

Vegetarians are sometimes considered the eccentric "odd bird," eating a "bird seed and grass diet." It is difficult to change a dietary pattern, even if it is unhealthy, when it means swimming upstream against social pressure and our old, programmed habits and belief systems. Nevertheless, it is necessary to examine one's programming and be willing to abandon what is no longer appropriate for maintaining one's state of total well-being of body, mind, and spirit. In this unfolding process, one learns to abandon what does not keep one in health and harmony. This gentle approach also helps to guide the rate of transitioning so it is in harmony with the body's physiological changes, the clearing of mind, and the subtle opening of spirit in one's life.

Planning one's own individualized diet and rate of transition requires some artful intelligence in the application of the principles and concepts I have shared. The process is real and basic rather than esoteric. It is a self-discovery process of trial and error to see what works to maintain the experience of the One. The hunger for the Divine can serve as a guiding light behind the appetite and guide one's choice of diet.

The place to start is with one's immediate dietary pattern. This involves learning to eat, by trial and error, the right amount of food that energizes the mind, body, and spirit. This will hopefully maintain and enhance the present flow of cosmic energy into the body, thus sustaining the present level of love communion.

One aid to the digestive system is to limit one's food intake to a maximum of three meals per day, with only juices or an occasional piece of fruit between meals. The exception to this is if one has hypoglycemia, which requires frequent snacks until the condition is stabilized or cured.

Chewing food well and creating a peaceful, joyful atmosphere in which to eat or digest the food will immediately improve digestion. There are several major stages of dietary transition. Each stage may take as little as one season in a yearly cycle. The concept of "transitioning" allows one to be receptive to the continued progress of one's evolutionary growth no matter what the time frame.

Four Transition Stages

More detail will be provided about these stages in this section, but for now it is sufficient to foreshadow this material by way of a brief description of these four dietary stages. Stage one is a transition from all bioacidic foods to natural, whole, organic foods. This means letting go of all processed, irradiated, chemicalized, pesticide-ridden and fungicide-containing, adulterated, fast, and junk foods and other sorts of "Hostess Twinkie" type foods. In this stage we also begin to give up red meats.

The second stage is letting go of all flesh foods, such as poultry and fish. It also includes not eating eggs.

Stage three is a vegetarian diet with the inclusion of dairy at the beginning and the moving to an 80% live food intake by the end.

Stage four is vegetarian without dairy and may be as much as 95-100% live foods by the end of stage four. Not eating flesh or any dairy products is not technically defined as a vegan because to be a true vegan means the absolute avoidance of any animal products in the total lifestyle. This includes the avoidance of leather clothing, honey, and gelatin capsules.

Preview of Chapter 18
Stage One: I Have No Beef With This

The first conscious eating stage is not becoming vegetarian. It is simply becoming conscious of what you are eating, from pesticides to nitrates. It is learning to read labels and ask the right questions to protect yourself. In this stage junk foods and commercially produced foods are given up for the most healthy and cost-effective organic foods. One also gets a chance to look at the viral, bacterial, and parasitic dangers of eating beef and chicken. In this stage, we let go of red meat. The time for action has begun. Are you ready to make this first step in the commitment?

   I.   Biocidic food

  II.   Protecting yourself from chemicalization

      A.   Major source of pesticide exposure comes from animal foods

      B.   Avoid commercial foods to be safe

 III.   Learning to read labels is good for your health

 IV.   Au natural—buy organic

  V.   Dangers of eating flesh

      A.   Chemicals in factory-farmed animals

      B.   Estrogen-injected animals—problems manifested in people who eat that flesh

      C.   Leukemia in children linked to diseased milk

      D.   Detrimental effects of fats in the diet

      E.   Unhealthy chickens and chicken processing

Chapter 18

Stage One: I Have No Beef with This

The first stage in the transition process is mental acceptance and an understanding that a dietary reorientation is necessary. This means significantly dropping one's intake of tamasic, health-destroying, biocidic foods. Giving up biocidic foods—processed, commercially grown, fast food and junk foods—means no longer offering oneself up as a sacrificial guinea pig to the pesticide, herbicide, additive, fungicide, food processing, food irradiating, microwaving, fast food, and junk food industries for experimentation. Stage one eliminates such deleterious foods as white sugar, white bread, candy, T.V. dinners, soft drinks, any meats that have been treated with nitrites and nitrates, pasteurized milk and cheeses, baked goods containing refined oils, foods containing additives, and prepared foods that have been stored in the refrigerator for more than two or three days.

Actually, almost all cooked foods become biocidic approximately twenty-four hours after preparation. Whether it takes one to four days to become contaminated with bacteria or mold is not the point, for all stored foods have lost their vital energy even if kept in the refrigerator. This is significantly less so if the food is quick frozen. As early as 1930 Dr. Kouchakoff found that the intake of processed foods so disturbed the white blood cell pattern of the immune system that it looked the same as a white blood cell pattern that is seen with infections. Eating highly processed, nitrate-, pesticide-, and additive-filled meats, like hot dogs and salami, gave the white blood cell pattern that one typically sees with severe food poisoning. Pesticides, herbicides, and additives in the foods have been linked with cancer, weakened immune system, allergies, neurotoxicity, hyperactivity in children, and brain allergies.

Another category of common pathological effects from these toxins is varying levels of neurotoxicity to the brain and rest of the nervous system which has more subtle symptoms, such as reduced mental functioning, decreased mental clarity, and poor concentration. Although the hard statistics of cancer are mentioned frequently in the discussion of pesticides, increased cancer rates is just one of the most extreme results of toxins in our food and water.

Unless one eats organic fruits and vegetables, one is continually exposed to pesticides. One of the most significant effects of an organic vegetarian diet is the tremendous health benefits of stopping the chronic poisoning from pesticides. In 1985, nearly one thousand people in the Western United States and Canada were poisoned by the pesticide Temik in watermelon. People had a variety of illnesses, including grand mal seizures, cardiac irregularities, and even several stillbirths. Recently the dangers of alar in apples were exposed. In 1987, the National Academy of Sciences concluded that in our lifetime pesti-

267

cides in American food may cause more than one million additional cases of cancer in the United States. Laurie Mott and Karen Snyder of the National Research Defense Council (NRDC) reported in the *Amicus Journal* that each year 2.6 billion pounds of pesticides are used in the United States and nearly all Americans have residues of the pesticides DDT, chlordane, heptachlor, aldrin and dieidrin in their bodies. A 1987 Environmental Protection Agency Report indicated that because of the massive agricultural use of pesticides, at least twenty pesticides, some of which are cancer-causing have been found in the ground water of twenty-four states. Between 1982 and 1985, the FDA detected pesticide residues in 48% of the most frequently consumed fresh vegetables and fruits. In 1975, the sixth annual report of the Council on Environment stated that dieldrin, which is five times more potent than the outlawed DDT, was found in 99.5% of the American people, 96% of all meat, fish, and poultry, and in 85% of all dairy products. Dieldrin is one of the most potent carcinogens known. It has caused cancer in laboratory animals at every dosage ever tested, no matter how infinitesimal the dose. Low level exposure in humans has been known to cause convulsions, liver damage, and destruction of the central nervous system. Fortunately dieldrin was banned in 1974, but who knows how lethal the next new line of pesticides may be. It's a form of American roulette. The drug companies are the only winners.

Dioxin (2, 4, 5-T), an active component of agent orange, is considered by Dr. Diane Courtney, head of the Toxic Effects Branch of the EPA's National Environmental Research Center, to be the most toxic chemical known. According to *A Diet for A New America,* millions of pounds of 2, 4, 5-T have been sprayed on American soil. The EPA has officially recognized that cattle which graze on land sprayed with dioxin accumulate it in their fat. According to pesticide authority Lewis Regenstein, those who eat beef get a concentrated dose of dioxin that has been concentrated as it moves up the food chain. Dioxin has been shown to produce cancer, birth defects, miscarriages, and death in lab animals in concentrations as low as one part per trillion. It is no wonder, according to David Steinman in *Diet for a Poisoned Planet,* that deaths from cancer in this country have risen from less than one percent in the beginning of the nineteenth century to one in four American men and one in five American women. Although there are other factors besides herbicides and pesticides that play a role in increasing the incidence of cancer, such as nuclear radiation and cigarette smoking, I wonder how much the cancer rate would drop if we stopped actively putting these and all the other pesticides in our food chain. Even if their toxicity is discovered and they are banned, once they have been introduced into the environment, the chlorinated hydrocarbon pesticides are extremely stable compounds that do not breakdown for decades or longer.

I do not feel scientists have discovered the full extent of the damage pesticides have already done to the nation's health. There are some indications suggested by the types of cancers that are statistically emerging that they are originating from the specific effects of certain pesticides. According to *Diet for a Poisoned Planet,* between 1950 and 1985, urinary bladder cancer has increased by 51%; kidney and renal pelvis cancer have increased by 82%. These types of cancers are directly associated with toxins in the drinking water. Testicular cancer, which occurs in significant proportion among farm workers and manufacturers of pesticides, has increased 81%. In 1985, nonHodgkin's lymphoma, which is linked with pesticide exposure, increased by 123%. The Surgeon General's Report on Nutrition and Health in 1988 estimated that as many as 10,000 cancer deaths annually could be caused from the chemical additives in food. This estimate does not even include pesticides. It is extremely difficult to know the exact percentage of the cancer increase due to pesticides, additives, and other environmental factors in our food, water, and air, but it most likely is significant.

In addition to the single pesticide factor effect which can be directly tested in the laboratory, there is often a more powerful synergistic effect from the multiple use of different toxins working together in the environment. This synergistic effect is difficult to assess. The cumulative effect of widespread, chronic, low-level exposure to multiple pesticides is only partially understood. One National Cancer Institute study found that farmers exposed to herbicides had a six times greater risk than nonfarmers of getting one specific type of cancer. Research at the University of Southern California discovered in 1987 that children living in homes where household and garden pesticides were used had a sevenfold greater chance of developing childhood leukemia. *The Amicus Journal* article entitled *Pesticide Alert* reported that in 1982 a congressional report estimated that between 82-85% of pesticides registered for use have not been adequately tested for their ability to cause cancer. In addition, 60-70% of pesticides were not tested for creating birth defects, and 90-93% were not tested for the possibility of causing genetic mutations.

In addition to the absence of single factor data, there is almost no data to show how these pesticides work when combined. In the *Journal of Food Science,* one of the few studies on the synergistic effect of pesticides reported that when three chemicals were each tested separately on rats, there was no obvious ill effect. When two of the three chemicals were added together, the health of the rats diminished. When all three were used synergistically, the rats all died within two weeks. This synergistic pesticide porridge of our food and water is probably creating the most overall damage to the health of all living forms in our environment. People who do not use purified water or organic food are exposing themselves significantly to this danger. The lack of available data on the health-destroying effects of pesticide use, both individually and synergistically, suggests the EPA has to be regulating more out of ignorance than from knowledge. Over 110 different pesticides were detected in all foods between 1982 and 1985.

Of the 25 pesticides detected most frequently in our foods, nine are known to cause cancer. This is a serious situation.

You Can Protect Yourself Against Food Chemicalization

Since there is very little real control and monitoring by the U.S. government or by the chemical companies, the responsibility for our health lies with us, as it always has. One has to avoid excess exposure to these poisons the best one can. According to the Pesticide Monitoring Journal published by the EPA, **the major source of pesticide exposure comes from foods of animal origin.** *A Diet for New America* points out that 95–99% of all the toxic chemical residues comes from meat, fish, dairy, and eggs. One can substantially avoid this high toxic exposure by choosing to eat vegetarian foods, such as fruits, vegetables, nuts, seeds, and grains, which are lower on the food chain and thus have less accumulation of these poisons. *The New England Journal of Medicine* has published a study that found that the **breast milk of vegetarian women has only one or two percent of the pesticide contamination as that of the national average for breast-feeding women on a flesh-centered diet**. This is a significant indication of how much effect one can have on one's pesticide exposure by becoming vegetarian. It is possible to further decrease exposure by only eating organically grown vegetarian foods. Sometimes, one is in places where it is not possible to obtain organic, vegetarian foods. It is still a safer choice to eat commercially grown fruits, vegetables, grains, nuts, and seeds rather than flesh foods. The body can detox a little pesticide exposure, but becomes overwhelmed if the exposure is chronic or too high.

David Steinman, in his book, *Diet for a Poisoned Planet,* has done an enormous amount of work in studying exactly which fruits, vegetables, nuts, seeds, and grains have the lowest toxic residues. He analyzed foods for more than one hundred different industrial chemicals and pesticides, using laboratory detection limits that were five to ten times more sensitive than the normal FDA detection standards. He did this by taking his food samples from four different geographic regions, analyzing them exactly as they would be eaten, and repeating this for four years ending in 1986. This gave him a total of sixteen samples per food to analyze and average. Each of the foods was rated according to which toxins were in each food and how many toxic residues were present. The combination of these two figures were factored into a cancer risk assessment. These findings were placed into three categories according to their safety. Safety was determined by the amount of pesticide residues and their cancer risk assessment. What I label as "relatively safe" are commercial foods which have minimal toxic effects. The next category, "marginally safe if eaten sparingly," is for foods to be avoided regularly. The third category is for commercial foods so potentially toxic that it is best to completely avoid them. I've turned his data for fruits, vegetables, nuts, seeds, and grains into several graphs shown on the following pages. Using these charts will minimize one's toxic exposure if, and when, organic produce is not available (see figs. 18, 19, 20, 21).

The best way to be safe, of course, is to avoid commercial foods. If enough people care about themselves and their children to only buy organic foods, the law of consumer demand on the market will force a shift that will increase the amount of organic farming and make more organic foods available at lower prices. Fortunately, a subtle shift toward organic farming and produce is happening in many parts of the U.S.

Learning to Read Labels is Good for Your Health

When one does decide that food quality and health are important, one enters into a whole new world of organic food and the healing lifestyle which goes along with it. There is great delight in learning to eat whole, natural, organic foods. Part of this dietary shift requires learning to read labels. One has to be clever at this. The *U.S. News and World Report* 6/18/90 issue points out that the FDA found 47% of domestic, and 76% of foreign, foods did not live up to the nutrient billing that was on the product label. I want to caution that shopping in a health food store does not mean one should not read labels. Not everything in a health food store is necessarily healthy.

The word "natural" these days can mean almost anything. The safest thing is to look for the words "certified organic." By insisting on organic foods whenever possible, we are not only protecting ourselves and our families but are also encouraging support for organic farming, and, therefore, are directly supporting the regeneration of our degenerating soils. A Harris poll showed that 80% of Americans want organic fruit and vegetables and over half are willing to pay for the small added cost of buying organic. Not only is organic food safer, but because it is grown in organically prepared soils, some initial research has suggested the organic food usually contains greater concentration of nutrients, such as vitamins, minerals, and enzymes, than pesticide-grown foods. For example, in the Firman Bear Report on research done at Rutgers University, organically grown foods were much richer in minerals than the "look alike" commercial produce. For example, organic tomatoes had more than five times more calcium, twelve times more magnesium, three times more potassium, 600% more organic sodium (organic sodium does not necessarily increase blood pressure like table salt), sixty-eight times more manganese, and 1900 times more iron. Organic spinach had more than double the calcium, five and one half times the magnesium, more than three times the potassium, seventy times the sodium, one hundred and seventeen times as much manganese, and eighty-three times the iron. Organic lettuce had three and one half times the calcium, three times the magnesium, three times the potassium, thirty times the sodium, one hundred and

Figure 18 - Commercial Vegetables

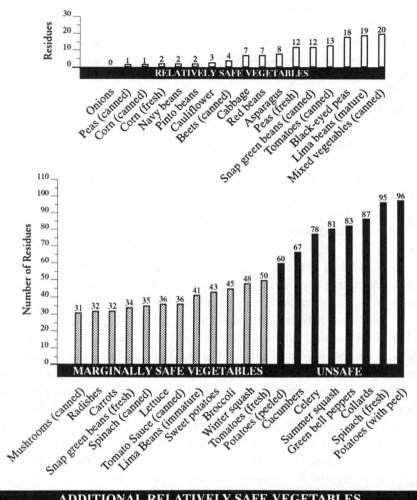

Alfalfa Sprouts	Asparagus	Adzuki beans	Bamboo shoots (canned)	
Bean sprouts	Beets (fresh)	Brussels Sprouts	Cassava	Chives
Cilantro	Daikon	Fava beans	Fennel root	Garlic
Jicama	Kidney beans	Leeks	Mushrooms (fresh)	Radicchio
Rapini	Red chard	Rhubarb	Shallots	Snow Peas
Watercress	Yams			

ADDITIONAL MARGINALLY SAFE VEGETABLES IF EATEN SPARINGLY

Artichokes	Bok choy	Cherry Tomatoes	Chili Peppers	Choysum
Dandelion greens	Dill	Eggplant	Endive	Escarole
Green peppers	Jalapeno peppers	Kale	Kohirabi	Lentils
Mung beans	Mustard greens	Okra	Parsley	Parsnips
Poblano peppers	Pumpkin	Pursiane	Red peppers	Rutabagas
Serrano chiles	Soybeans	String beans	Swiss Chard	Tomatillos
Turnips				

Figure 19 - Commercial Fruits

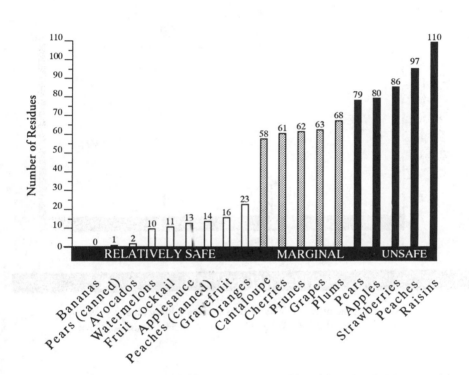

ADDITIONAL REALATIVELY SAFE FRUITS

Bitter Melon	Coconut	Dates	Figs	Guavas	Lemons
Limes	Papayas	Passion Fruit	Pineapples	Plantains	Tangerines

ADDITIONAL MARGINALLY SAFE FRUITS IF EATEN SPARINGLY °

Apricots	Blackberries	Blueberries	Casaba	Cranberries	Crenshaw Melon
Currants	Feiojas	Honeydew	Kiwi Fruit	Kumquats	Nectarines
Persimmons	Pomegranates				

Figure 20 - Commercial Nuts and Seeds

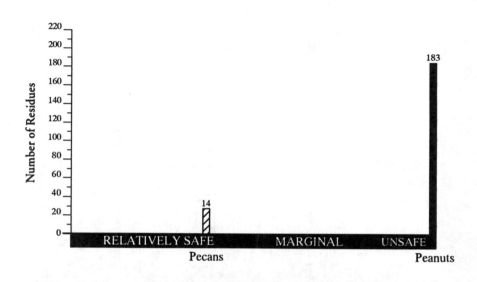

REALATIVELY SAFE

Almonds	Chinese pine nuts	Watermelon seeds	Pistachios	Walnuts
Sesame seeds	Sunflower seeds	Water Chestnuts	Hazelnuts	Flax
Pumpkin Seeds				

MARGINALLY SAFE IF EATEN SPARINGLY

Lycee nuts   Radish seeds

Figure 21 - Commercial Grains

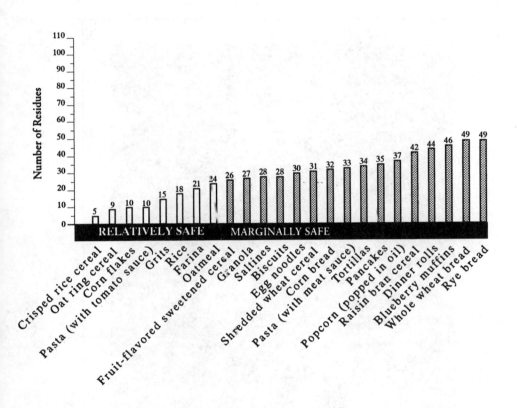

Data for graphs, Fig. 18-21, from *Diet for a Poisoned Planet* by David Steinman.

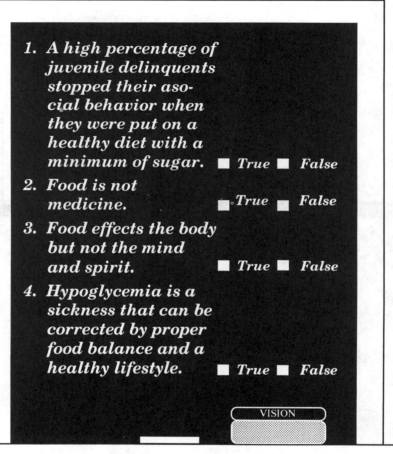

1. **A high percentage of juvenile delinquents stopped their asocial behavior when they were put on a healthy diet with a minimum of sugar.** ■ *True* ■ *False*

2. **Food is not medicine.** ■ *True* ■ *False*

3. **Food effects the body but not the mind and spirit.** ■ *True* ■ *False*

4. **Hypoglycemia is a sickness that can be corrected by proper food balance and a healthy lifestyle.** ■ *True* ■ *False*

VISION

BLACKBOARD QUIZ

1. T   2. T   3. F   4. T

SOME MARGINALLY SAFE
COMMERCIAL VEGETABLES

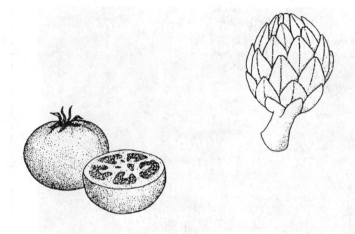

Marginally safe commercial vegetables, eat sparingly

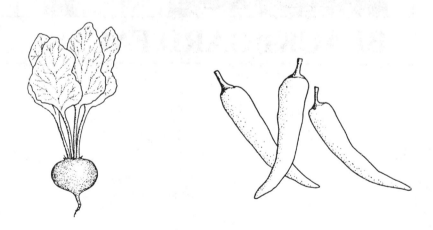

The average American meat eater consumes in a lifetime:

A. Eleven beef steers

B. One calf

C. Three lambs

D. Twenty-three hogs

E. Forty-five turkeys

F. Eight hundred and twenty-six fish

Do you want your body to be an animal GRAVEYARD?

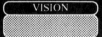

BLACKBOARD FACTS

Avoid eating when you are:

> *Sad*
> *Angry*
> *Under Stress*

Remember: food is love and life is love.

*Eating when calm and able to focus
on your food is a way to love yourself*

VISION

BLACKBOARD FOOD FOR THOUGHT

sixty-nine times the manganese, and fifty-seven times the iron. **The overall estimate of the Rutgers research suggested that organic foods had 87% more minerals and trace elements than food that was commercially grown.** Although organic foods may cost a little more, mineral for mineral, they are more than worth their price. Dr. Paavo Airola, the world famous nutritionist, mentions that research shows certain antimalignancy factors are present in organically grown foods.

Au Natural

Dr. Paavo Airola, in his popular book, *How to Get Well,* points out that it has been scientifically proven that one's health and longevity is directly related to the naturalness of the food one eats. He points out that in areas where indigenous people have been found to be eating whole, natural, unprocessed foods, they experience good health and longevity. When denatured, refined, processed, and canned foods, such as white flour and white sugar, are introduced into these cultures, acute and chronic degenerative diseases become rampant. Knowing this, one can make a choice to reverse this process of chronic, degenerative disease by starting to eat whole organic foods.

Part of making this shift involves buying one's food in different places. It means getting familiar with health food stores which have organic produce sections, finding supermarkets which have added organic produce sections, or even asking your local supermarket to add an organic produce section. In certain parts of the country, farmers' markets are frequented by organic farmers selling their produce at prices extremely competitive to commercially grown produce. If one can find organic produce at local farmers' markets, it is worth talking to the organic farmer about how his or her soil is prepared. This way one develops a feeling for the meaning of organic produce and also gets to know the person who is producing the food. This is a way to personalize the process of food "gathering." The food and the food provider are no longer anonymous with this approach.

Shifting to a More Healthy Diet

Stage One is also a time to begin thinking about the acid-base ratio of the foods one eats and its effect on the body, the practice of food combining, doing regular exercise, and cultivating healthy eating patterns. Eating more fruits, vegetables, grains, legumes, nuts, seeds, and raw dairy as the central focus of one's diet is a big departure from the traditional concept of the typical American diet, but most everyone finds this new world of health-giving foods exciting and rewarding. After an initial adjustment phase, these foods generally taste better in the long run. Stage One can be considered the first major step in one's gradual re-education to healthful eating patterns.

Dangers of Eating Flesh

Stage One includes dropping red meat from the diet. If one is not ready to completely let go of red meat, one may consider eating organically raised flesh foods until one is ready. Letting go is much easier to do if one is well-informed about the health dangers of red meat, not to mention the moral issues connected to eating meat, which have already been addressed in a previous chapter. The first thing to keep in mind is that farm animals, primarily cattle, chickens, eggs, and milk, are not of the same quality or as safe as they were one hundred years ago. In the olden days, the animals were a lot healthier because their food was largely unadulterated since most of them were "free range" animals.

The livestock industry has depersonalized today's farm animals into "products" that are mass produced in an assembly line fashion. Farm animals have a considerably higher percentage of fat nowadays because of a lack of exercise and the chemicals and hormones added to make the animals grow bigger and faster in as cheap a way as possible. In 1975, the World Conference on Animal Products reported that **factory-farmed animals have about thirty times more saturated fat than those who were pasture-raised.** Since World War II, these farm animals have been inundated with an insidious brew of pesticides, hormones, growth stimulants, insecticides, tranquilizers, radioactive isotopes, herbicides, antibiotics, and other assorted drugs and colorants. All these substances are considered legal. Other illegal hormones are also still being added to increase weight.

There are so many problems associated with eating flesh and animal by-products, such as milk and eggs, that it would literally take another book in itself to describe these hazards. A few outstanding pieces of information must be mentioned, however. For example, Dr. Saenz, a pediatrician, reported an epidemic of premature sexual development that was connected to the eating of animal products. This was reported in the February 1982 issue of *Journal of the Puerto Rico Medical Association.* The segments of the population primarily afflicted were female children from age one and up. What happened was that infants and young children began to develop mature breasts and uteruses, vaginal bleeding, and other signs of puberty. One fourteen year old boy was reported to have mature female breasts that needed to be surgically removed. Dr. Saenz's findings showed that the appearance of abnormal breast tissue in infants was related to local, whole milk consumption. In the older children, it was related to consumption of whole milk, beef, and chicken flesh from animals which had been given estrogen to increase their weight. The doctor consistently found that when these foods were removed from the diet, the symptoms usually disappeared within a short time. According to *A New Diet for America,* one English medical journal reported that hormone traces in chemically fattened livestock were causing British school girls to mature sexually at least three years earlier than the previous national average. There is reason to believe that to some extent this high estrogen intake from beef and dairy products happens in the U.S. as well.

Modern science has found a variety of diseases and parasites that can be transferred from animals to man, such as trichinosis, toxoplasma gondii, fungi, and even viral infections and salmonella, which is the main cause of acute dysentery. There is also the problem of severe infections from antibiotic-resistant bacteria growing in the meat from the heavy use of antibiotics in livestock.

Dr. Rudolph Ballentine points out in his book, *Transition to Vegetarianism,* that over 40% of adults have been exposed to toxoplasmosis. In children, toxoplasmosis has been known to cause blindness and mental retardation in newborns. Most toxoplasmosis infections come from meat and some may also come from cats. In the *Cancer Journal for Clinicians,* an article by Kin Shim, M.D., reported that one hundred percent of monkeys fed milk from leukemic cows developed leukemia within a year. In Denmark it was found that child leukemia was connected to the consumption of cow's milk that was taken from Danish cows that had leukemia. Twenty percent of the cows in Denmark have leukemia. The hypothesis is that a leukemia-inducing virus is transferred from cows, through their milk, to the children. The monkey leukemia infection suggests the same route of infection as the children of Denmark. All this animal, food-related disease brings up the question as to how long must people experiment with themselves as human "guinea pigs" before waking up to the dangers of eating flesh foods and dairy products?

To eat animals and fish in today's world is to take on the psychology of victim consciousness. Once informed of the dangers, it is hard to separate the eating of flesh food from a passive form of a death wish.

What if it were possible to consistently get organically grown beef and poultry? Would it be worthwhile to eat beef and chicken for our nutritional well-being? Nutritionally, meat is relatively high in iron, B_{12}, and protein. However, it is not a balanced food and is almost totally lacking in vitamins A, C, and E. Flesh foods are also low in minerals, such as calcium, and high in phosphorous. The phosphorous to calcium ratio is 20/1. The U.S. Army Medical Research and Nutrition Laboratory in Denver, Colorado has found that the more meat one eats, the more B_6–deficient one becomes. A high-protein diet seems to cause severe deficiencies in B_6, calcium, magnesium, and niacin. High flesh food intake also increases the ammonia, which has been found by Dr. Willard J. Visek of Cornell University to be implicated as a carcinogenic agent. High ammonia in the system is also toxic to the nervous system.

DANGERS OF A HIGH-FAT DIET

1. *Clogged arteries, high blood pressure, fatigued hearts, and heart attacks.*

2. *Clumps red blood cells causing slower blood flow to brain and all tissues.*

3. *Makes diabetes worse.*

4. *Impairs function of liver.*

5. *Slow digestion.*

6. *Slows the mind because of sluggish circulation.*

VISION

BLACKBOARD FATS

A most significant problem associated with flesh eating is the fat associated with a high meat diet. By eliminating the high fat intake associated with the high flesh diet, it is estimated that 90% of the deaths from colon cancer in the U.S. would dramatically be reduced. The rate of cancer for meat eaters is 4.3 times greater for cancer of the colon. Heart disease, according to the 1961 Journal of the American Medical Association, would be drastically reduced by 97%. Cancer and heart diseases are the two leading causes of death in this country. In beef, pork, and lamb, the percentage of calories that come from fat is 75% to 85%. Chicken is right up there with 60% of the calories coming from fat. Turkey has 55% of the calories in the form of fat. It is significant that these fatty foods are consumed in heated, cooked form.

Cooked fats, especially of animal origin, are positively harmful to health. The average American diet contains around 40-45% of calories in the form of cooked fats. This high percentage of cooked fat in the diet is associated with the increased diseases of heart, cancer, and other chronic, degenerative diseases.

Although nuts and seeds have oil contents as high as the fat contents in some flesh food, because these plant-based foods do not contain cholesterol or store ingested estrogen and other chemicals in their oil as do animals, these foods are much safer and healthier. Nuts and seeds can be eaten raw, preferably soaked. When they are eaten in this form, the naturally occurring, fat digestive enzyme— lipase—helps to digest the oils in the nuts and seeds.

There seems to be a dramatically different effect of raw versus cooked fat in the diet. It actually holds true for raw meat as well. Raw meat, like live fruits, vegetables, nuts, seeds, and grains, possesses viable fat digestive enzymes which are not destroyed unless heated. I am not suggesting that we start a raw, flesh food fad, however. **The real issue associated with fats and their linkage to cardiovascular disease may not simply be the amount of fat in the diet, but whether the fat is raw or cooked.** The well-respected, nutritionally oriented physician, Henry Bieler, M.D., in his book, *Food Is Your Best Medicine,* makes exactly the same point in his discussion of cardiovascular disease. In his book he says:

> "Overeating of fats and oils, as long as they are in their natural state, cannot cause arterial disease....It is only when unnatural fats, or fats which have been altered by being overheated, are consumed as food that the trouble arises."

The Fat of the Land is not so Dangerous if it's Raw

To complete the discussion of fats, oils, and raw foods, one needs to be familiar with the terms "cis isomer" and "trans isomer." Isomers are two compounds that have the same atoms but which have different chemical and physical properties because they are structurally organized in a different way. The cis form is the biologically active form of fatty acids and it is organized in a curved structure. The trans form is the biologically inactive form and it is organized with a straight structure. The cis form of the essential fatty acids can be biologically processed by the body to form the biologically active fatty acids and prostaglandins. The trans form cannot be biologically processed in an effective way by the body and essentially clogs the metabolic pathways. The cis form of fatty acids are found in the live, whole foods and to a lesser extent in low heat-processed, extracted oils.

Dr. Douglass of the Kaiser Permanente Hospital in Los Angeles reports that not only does cooking fats change the molecular configuration of fatty acids from what is called a "cis" to a "trans" configuration, but also pressing and hydrogenating changes fats from the curved cis formation to a straight trans formation. This trans configuration of the fatty acids goes into the molecular configuration of our cell membranes just as the normal cis formation does. The result is that the trans fats partially blocks respiration function of the cell membrane. This seems to be associated with a less efficient cell function and even cancer. Many studies, for example, have shown that fried fats are highly carcinogenic. This is one reason why no margarine exists that is healthy to eat because every brand contains processed fats which have a high percentage of trans fatty acids.

Another major difference between processed and raw fats is the enzyme content. Studies on the Eskimos who eat raw blubber by the pound show no significant incidence of hardening of the arteries or other forms of circulatory disease, including hypertension. On the other hand, Eskimos of the same genetic background who had taken up modern civilization's habit of cooking their food, and who kept the same high-fat diet, had a high percentage of cardiovascular diseases. In addition to the difference between cis and trans structures, another major difference is the active lipase found in the raw blubber. Lipase is the enzyme needed to digest fat. In the raw form, the fat contains a significant amount of lipase to help with its own digestion. All throughout nature, when the raw fats of an animal, or raw oils of plants, are eaten along with their associated enzymes, no harmful effect on the arteries or heart seems to result (fats that come from animal sources are opaque; oils that come from plant sources, with the exception of coconut oil, are translucent). This doesn't contradict the studies on high fat intake and their association with cardiovascular disease because the studies were all done primarily with cooked fats in which the lipase is destroyed

HOW TO AVOID
DANGERS OF FATS

1. *Eat primarily low-fat foods like vegetables, fruits, and grains.*

2. *Meet your daily oil and fatty acid needs with unprocessed, un-cooked, whole foods, such as raw seeds, nuts, and avocados.*

3. *Avoid pressed and extracted oils and fatty foods which have been cooked, fried, hydrogenated, or irradiated.*

4. *Avoid cooked foods with high fat content, such as flesh foods, eggs, fried foods, dairy, mayonaise, ice cream, pizza, cookies, and candies.*

5. *Avoid a high-salt diet because it creates a craving for fats.*

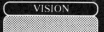

VISION

BLACKBOARD FATS

and the fat molecular structure is changed. The nutritionists who are strongly urging low-fat diets seem to have overlooked this major difference between cooked and raw fats. What this means is that vegetarians who have raw avocados and raw, soaked, or sprouted nuts or seeds do not have to be as concerned about atherosclerosis; however, beware that an excess of even raw oils in the diet may cause some problems, such as red blood cell clumping, decreased blood flow in smaller vessels, and less oxygen getting to the tissues.

All types of processing of oils tends to destroy the lipase, not just cooking them. For example, olives and coconuts have plenty of lipase, but their oils have none. In general, oils as they occur naturally in plants, as in sunflower seeds and avocados, have all their nutrients and enzymes intact, whereas the extracted oils, even if cold pressed, are missing many nutrients and their associated enzymes. The usual form of heat-processed, polyunsaturated oils containing the omega-6 and omega-3 fatty acids, such as safflower and other vegetable cooking oils, may have 20-50% of their fatty acids in the trans form. Other foods high in processed, polyunsaturated, fatty acids are bakery goods, processed meats, soups, candies, cookies, and fried foods. These heat-processed polyunsaturated fatty acids may actually lead to a deficiency of essential fatty acids because we fill ourselves up with these trans fatty acids instead of the raw, active, cis essential fatty acids. Research reported in the March 1971 issue of *Lancet* has also shown that these heat-processed, polyunsaturated, fatty acids, although linked to decreased heart disease to some extent, have been associated with the near doubling of cancer rates as compared to control people in the study who were on a low intake of polyunsaturated fatty acids. The fact that cancer rates increased may be because of the effect of the high amount of trans fatty acids produced in the processing and because of the increase in free radical production from the heating of the polyunsaturated fatty acids from the cooking and processing of the oils.

Until some research is done to prove otherwise, the main danger of fats and oils, however, is from being cooked, irradiated, hydrogenated, fried, or even cold pressed. Oils in small to moderate amounts seem to be quite safe if they are ingested in their natural form in whole, uncooked foods. This is not an invitation to push the raw oil and fat intake up to 40% of the diet, as we see in the typical American diet. Although there is not enough research to document exactly how much uncooked food is safe that is high in fat or oil, my general feeling is 10-20% of calories from fat in the diet is healthy and safe. The percentage varies with each person according to their constitution. A diet that is approximately 10% calories from natural, whole, uncooked, high-fat or high-oil foods will be healthier for kapha and pitta constitutions; a diet that will be healthier for vata constitutions will be closer to 20%. Aside from nuts and seeds and a few high-fat fruits or vegetables, like avocados, a vegetarian diet of fruits, vegetables, grains, beans, and legumes has a minimum of oil. In other words, a normal vegetarian diet is a low-oil diet.

A High Flesh Food Diet is an Unhealthy, Low-fiber Diet

Another problem associated with a high flesh food diet is the low fiber content. Red meat, poultry, fish, eggs, and cheese are essentially devoid of fiber. The lack of fiber is associated with a sluggish digestive tract. A sluggish colon produces such symptoms as constipation and accumulation of toxins in the colon. One of the beneficial functions of fiber is to help remove toxins from the colon. For example, fiber removes toxins secreted by the liver and bile and also removes the cancer-causing bile acid breakdown products. If these toxins and bile acid breakdown products are not removed, they often are reabsorbed into the system through the colon. Also, certain bacteria grow on the bile acids and produce a cancer co-factor that is associated with cancer of the colon. Dietary fiber is also important for removing other toxins and radioactive, breakdown products from the colon. Fiber is needed for normal bowel functioning. I often see people, who have had difficulties with constipation and gas, develop normal bowel functioning when they switched to a high-fiber, vegetarian diet.

Many people switch to poultry when they stop red meat. Unfortunately, poultry, which has a similar profile of dangers as red meat, has some outstanding problems of its own: high incidences of salmonella and campylobacter infections. According to *Advances in Meat Research,* by Pearson and Dutson, over 80% of chickens, and 90% of turkeys, are infected with campylobacter. These bacteria cause an intestinal infection similar to salmonella. These organisms have become antibiotic-resistant because of the high use of antibiotics in poultry. This means that when they cause an infection, antibiotics will not work effectively to kill them.

According to the Project Censored ratings, a news report in the June 8, 1990 *Pacific Sun,* the "fowl" play in the chicken industry was voted one of the ten most underreported stories of 1989. In their article it is pointed out that the incidence of bacterial salmonella infection is now two and one half million cases per year, including an estimated one half million hospitalizations and nine thousand deaths. They point out that the epidemic is caused by a huge leap in consumer demand for "healthier food" called chicken, as they switch from red meat, and by a massive failure of the U.S. Department of Agriculture to be able to inspect the chicken. The new decrease in USDA staff has lead to an increase in contaminated chicken slipping through en mass. The article states:

> "The USDA has placed gag orders on inspectors and destroyed documents disclosing that the agency has approved massive amounts of contaminated food."

The words "all natural ingredients"
should not let you forget to pay atten-
tion. Take the time to read the labels.

VISION

BLACKBOARD FOOD FOR THOUGHT

In the *Pacific Sun* article, Dr. Carl Telleen, a retired USDA veterinarian, revealed how:

> "...chicken carcasses contaminated with feces, once routinely condemned or trimmed, are now simply rinsed with chlorinated water to remove stains."

According to Telleen,

> "Thousands of dirty chickens are bathed together in a chill tank, creating a mixture known as "fecal soup" that spreads contamination from bird to bird."

This creates what Telleen calls, "instant sewage." Reading about articles like this makes it easier for many of the readers still eating poultry to make the transition away from poultry a little faster.

In addition to these two potent bacteria, there may be a virus-bacteria type of organism that has been found in chicken tumors that seems to be transmittable to humans. This organism is thought to be identical to the microbe found by Dr. Peyton Rous in chicken tumors. He showed this virus is transmittable. For this pioneering work he received a Nobel Prize in 1966. The extent to which this microbe might be associated with human cancer is still debatable. As discussed earlier, the work by Virginia Livingston Wheeler, M.D., strongly suggests that most chickens are at least microscopically infected with cancer and that this chicken cancer, as with the Rous virus, may be transmittable to humans.

As the awareness of moral and health consciousness continues to awaken in our world, it will become easier and easier to give up flesh foods. In making the transition through stage one, and for that matter, through any of the four stages, it is important to move slowly enough so that one can fully integrate each step of the way to facilitate a permanent change. Fasting from flesh foods for one week four times a year helps to support one's transition away from flesh foods.

1. *Eating additive-, nitrate-filled foods like hot dogs and processed deli meats can give the same white blood cell pattern that one sees with severe food poisoning.*

2. *Unless one eats organic fruits and vegetables, one is continually exposed to pesticides, herbicides, and other assorted toxins.*

3. *The Surgeon General's Report on Nutrition and Health in 1988 estimated that as many as 10,000 cancer deaths annually could be caused from chemical additives in food.*

4. *Forty-seven to seventy-six percent of food manufacturers do not live up to the nutrient information that was produced on the product labels (News & World Report 6/18/90).*

5. *Not everything in a health food store is necessarily healthy.*

VISION

BLACKBOARD FACTS

Preview of Chapter 19
Safe and Healthy Public Water, a Nostalgic Wish

Safe and healthy water is becoming increasingly difficult to get because of the high degree of water pollution throughout the world. In this chapter we discuss this issue and the ways we can create healthy water for ourselves. You will also get a chance to play biochemist again as we consider a new biological energy associated with water colloid systems. It is called zeta potential. Are you ready to consider the seriousness of our water problem? Are you ready to do something to protect you and your family?

I. How did all of this water pollution begin?
    A. The beginning of our tainted water supply
    B. Cancer increase with water consumption

II. Finding or making healthy water
    A. Bottled, mineral, filtered, distilled water advantages and disadvantages
    B. Charcoal filtering
    C. Reverse osmosis
    D. Water distillers

III. Structured water and zeta potential
    A. Liquid crystals in water—what they do
    B. Surface tension of water
    C. Our blood's colloid system and water

IV. Factors which decrease zeta potential

Chapter 19

Safe and Healthy Public Water, a Nostalgic Wish

Just as consuming organic foods is a way to avoid ingesting toxins into one's body, becoming aware of the quality of water one drinks and uses is becoming increasingly essential in today's polluted world, since water can be a major source of toxins. According to *Diet for a Poisoned Planet*, less than one percent of the earth's surface water is safe to drink. In some places of the United States and other countries, the term "drinking water" for tap water should be considered nothing more than a nostalgic euphemism. In order to best understand which water is safe to drink, bathe in, and prepare food with, one needs to know more about water pollution, how to purify water to make it safer for use, and also what form of water is healthiest to drink.

Second to oxygen, water is our most important nutrient. Without it, we would not be able to survive. Water comprises 90% of a baby's body and around 65-70% of an adult's. According to Patrick and Gael Crystal Flanagan, authors of the *Elixir of the Ageless,* our muscles are composed of 75% water, our brain is composed of 90% water, our liver is 69% water, and even our bones are 22% water. They point out that in a lifetime people drink an average of 7,000 gallons, or 58,333 pounds, of water. Water is a major component of all our foods. Cooked grains are 70% water.

In general, fruits contain the highest amount of structured water, approximately 85%, and vegetables contain slightly less, although some vegetables, like carrots, contain 88% water The water in the cell structure of raw plant foods is the most biologically active available. This biologically active water is termed "structured" water. Structured water either already contains, or has the capacity to contain, more energy than water, such as distilled or spring water. Researchers have found that in structured water the angle of the molecular bonding between the hydrogen and oxygen atoms is different than uncharged, unstructured water. One can unstructure water simply by heating it (more on structured water in a latter section of this chapter).

The problem of water pollution is very much in people's awareness nowadays. Since one can smell, taste, and see water of questionable quality, the water problem is more accepted as a problem because it is harder to ignore than invisible poisons in the food. Water that is visually oily, has a smell, or has an oily taste, may be polluted with industrial wastes. If water smells like rotten eggs it may be intermingling with sewage. A metallic taste in water may indicate high lead or manganese levels. If the water is cloudy, it may indicate too much potentially dangerous organic matter or that the water is inadequately purified. A blue-green color may suggest a high copper level. If there is too much chlorine, one's stainless steel sink may become pitted or turn black. Color, taste, odor, and stains on fixtures indicate a high level of contamination. Lower, yet still very toxic, levels of contaminants are often colorless, tasteless, and odorless. A complete water analysis for microbial, inorganic, and organic contamination may be the only way to find out the quality and safety of one's water.

Radiation is one of the more deadly contaminants in water. Naturally occurring forms of radiation that are found in water supplies around the country come from uranium, radium, and radon that comes in contact with the ground water. According to *Diet for a Poisoned Planet,* radium in the drinking water is one of the most important causes of birth defects and a cause for increased cancer. In Florida, elevated radium in the water has been associated with increased rates of leukemia. In Iowa, an increased rate of cancer of the lung and bladder among males, and breast and lung cancer among females, was discovered in population centers where the radium in the water supply was greater than five picocuries per liter of water (the federal standard for maximum allowable radium in the water). Childhood leukemia rates were found to be nearly double in North Carolina and Maine in areas where the drinking water had high radium concentrations. Maximum radon levels in the water should not be greater than ten picocuries per liter. Since radon will leave water as a gas, an aeration unit to remove the dissolved radon gas from the water before it enters the home is an effective solution to the problem of radon contamination. Reverse osmosis water purification systems can remove uranium and radium. Activated carbon filters will remove radon. We will discuss these and other water purification methods later in the chapter.

In addition to naturally occurring radiation, the public now has to contend with radiation spills from several food and medical supply irradiation plants that have been built in this country. For example, in Dover, New Jersey, in 1974, the International Neutronics irradiation facility had a cobalt-60 spill which they tried to "clean-up" from their radiation plant by dumping 5,700 liters of cobalt-60 contaminated water down the bathroom drains into the public sewer system.

The water that the general public uses comes from two sources: underground sources, such as springs and wells, and surface water, such as river and lakes. Presently, both these sources are becoming more and more polluted as toxic chemicals, acid rain, raw sewage, agricultural herbicides, pesticide runoff, chlorination, fluoridation, sewage landfills, and radioactive wastes are either dumped into, or seep into, these two types of water sources. One of the best-known examples of toxic water pollution to date is the infamous Love Canal, where, according to the New York Times in 1984, thousands of tons of toxic chemicals were dumped, including 60 pounds of the deadly poison, dioxin.

How did this all begin?

The tradition of putting additives in water by dumping questionably safe chemicals in the water started unwittingly with the addition of chlorine to water to protect us against waterborne diseases such as cholera, typhoid, dysentery, and hepatitis. Unfortunately, chlorine is a volatile chemical which likes to combine with the various industrial pollutants dumped into waterways. When chlorine combines with certain other chemicals it forms a class of toxic chemicals called tri-halo-methanes (THMs). Some examples of THMs are carbon-tetrachloride and chloroform. If this were not enough, the dumping and washing off of pesticides from the land brings many other chlorinated hydrocarbons into our waters, such as DDT, PCBs, and dioxin.

The pollution situation is so out of control that in monitoring cancer rates in Philadelphia, one can correlate the different rates and types of cancer in the population depending on which river the people lived near. According to Steve Meyerowitz, in his book, *Water,* the Environmental Cancer Prevention Center found that residents drinking from the west side of Schuylkill River had 67% more cancer deaths from esophagus cancer than those on the east side. Those drinking from the Delaware River on the east side suffered 59% more deaths from cancer of the brain, 83% more malignant melanoma, and 32% more colorectal cancers than those on the west side. This is just one of many studies that links specific water pollution to an increase in cancer rates.

The increase in specific cancers, and cancer in general, to epidemic proportions in the United States and other industrialized countries is not a question of just negative psychological "cancer-producing attitudes" held by isolated individuals. It is difficult to assess the precise degree to which our polluted waters are causing disease, genetic mutation, developmental abnormalities, and birth defects; however, no one today could coherently argue that this isn't a frightening and very real problem. An herbalist friend of mine once said, **"Pay attention to your elimination or it will eliminate you."**

Unfortunately, we are barely paying attention to our elimination. Even when the Environmental Protection Agency has set standards of quality to protect our drinking water (as it did in 1979 by limiting THMs in drinking water to 0.1 parts per million), according to *Water,* by Meyerowitz, the waterworks operators sued the EPA to rescind its protective standard. Meyerowitz points out that a congressional study in 1982 showed that many waterworks operators simply ignore the standards anyway. It seems that whenever the question of health versus profit comes into play, the choice by those in charge of disposal and storage of toxic wastes seems to be profits over health. For example, the New York Times, in October 1984, describes one congressional survey in 1983-84 on the disposal of toxic wastes that concluded that less than 20% of over 6,500 disposal and storage sites were actually in compliance with the law and that the

EPA had been deficient in upholding standards for protecting underground water supplies. Another New York Times article in November 1984 describes a General Accounting Office investigation in 1983 that found 146,000 violations of the 1980 Safe Drinking Water Act. It pointed out that the EPA only referred 21 cases for enforcement in the ten-year history of the Act. The Natural Resources Defense Council reported, in a letter from its executive director, John Adams, that one third of the United States' large waste water dischargers were in violation of the Clean Water Act.

The point of this information about unrestrained water pollution becomes obvious. Since governmental agencies are not able to, or are unwilling to, enforce the laws to protect the quality of our water, and business people are choosing not to act responsibly for the greater public health and well-being, it follows that **we need to take individual responsibility to protect ourselves from polluted and toxic water.** The best way to do this is to take control of our own drinking and cooking water, and if you can afford to, your own bathing water as well, since toxins can be absorb into the body through the skin.

The book *Diet for a Poison Planet* mentions a water testing company that I also recommend for a complete analysis of your water supply: **Watercheck National Testing Laboratories, Inc., 6555 Wilson Mills Road, Cleveland, Ohio, 44143, phone: 216-449-2525.** They can test for the following contaminants: microbiological; coliform; inorganic chemicals-metals; inorganic chemicals-other; organic chemicals-trihalomethanes; organic chemicals-volatiles; pesticides; herbicides; heavy metals; and PCBs.

When one asks oneself if it is worth it to pay attention to water, I cite a recent California Department of Health Study that showed that California women who drank bottled water or filtered water had significantly lower rates of spontaneous abortions and babies with significantly less birth defects than those who drank tap water. Though there might be other factors responsible, who wants to take a chance when life itself is at risk?

Finding Healthy Water

Alternative sources of water are: bottled, spring, and mineral water; filtered water; distilled water; and water purified by various types of purifiers, such as ozone purifiers, carbon block purifiers, and reverse osmosis systems. Each has its advantages and disadvantages. Bottled, spring, and mineral water that are packaged in plastic containers absorb chemicals from the plastic container into the water. The plastic taste in the water can be detected without much difficulty. If one is going to buy water from stores, it is much better to purchase water in glass bottles. Mineral water and spring water differ in that the mineral waters often come from therapeutic springs and generally have more minerals than spring water. Water that has 500 million parts per dissolved solids is defined as mineral water.

Some of the mineral waters are naturally carbonated and others are synthetically carbonated with carbon dioxide. In the human body, carbon dioxide is a waste product of cellular metabolism which, when combined with water in the system, makes carbonic acid. This carbonic acid makes our system more acidic. For some people it also creates gas and bloating. In other words, carbon dioxide in water is not particularly healthy, although it is considered fashionable.

Some mineral waters may be extremely high in a particular mineral or several minerals that could potentially create an imbalance in some people if consumed in sufficient quantity over time. One of the biggest problems with bottled water is that one really doesn't know what's in the bottle or if the bottle has been mislabeled to appear as if it is spring water. Some bottlers treat their water with ozone, deionization, or even chlorine in order to purify it. Some "spring water" is simply purified, city tap water. In India, I stopped drinking bottled water because, as a physician, I saw too many people who got sick after drinking bottled, "purified" water, which in some cases was just untreated water put into a clean bottle. Trying to stay with more well-known name brands is a good idea, but not a 100% guarantee of anything. A few years ago, Perrier caught some unscrupulous individuals bottling New York City tap water and selling it as Perrier water. It is best to read the label and choose a company that has a solid reputation. Brands labeled "drinking water" may be just tap water, although almost all bottled water is highly filtered. Look on the label to see if the water has been drawn from a spring or an artesian well.

Compressed, activated, charcoal block filters are an inexpensive way to get protection from the carbon-based, organic pollution, pesticides, herbicides, insecticides, PCBs, cysts, heavy metals, asbestos, VOC (volitile organic chemicals), and THMs in our city water. They also eliminate chlorine and foul odors. They do not, however, absorb inorganic mineral salts such as chloride, fluoride, sodium, nitrates, and soluble minerals. For this reason, they are best for city water systems but not for well water systems which have a potential to be polluted with high amounts of nitrates from agricultural wastes. A concern regarding granular charcoal filters is their tendency to be a gathering ground for bacteria, yeasts, and molds, and their inability to remove pollutants found in some drinking water. Some of the more sophisticated charcoal filters do have a reverse wash system in an attempt to compensate for this. Another problem with charcoal filters is that the charcoal can break down with age or from hot water and release their contaminants back into our drinking water. The best way to avoid this is to pay attention to any change in taste, smell, or color of the water, or a reduction in water flow rate. Duane Taylor, a water expert from North Coast Waterworks in Sonoma County, in a personal communication, suggested that the main problem with charcoal filters is that the user does not replace the filter often enough. He recommends purchasing a filter unit which will stop the flow and make the user change the filter when its filtering capacities are used up. If one does not have such a filter, then he recommends changing the filter at 75% of the manufacturer's suggested lifetime. If one waits until there is already a taste change, decrease in rate of flow, or smell to the water, the filter may already be dumping contaminants back into the water. Activated carbon is rated based on its ability to remove iodine and phenols. The iodine number should be greater than 1000 on the measuring scale and the phenol number should be 15 or less. Another important consideration for carbon filter effectiveness is the contact time of water with the filter. The slower the flow rate and the more carbon there is in the filter, the better job the filter does.

Reverse osmosis (R.O.) is one of the best systems to get pure water without using up a lot of energy. Reverse osmosis units (R.O.s) are able to remove bacteria, viruses, nitrates, fluorides, sodium, chlorine, particulate matter, heavy metals, asbestos, organic chemicals, and dissolved minerals. They do not remove toxic gases, chloroform, phenols, THMs, some pesticides, and low molecular weight organic compounds. When combined with an activated carbon filtration system, however, they can remove the entire spectrum of impurities from the drinking water, including organic and inorganic chemicals. Many R.O. units now have pre- and postfilters which take care of any residual impurities that the R.O. unit does not take out.

In R.O., the water to be filtered is forced through a semipermeable membrane by the moving elements from more concentrated to less concentrated solutions. The membrane is permeable to pure water but not to most of its impurities. If conditions are right for sufficient water pressure and the water is not excessively hard, almost no energy is needed for the operation of R.O. systems. A pressure pump is needed if the total dissolved solids are greater than one thousand parts per million. The water is as pure as distilled, yet it is not heated as in distilled water, and therefore not destructured, which is a great advantage. Sometimes a pressure pump is needed for extremely hard water and this does require electrical energy. The main problem with an R.O. unit is the fragility of the semipermeable membrane. Some membranes can be destroyed by chlorinated water, highly alkaline water, or temperatures over 100 degrees Fahrenheit. If the water is chlorinated, a cellulose membrane is needed. A polymer membrane can be used if the water is not chlorinated.

In my home we use an R.O. unit, and have had the membrane break in less than the expected three years. For this reason, it is good to check the water supply regularly. Newer and stronger membranes are now available on the market, but we are still in the habit of checking the water purity every four months and/or whenever there is a change in the taste. While R.O. units are similar in appearance and claimed performance, there are many complex, interdependent choices regarding pretreatment, membrane choice, and post-treatment systems. To select a system that fits your water filtration needs and to develop the best maintenance plan, it is best to talk with someone who has some in depth knowledge of the many factors involved. If properly done, an R.O. unit may be the most energy-efficient and best way to protect your water. In the past, R.O. units required a lot of water to work properly, which is a disadvantage, particularly during times of drought. Some of the newer models have now been designed to operate with a minimal water usage.

Water distillers, although generally more expensive, remove most everything from the water including: bacteria, fluoride, nitrates, radionuclides, and organic and inorganic toxins; heavy metals, such as lead, mercury, and cadmium; and soluble minerals, such as calcium and magnesium. Some toxic organic compounds, such as THMs and dioxin, have the same, or a lower, boiling point as water and therefore are not filtered out by the distillation process. Some of the more expensive distillers have built in preboiler or postboiler filters as options which eliminate this problem. There are two major problems with water distillers. One is that they are energy intensive and expensive unless one has a solar water distiller. The other problem is that distilled water is dead, unstructured water that is so foreign to the body that one actually temporarily gets a high white blood cell count in response to drinking distilled water. It is, however, possible to revive this dead, destructured water by the use of a product called Crystal Energy, which will be explained in the following section.

Structured Water

A key to understanding water is the concept of structured water. As was well-documented in *Spiritual Nutrition and The Rainbow Diet,* the more structured water there is in one's biological system, the better the enzyme systems carry out their metabolic processes and the easier it is for vitamins and minerals to be assimilated into the cells. Another way to understand the concept is that the more structured the water is, the higher its SOEF energy.

Structured water means that the water molecules in the water are more fully organized. When the water becomes structured, individual water molecules become grouped into high-energy, liquid crystalline units or crystal-like shells. In structured water, the actual bond angle of the two hydrogen and one oxygen atom in a basic water molecule is different than unstructured water. According to Patrick and Gael Flanagan, the most stable water crystal cluster has eight molecules. Intermixed with these liquid crystal structures are free, individual water molecules which are not bound to any other water molecules. When water is highly structured, it contains a high percentage of these liquid crystal units. Most water in healthy biological systems is highly structured. In lakes, streams, and oceans we have mostly unstructured or bulk water. As water is cooled to the freezing point, the number of liquid crystals is increased and it becomes so structured that it forms an ice crystal.

The general findings of several researchers suggest that the more structured the water, the more life energy it can hold. The more structured the water in a biological system, the better the individual cells function. This seems to be true for all levels of our biological systems where water exists, such as in the blood, and in interstitial and intracellular fluids. The research cited in *Spiritual Nutrition and the Rainbow Diet* suggests that the more structured, intracellular water there is, the more balanced and concentrated intracellular ions there are, such as calcium, potassium, and sodium. Nuclear, magnetic resonance studies reported by Carlton Hazelwood have shown that the intracellular water of cancer cells has significantly less structured water than normal healthy cells. Norm Mikesell has reported that when there is a decreased amount of intracellular structured water, the healthy intracellular ratio of sodium to potassium is disrupted. He concludes, as I do, that a decrease in intracellular, structured water is associated with a decrease in the general quality of health.

When the living organism takes in "bulk" water, it must first structure the water so it can be utilized by the system. High energy colloids, or particles with a high electrical charge, act as "energy seeds" that attract the free water molecules to form liquid crystal hydration shells. There are many types of colloids in nature. The most stable of the colloid systems found in nature are those found in living organisms. They are coated by neutrally charged polymers made of albuminoid or fatty acid type materials. The Flanagans point out in their book, *Elixer of the Ageless,* that this type of colloid is the same type of colloid found in the famous Hunza water. This is the water that the Hunzas drink from their natural glacial streams. Some believe that this colloidal water of the Hunzas, who are known for their longevity of up to 130 years, is the key, or at least one key, to their incredible health and vital longevity.

With precise instruments the Flanagans have also verified water can be structured by sunlight, crystals, magnets, or the energy from our hands. What they also found was that this structured effect would persist as long as the water was not disturbed in a turbulent way such as pouring into a glass to drink or by actually drinking it. Fortunately, they were able to invent a colloid solution, based on their understanding of the Hunza water, that would structure water in such a stable way that it would not be disrupted by mechanical, electrical, or even microwave ovens.

In their research the Flanagans also found that the surface tension of the water was an excellent measure of the free energy of the water molecules. The more zeta potential, or free energy, a liquid has, the lower the surface tension. Unstructured water, such as distilled water, has a surface tension of 73 dynes/centimeter. Carrot juice, which has the lowest surface tension of all the juices (no data is available on wheatgrass), has a surface tension of 30 dynes/centimeters. After sitting overnight its surface tension rises to 68, and after 24 hours it reaches the 73 dynes of unstructured dead water.

300

The most healthy liquids are those which have the highest zeta potential or free energy. They are the most structured. A high concentration of anions (negative ions) in water is also associated with health because anions increase the zeta potential of the blood, the interstitial fluids, and the intracellular fluids. In *Elixir of the Ageless,* research is presented which shows that when cations (positive ions) are introduced into fluid systems, this diminishes the activity and function of our biological colloids, and hence, decreases the zeta potential. When this zeta potential is decreased, our biological systems, which depend on the integrity of the fluids, begin to function less well. In carrot juice, when the zeta potential is decreased and the colloidal particles lose their charge, the carrot colloidal system loses its integrity and collapses. The physical evidence of this collapse is the "goop-jell" that we often see in carrot juice several days after it has been made. When we talk about the blood's colloid system collapsing, one can visualize this carrot juice goop as an example of a collapsed colloid system. A colloid collapse in the cells and extracellular fluids impairs the transfer of nutrients into the cells and the excretion of toxins from the cells.

When the zeta potential decreases in the blood, the red blood cells tend to aggregate, blood viscosity or thickness increases, and the red blood cells lose their discreteness. This process can readily be seen with a special microscope known as a dark field microscope. This sludging effect has been associated with general poor health and lack of oxygen in the tissues. In summary, what decreases biological colloid activity, and therefore zeta potential, also seems to be associated with a lower energetic cellular functioning of the living organism. This obviously creates a lower quality of health.

Factors Which Decrease Zeta Potential

The next step in our discussion is to use our understanding of structured water, biological colloids, and health to determine what factors decrease biological colloid activity, and therefore, zeta potential. The Flanagans, who are two of the premiere researchers in this field, have found that ELF (extremely low frequency) signals from hair dryers, T.V. sets, computers, washing machines, and clothes dryers all decrease colloid stability. They have also found that any type of food processing, such as cooking, microwaving, and food irradiation, breaks down the protein coatings of the biological colloid particles in the fluids of the food that is being processed. The result is the destruction of the zeta potential of the foods. The zeta potential may be the energy referred to as the "life force" in enzymes and live foods, as well as a measure of their SOEFs.

Cooking foods causes a destructuring of the biological fluids in our food. In essence, cooking causes a death of the colloid energy system in the food. Devoid of its colloidal life force, the food is essentially dead. Live food, on the other hand, has a high zeta potential and colloid structure.

301

It is important, then, to be aware of what factors can destroy the zeta potential of our biological colloidal system. According to the Flanagans' research, aluminum can cause severe destruction of the colloidal property of our biological fluid systems. Aluminum is used in some baking powders, antacids, deodorants, cookware, and canteens. The aluminum cans used in the soft drink and beer industries may leach aluminum ions into the liquid, despite the plastic lining inside. Aluminum silicate, as found in natural clays such as bentonite, is the only aluminum that the Flanagans found to be safe. Perhaps the biggest problem associated with aluminum is its use in water purification plants. According to the Flanagans, most purification systems add too much aluminum. The result is that the excess aluminum ions end up in tap water. The municipal water systems also routinely add cationic mineral salts which show up in the tap water. A high amount of cations (positive ions) in the water of any sort also destroys zeta potential. Aside from the aluminum beer cans, the beer itself, because it contains large amounts of cationic minerals, drops zeta potential. Although beer is the worst offender of the alcohols because it is packaged in aluminum, even small amounts of alcohol will also cause a coagulation of the liquid colloid system in our body. A high-salt diet will also diminish the zeta potential of our blood and other biological fluids.

The best approach to maintaining a high zeta potential in our fluid colloid system so that our life fluids stay in a high-structured, high-energy, healthy state is to take in fluids and foods that increase the zeta potential rather than decrease it. The best diet for this is one abundant in live foods, especially if they are high in structured water (high zeta potential colloid liquids) and anionic electrolytes. Raw fruits and vegetables and fruit and vegetable juices fulfill this prescription.

After this brief but involved survey of colloidal chemistry described above, one begins to see that there is a natural order to things that makes life simple and healthy. **If we choose to live according to the natural laws of nature, a high zeta potential is maintained without having to be biochemistry experts. One who eats raw foods and drinks structured water doesn't have to worry about zeta potential.**

The Flanagans have developed a stabilized, high zeta potential liquid crystal colloid product. Because it is made of microscopic-sized crystal colloids, they call it Crystal Energy. By putting eight drops per glass of water, this product reestablishes the zeta potential of the liquid, even if it has been previously dead, unstructured, distilled water. I recommend adding this, at one teaspoon per gallon, to distilled water or reverse osmosis water to restructure the water. Their research using a dark field microscope has shown that within five minutes after drinking a glass of this liquid crystal water, red blood cells will unclump.

By maintaining a high zeta potential in our blood, our interstitial fluids, and our intracellular fluids, we are less likely to have the zeta potential of our biological colloid systems disrupted or destroyed by the myriad of zeta potential destroyers to which we are exposed in our environment. The more energy in our system the higher are the SOEFs, and the better organized, and therefore healthier, are all our biological systems. This is true on the level of DNA/RNA replication as well as for all the cells, tissues, organs, and organ systems of the body. Even the cellular mineral balance becomes more ideal.

1. *In your lifetime you are going to drink 58,333 pounds of water— that comes to 7,000 gallons.*

2. *Water comes from two sources: underground water and surface water, such as rivers and lakes. For years thousands of tons of toxic chemicals have been dumped into our fresh water supply. Now much of our water is polluted.*

3. *Make sure the water you drink is pure by filtering it at the tap.*

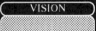
VISION

BLACKBOARD FACTS

Preview of Chapter 20
Stage Two: Not a Time to Go Fishing

There are no nutrients found in fish which cannot be found in safer and more healthy vegetarian sources. At one time it was thought that fish had the highest percent of omega-3 fatty acids which are known to prevent blood clotting. Flax seed has 18-24% as compared to 0-2% in fish. What fish do have in abundance as compared to vegetarian food is mercury, PCBs, salmonella, and hepatitis virus found in polluted waters. The toxicity in fish is so serious that some studies have found that babies whose mothers have eaten fish from Lake Michigan have lower birth weight and more neurological problems. There are no good reasons for hanging on to our old habitual flesh food patterns by continuing to eat fish and many reasons for letting go. This is the last step in the transition to a vegetarian diet. Are you ready to make this "off-fishal" transition into a new world of health and spiritual enhancement?

I.   Why fish had been considered a viable alternative to beef and chicken

    A. Fish are high in minerals

    B. Fish protect against certain diseases

    C. Omega-3 fatty acids

II.   Flax seed is a much better alternative to fish EPA

    A. Flax seed contains more omega-3 fatty acids than fish provides

    B. How to take flax

III. Dangers of eating fish—PCBs & mercury toxicity

Chapter 20

Stage II: Not a Time to Go Fishing

The key features of the Stage Two diet increase the amount of organic, health-promoting foods to about 90% and phase out fish and chicken from the diet. To have eliminated flesh foods from one's diet except for fish and chicken is a major step toward health. Usually, most people seem to naturally eliminate chicken first from the diet.

Fish, in many ways, seems to be a transition food in our culture. Sometimes fish are euphemistically referred to as "sea vegetables." This is a nice way to avoid acknowledging we are eating a living, breathing, moving, conscious animal form. Ecologically speaking, fish do not destroy topsoil as the poultry and animal industries do. Fish also possess several healthy nutritional aspects. Lean fish, such as flounder, haddock, and cod, have as little as one percent fat. This makes them a relatively fat-free source of concentrated protein. Marine fish are also good nutritional sources of selenium, iodine, and many trace minerals not found in poultry and red meat. They are high in vitamins A and D and also vitamin B$_{12}$. The fact that fish have these beneficial nutrients does not mean, however, that I recommend fish on a general basis.

Perhaps the most important nutritional attribute of fish is the high content of eicosapentaeoic acid (EPA), a derivative of omega-3 fatty acid commonly know as linolenic acid. The main omega 3-containing fish are mackerel, sardines, tuna, trout, and cold-water salmon. Researchers have found that diets high in EPA protect against heart disease, strokes, pulmonary embolisms, and peripheral vascular diseases, including gangrene. The high concentrations of EPA seem to act as a natural blood thinner and antisludge factor in the blood. Decreasing the clotting tendency of the blood is probably the main mechanism by which the EPA works to create less mortality from heart disease. It is generally recognized that EPA also decreases cholesterol and triglyceride levels.

There is a plant-based source of omega-3 fatty acids that rivals and surpasses fish sources on all counts. According to Donald Rudin, M.D., and Clara Felix, in *The Omega-3 Phenomenon,* flax seed is highest in omega-3 fatty acids of all foods. Flax seed omega-3 cuts blood cholesterol by 25% and triglycerides by 65%. EPA is also produced in the human body from one of the omega-3 "essential" fatty acids called linolenic acid. The word "essential" in this context means that the human body cannot produce linolenic acid by itself, but must depend on outside sources to supply it. Fish oils are known to have a high content of essential fatty acids, especially the omega-3 fatty acids, including the linolenic acid which is made into EPA by the body.

The fatty acids are components in every cell in the body and help to determine the biological properties of these cells. The World Health Organization suggests that three percent of the total caloric intake for adults should be from essential fatty acids. Children and pregnant and lactating women are advised to take six percent. The essential fatty acids provide energy to the body, maintain body temperature, insulate the nerves, enhance the immune system, and protect body tissues. The two principle forms of essential fatty acids for humans are the omega-6 and the omega-3 fatty acids.

The omega-3 and omega-6 fatty acids are the biological precursors to a group of highly reactive, short-lived, molecular, hormone-like substances known as prostaglandins (PGAs). The PGAs play a role in regulating the second-by-second functioning of every part of the body. Each organ produces its own PGAs from the essential fatty acids stored in that organ. The PGAs are critical for cell membrane function because PGAs become a part of the membrane construction themselves. PGAs help to balance and heal the immune system as well as help to reduce inflammatory reactions such as those seen in arthritis and allergic reactions. If there are dietary imbalances that lead to imbalances in the PGAs, then disease may arise. Although the research is not definitive, a ratio of omega-6 to omega-3 fatty acids of between 4/1 and 9/1 seems to be the best balance.

In the omega-6 series there is linoleic acid (LA), gamma linolenic acid (GLA), dihomo-gamma linolenic acid (DGLA), and arachidonic acid (AA). The omega-6 fatty acids are found in seed oils such as sunflower, safflower, corn, soy, and evening primrose. Peanut oil has some omega-6, as does olive, palm, and coconut oils. High amounts of GLA is found in mother's milk, primrose oil, borage, and black currant oil.

Fish are found to have high amounts of EPA and some moderate amounts of the precursors of the omega-3 series. Fortunately, vegetarians do not have to worry about sources of omega-3 fatty acids because flax seed, walnuts, legumes, and sea vegetables have high concentrations of omega-3 fatty acids. In the omega-3 series, there is alpha-linolenic acid (ALA), eicosapentaenoic acid (EPA), and docosahexaenoic acid (DHA).

The omega-3 series should constitute approximately ten to twenty percent of our fat intake. Some of the reported benefits of the omega-3s are: protection against heart disease, strokes, and clots in the lungs; anticarcinogenic activity against cancer tumors; diabetes; prevention and treatment of arthritis; treatment for asthma; PMS; allergies; inflammatory diseases; water retention; rough, dry skin; and multiple sclerosis. The omega-3s are reported to increase vitality, and contribute to smoother skin, shinier hair, softer hands, smoother muscle action, the normalization of blood sugar, increased cold weather resistance, and a generally improved immune system. Omega-3s are also important for visual function, development of the fetal brain, brain function in adults, adrenal function, sperm formation, and the amelioration of some psychiatric behavior disorders. It may take 3-6 months to see results.

Flax seed contains 18-24 percent omega-3 compared to
fish of zero to two percent. This is significant because many
think that they need to eat fish in order to get the omega 3-de
and artery protection. Abundant research on the subject in
simply not true. The vegetarian flax seed has many major ad
oil. The first is that the omega-3 is a basic building block in tl̲ ̲.̲.̲.̲.̲.̲.̲.̲.̲.̲ ̲body for
many body functions, only one of which is to make EPA. The fish oil doesn't
supply omega-3; it supplies the EPA–and therefore limits the body's options to
make what it needs from the omega-3. Thus, the omega-3 is a better nutritional
resource than the high-EPA fish oil. Another major difference is the fiber which
comes in the flax seed. Fish has no fiber and also is a highly concentrated food.
Unlike many other plants, flax seed has a special fiber called lignin which our
body converts to lignans. These lignans help to build up the immune system and
have specific anticancer, antifungal, and antiviral properties. High levels of
lignans are associated with reduced rates of colon and breast cancer. Just ten
grams, or about one to two teaspoons of flax seed per day raises levels of the
lignans significantly. A third advantage of the flax seed oil over fish, is fish and
fish oil is high in cholesterol. Three and one half ounces of cod liver oil contain
570 milligrams of cholesterol which equals the amount found in two egg yolks.
The fourth advantage of flax seed oil over fish is fish are often high in toxic
residues because they sometimes live in polluted waters. The fifth reason flax
seed is more propitious is that high levels of fish oil are rich in vitamin A and D,
which can be toxic in high doses. Please note that provitamin carotene, which is
converted by the body to utilizable vitamin A, cannot be toxic like animal-
sourced vitamin A.

How To Take Flax

Although some clinicians have estimated one regularly needs as much as
three tablespoons of flax seed oil per day, three tablespoons may be more a
therapeutic dosage instead of a maintenance dose. Dr. Rudin, another flax seed
researcher, uses 2 to 5 tablespoons per day. Researchers at Omega Nutrition,
who produce a high quality flax seed oil, feel that a healthy daily dose is closer
to one teaspoon of oil per day or three teaspoons of the flax seed in its whole form.
Flax seed oil from Omega nutrition seems to be the flax seed oil on the market
with the most enzymes preserved and the least amount of fatty acids changed
from cis to trans. Because their flax seed oil is so close to the natural state, it is
the one exception to using free oils in the diet.

When taken as a whole seed, the flax seed is best soaked, as with other seeds,
in order to deactivate the enzyme inhibitors. I have found it best to use them in
a blender with water, fruits, vegetables, or other seeds. Breaking up the soaked
seeds in a blender makes them easier to assimilate and minimizes the laxative

from the whole soaked seeds. One can also just grind the whole, dry flax in a coffee mill and take it directly. I feel that the addition of flax seeds to the diet is important for vegetarians, particularly live fooders. I have had several cases of people on a raw food diet that did not include flax seeds who had health problems which disappeared within a month after they began taking flax seed or flax seed oil. I consider flax seed an essential for a healthy live food diet. If one wants to take flax seed oil instead of the seeds themselves, the flax seed oil that should be used should be packaged in a light- and air-blocking container and should not have been heated to temperatures above 118 degrees during the processing and bottling. Once opened, it should be refrigerated and consumed within 3 to 6 weeks. In an unopened state it will retain its strength for four months.

Fishing in Polluted Waters

From a practical view, eating fish is potentially dangerous because of the widespread, ever-increasing pollution of the waters of the world. The biggest water contaminants are the PCBs and mercury. PCBs, along with dioxin, DDT, and dieldrin, are among the most toxic of chemicals on the planet. According to J. Culhane, in his 1988 article "PCBs: The Poisons That Won't Go Away," only a few parts per billion can cause cancer and birth defects in lab animals. The Tenth Annual Report of the Council on Environmental Quality sponsored by the U.S. government found PCBs in one hundred percent of all sperm samples. According to a *Washington Post* article in 1979, the PCBs are considered one of the main reasons that the average sperm count of the American male is approximately seventy percent of what it was thirty years ago. This same article also points out that twenty-five percent of college students are sterile today as compared to one half of one percent thirty-five years ago. Most toxicity experts agree that the main source of human contamination comes from eating fish from waters in which the PCB levels are high, which nowadays can be almost anywhere. The Environmental Protection Agency estimates that fish can accumulate up to nine million times the level of PCBs in the water in which they live. PCBs have been found in fish from the deepest and most remote parts of the world's oceans.

Fish and shellfish are natural accumulators of toxins, because they live and breathe the water in which they live. Shellfish, such as oysters, clams, mussels, and scallops, filter ten gallons of water every hour. In a month, an oyster will accumulate toxins at concentrations that are 70,000 times more concentrated than the water they are living in. The problem doesn't stop by not eating fish when one realizes that half the world's fish catch is fed to livestock. According to *A Diet for New America,* more fish are consumed by U.S. livestock than by the entire human population of all the countries in Western Europe. Periodic testing in the U.S. has found eggs and chickens highly contaminated with PCBs after being fed fish that were contaminated with PCBs.

Mercury toxicity from ingesting fish is another well-known source of illness. There are two forms of mercury that are the most dangerous. One is the quicksilver mercury and the other is methylmercury, which is about fifty times more toxic. Although there is a general agreement that mercury in plants is a less toxic form, experts do not agree as to whether the mercury in fish is stored primarily in the form of the more toxic methylmercury. In any case, children and adults who have eaten fish from mercury-contaminated waters from Minamata Bay, Japan in 1953, along the Agano River in Niigata, Japan, in 1962, and other locations in Iraq, Pakistan, and Guatemala, all have suffered either death, coma, or a variety of brain and neurological damage.

Aside from these more acute incidents of chemical factory mercury contamination, mercury contamination of fish is widespread. According to Rudolph Ballentine, M.D., mercury toxicity is being reported with increasing frequency by physicians as well as dentists. The two main contributing factors seem to be a diet high in fish and the common use of silver-mercury amalgams for dental work. Fish consumption alone may be enough to cause mercury toxicity. An article by the Canadian Medical Association in 1976 reported that Indians in Northern Canada, who ate over one pound of fish per day, had symptoms of mercury poisoning. A 1985 study in West Germany of 136 people who regularly consumed fish from the Elbe River found a correlation between the blood levels of both mercury and pesticides and the amount of fish eaten.

Fish and shellfish may also carry their own toxins. The most common of these toxins is ciguatera poisoning. The cigua toxin is both a neurotoxin and gastrointestinal toxin which may give symptoms of numbness and tingling to lips, nausea, abdominal cramps, paralysis, convulsions, and even death. A little less than one case in ten is fatal. Certain species of red snapper, pompano, jackfish, groupers, and eels may have the toxin. Certain shellfish, such as clams, mussels, scallops, and crabs, may take in a toxic substance in plankton at certain times of the year which may also cause a poisoning effect that is similar in severity to ciguatera poisoning. This poisoning is difficult to treat. I have seen at least one patient who was unable to work for several years after suffering such a poisoning.

Because there does not seem to be any fish available that are not potentially filled with toxins, one should consider carefully whether it's worth the risk to eat fish. In a study in the *Diet and Nutrition Letter of Tufts University,* it was reported that the more fish pregnant mothers ate from Lake Michigan, the more their babies showed abnormal reflexes, general weakness, slower responses to external stimuli and various signs of depression. They found that mothers eating fish only two or three times a month produced babies weighing seven to nine ounces less at birth and with smaller heads. Jacobsen, in a follow-up study that was reported in *Child Development,* found that there was a definite correlation between the amount of fish the mothers ate and the child's brain development, even if was only one time per month. He found that the more fish the pregnant mothers ate, the lower was the verbal I.Q. of the children. Children are usually the most sensitive to toxins, and they are prime indicators of what may be happening to adults on a more subtle level. A Swedish study in 1983 found that the milk of nursing mothers who regularly ate fatty fish from the Baltic Sea had higher levels of PCBs and pesticide residues than even meat eaters. Lactovegetarians were found to have the lowest pesticide residues in this study.

The sanitation problem associated with fish and shellfish must also be considered. Once the fish or shellfish are caught en mass in the trawler nets, the crushing pressure on the fish causes the intestinal contents to be squeezed out, contaminating the rest of the catch. Also, the fishing net is oftentimes dragged across the bottom of the ocean where the sediment is highly contaminated with toxins and bacteria. In the book, *Basic Food Microbiology,* it is reported that the contamination from the sediment results in a bacterial count that ranges up to a million per gram. This is a very high count; salmonella, for example, in counts as low as one to ten bacteria per gram, have caused infections in humans. Salmonella is not so much a problem with shrimp, but more with bottom-feeding fish and shellfish in coastal waters which have been polluted by sewage. By the time fish have reached port, most have suffered considerable contamination and microbial growth. The task of processing, which involves gutting and filleting, further spreads the contamination. The inspection of fish for contamination is more thorough than government inspection of beef and poultry. Sixty percent of the fish are inspected by the National Seafood Quality and Inspection Laboratory. Shellfish are inspected under a special surveillance agency set up after a typhoid breakout in 1925.

Not only do the bodies of fish become the depositories of chemical toxins, but they have the propensity to concentrate microorganisms as well, especially salmonella and hepatitis. In *Basic Food Microbiology,* it shows that seven to twenty percent of shellfish and forty percent of the mussels collected from five separate collecting stations were contaminated with salmonella. Some, but not all, of this bacterial and viral contamination can be avoided if the shellfish are cooked. For example, in *Transition to Vegetarianism,* Dr. Ballentine reports that a bacterial count of over a million per gram was found in crabs that were boiled for thirty minutes.

I have presented many reasons why one would want to give up fish. There are no nutrients found exclusively in fish that cannot be found in safer, healthier, vegetarian sources. Although once considered a healthy food, modern-day pollution has made all seafood risky to eat. The biggest reason of all not to eat fish is to love oneself more than being addicted to old eating patterns of culture and convenience.

310

Unless one tends to overeat, a vegetarian diet will leave one feeling lighter than a flesh-centered meal. Feeling lighter indicates there is less strain on the digestive system and more energy available to the body and mind.

Feeling lighter always feels good! It is a way of loving yourself and being in the light.

VISION

BLACKBOARD FOOD FOR THOUGHT

Preview of Chapter 21
Stage III: Developing a Vegetarian Diet

Stage III is the first step into vegetarianism. It is a major lifestyle change and needs to be experienced in that light. There may be some minor psychological shifts as well as a slow detoxification process that is initialized. By moving into it slowly and peacefully these changes will have a minimal impact. The two best-known diets for a beginning vegetarian are the Airola Diet and macrobiotics. Both these diets will be discussed. You may settle into either of these two diets and be quite comfortable. The conscious eater diet includes these and, by the end of Stage III, takes you a little further for optimal health. It allows you to do building or cleansing, heating or cooling, balance yin and yang, and acid-base. In this chapter you are also introduced to the concept of biogenic and bioactive foods and fermented foods. The questions about dairy products, calcium balance, fiber, oxalates, and phytates are also addressed. In beginning a vegetarian diet, give yourself four to six months to make the transition. Are you ready to change to a diet which will significantly improve your health and aid your spiritual well-being?

   I. Developing a vegetarian diet

  II. Biogenic foods

 III. The psychology of the transition to vegetarianism

 IV. Holy cow! Pros and cons of dairy products

  V. The Airola Diet

 VI. The Macrobiotic Diet

 VII. Fermented live foods

VIII. Nuances of the Stage III Diet

Chapter 21

Stage III: Developing a Vegetarian Diet

The transition to a vegetarian diet is a major life step. People come to vegetarianism in many different ways. Some choose it for ethical reasons, others to minimize cruelty to animals, others for health reasons, some to help preserve the ecology or to create an atmosphere for world peace, and some make the change for specifically spiritual reasons or to enhance their meditation. For many the change may be motivated by a combination of all of these reasons. Whatever the reason, it is a transition worth understanding so it can be done gracefully and in the most healthy, harmonious, and peaceful way. By making the changes gradually, one gives the body, mind, and circle of family and friends a period of adjustment that supports the transition. This approach helps to guarantee a sustained shift to a vegetarian way of life.

Most often, when one stops eating all red meat, poultry, fish and other seafood, and eggs, one naturally shifts from a high-protein, high-fat, low-fiber, low-complex carbohydrate, high-pesticide diet to a low-fat, low-protein, high-natural carbohydrate one. This high-, natural-, complex-carbohydrate and low-protein diet is the one recommended by the highly prestigious International Society for Research on Nutrition and the Diseases of Civilization.

Not everyone makes such a smooth shift from a flesh-centered to a vegetarian diet. There is a tendency for some people, under the illusion they are eating a low-fat and low-protein diet, to think that because they stopped eating the highly concentrated protein of flesh foods, they can begin eating large amounts of dairy, oily foods, tofu, and roasted nuts and seeds. These foods are high in cooked fats and protein and should not be eaten in excess either. The general findings of the cross-cultural studies suggest that a diet high in natural complex carbohydrates and low in protein creates the best health, vitality, and longevity. Many of the cultures which are noted for their longevity eat only one-half to one-third the protein that the western nations eat. A diet high in complex natural carbohydrates includes fresh fruits, vegetables, nuts, seeds, legumes, and grains. This is the essential diet followed by many long-lived people such as the Hunzas, many of whom live close to one hundred years or more, and the Russian Caucasians, called Abkhazians, who have seven times more centenarians per million than the U.S. Although the Abkhazians eat some meat, according to Paavo Airola, most of their centenarians are vegetarian. Other long-lived cultures, such as the Bulgarians and Vilcabamban Indians, also follow a similar diet. Americans, who are the world leaders in cancer, heart disease, arthritis, obesity, high blood pressure, multiple sclerosis, mortality rates, miscarriages and birth deformities, eat more meat, more protein, and probably more cooked fat than any other nation.

Biogenic Foods

Raw or sprouted seeds, nuts, grains, and grasses are the most potent life force foods. They are called biogenic foods. These foods contain the secret of life itself, the germ, which contains the reproductive power for the perpetuation of the species. They contain the spark of life which sparks the life of those who eat them in their live form. These foods have all the nutrients essential for bountiful human health and longevity. When sprouted, many of the nutrients are increased and the nuts, seeds, and grains become considerably easier to digest. When most seeds and nuts are soaked and sprouted, naturally occurring digestive enzyme inhibitors are washed away and the proteins, lipids, and complex carbohydrates become predigested into free amino acids, free fatty acids, and simpler carbohydrates. Cooking may destroy these enzyme inhibitors, but it also disrupts the SOEFs, destroys vitamins, mineral complexes, and food enzymes, and coagulates the protein. Many of the grains contain complete proteins, essential fatty acids, and many vitamins and minerals. They are a high-quality source of vitamin E, lecithin, and most of the B-complex vitamins. They also are high in fiber which is so vital to our health. The increase in biogenic foods is part of Stage III.

Bioactive Foods

These are fully mature foods that are live, but not the super high life force foods as biogenic foods are. They are excellent foods and very much a part of Stage III. The difference between biogenic and bioactive foods is the difference between the high vitality of a young child who is rapidly growing verses the vitality of a healthy adult. Bioactive foods include all of the vegetarian foods, such as vegetables, fruits, mature seeds, nuts, grains, beans, and legumes.

Vegetables, including sea vegetables such as dulse and kelp, are also extremely important to our health. They are excellent sources of minerals, such as calcium and iron, as well as enzymes and vitamins. They contain complete proteins which, according to Paavo Airola, often have a better net protein utilization value than proteins from animal sources. One acre of leafy greens contains twenty-five times the amount of protein as one acre devoted to livestock. Vegetables serve both as cleansers and builders for the body.

Fruits are nature's sunshine and pure gifts to us from Mother Nature. They are nature's solar collectors and can be thought of as condensed sunlight. Most fruits are rich in vitamin A and C and a varied assortment of essential minerals. They are the highest of all foods in boron, which is important in preventing osteoporosis. They are not only nutritive but also good detoxifiers and bowel cleaners. They contain a higher amount of structured water than any other food and are high in energetic radiations arising from the four elements of air, sun, earth, and water.

Legumes, such as soybeans, peanuts, and kidney beans, are powerful building foods which are high in protein. According to the Max Planck Institute, about fifty percent of the protein is coagulated when any protein is cooked, so soy and other legumes that need to be cooked are, for this reason, not the best protein as compared to those of nuts, seeds, and grains which can be eaten raw or sprouted.

Soybeans have provided a source of high protein in Asian countries for many thousands of years. Because of their strong inhibitory enzymes, they must be sprouted or cooked before they can be safely consumed. They are high in fiber and lecithin. They also give a good supply of vitamins. If not cooked, they also provide a good source of vitamins, especially the B vitamins.

A vegetarian diet is always less toxic than animal foods, even if the vegetarian food is not organic food. According to pesticide authority Lewis Regenstein, meat contains fourteen times more pesticides than plant foods and dairy contains five and one half times more. Regenstein points out that FDA studies also show that red meat, poultry, fish, and dairy contain pesticides more often, and in greater amounts, than plant foods. In 1975, the Council on Environmental Quality reported that 95% of the nation's DDT ingestion was from animals. John Robbins states that this same percentage holds true for other pesticides also.

Shifting to a Vegetarian Diet

Two of the most popular vegetarian diet patterns are Airola's dietary approach and the macrobiotic approach. One general reason they are both so health-promoting is by an act of omission. A vegetarian diet, even if it includes some dairy, automatically decreases the incidence of cancer, heart disease, high blood pressure, osteoporosis, rate of aging, and other chronic degenerative diseases. A transition to a nonjunk food, vegetarian diet, such as the Airola or macrobiotic diets, in which all fast and highly processed, deep-fried or irradiated foods, white sugar, white bread, T.V. dinners, french fries, and pastries are eliminated, will bring even greater benefits to health. If done properly, the transition to a vegetarian diet will almost always increase one's sense of well-being, vitality, and endurance.

The Psychology of the Transition to Vegetarianism

The typical American dinner plate features an animal food with various minor vegetable side dishes surrounding it. When one switches to a vegetarian diet, psychologically, there is a shift from a central meat item on the plate to a more balanced feeling in which all that one eats gets equal attention and value. Unless one tends to overeat, a vegetarian diet will leave one feeling lighter than a flesh-centered meal. This is a new sensation that one will get used to after awhile and begin to enjoy. Feeling lighter usually indicates there is less strain on the digestive system and more energy available to the body. After eating, one is less likely to feel sleepy and the mind will tend to be clearer. The blood stream stops becoming flooded with saturated fats as well as toxins that come from the cells of the deteriorating fish, poultry, or red meat animals. A clear mind and good health is also associated with a clear blood stream. All these benefits will accrue to one who becomes a vegetarian.

A vegetarian diet does not tend to numb the emotions, mind, spirit, or subtle physical sensitivity like a flesh-centered diet may. The result is that in the process of the transition one becomes more sensitive and more in touch with feelings and the subtle energies of the life process. Most people find that it makes it easier to meditate as well.

To compensate for the accustomed heavier feeling that one was used to on a flesh-centered diet, sometimes in the beginning, one will be drawn to heavier, cooked meals, such as cheese dishes, lentil loaves, and tofu arrangements which resemble meat dishes. This is often the kind of food featured in vegetarian restaurants. Many feel comfortable with this level of vegetarian diet and do not proceed onward. Ethnic dishes, such as vegetarian lasagna, Chinese food, Mideastern dishes, et cetera, often fit in well with Stage III because they are culturally accepted and familiar.

Another common tendency is to eat a lot of dairy, nuts, and seeds in order to "compensate" for the fear of not getting enough protein and that sense of not feeling as full as when one ate heavier meat dishes. Many people, including myself, went through this phase in the late sixties and early seventies. Nowadays, the protein scare has been diffused so not as many people worry about not getting enough protein on a vegetarian diet. Although I felt better and healthier on my new vegetarian diet than when I was on an animal diet, when I was eating these heavy cooked vegetarian foods, I actually gained a little too much weight until I figured out that what was going on. By cutting down on dairy intake and my frequent snacks of nuts and seeds, I felt even better.

Because Stage III eliminates all animal products, it is natural for one to begin to eat a lot more grains, beans, fruits, vegetables, raw nuts and seeds, sea vegetables, soaked and sprouted grains, legumes, nuts and seeds, and raw dairy. Most of these foods are high in fiber, whereas all flesh foods, dairy, and eggs have essentially no fiber. A vegetarian diet increases all types of dietary fiber and consequently produces a cleaner, less toxic bowel condition. On a healthy vegetarian diet there is usually no longer a need to supplement one's diet with oat or wheat bran fiber to assist bowel regularity. In fact, to continue adding fiber to the vegetarian diet can produce an excess of fiber and may even cause digestive difficulties and gas.

Vegetarians Get More Fiber

Fiber is defined by its indigestibility. The two main types of fiber are cellulose and pectin. Humans do not produce the digestive enzymes to break down either of these. A third type of fiber which is closely related to cellulose is called lignand. The percentage of fiber in a plant increases with its age. Fiber is commonly found in stems, peelings, and hulls. An excess of lignand and cellulose can be irritating to the bowels and can also produce gas. Supplemental bran is primarily this type of combined fiber. Cellulose fiber is good for bulking the stool and also binding carcinogenic and radioactive chemicals. It is the other fiber type, pectin, primarily found in fruits, which is what binds the bile salts and takes them out of the system. The more bile salts taken out of the system, the less bile salts are available to be reabsorbed to make cholesterol. Another disadvantage of consuming too much of both types of fiber is that an excess of fiber tends to bind minerals and keep them from being absorbed into the system. In order to minimize the mineral loss from fiber, one may want to remove the tough, woody parts of vegetables and fruits, such as the stems, peelings, and hulls. It took me a while to figure this out because I had been attached to the idea of eating the whole plant. Once I began to eliminate the excess and tough plant roughage, particularly stems, I found it easier on my digestion. If people are suffering from sore bowels, juicing the fruits and vegetables is another way to minimize the roughage and maximize the assimilation of minerals and vitamins.

Phytates and Oxalates

The significance of phytates and oxalates in the vegetarian diet needs to be clarified. The very earliest research suggested that in some grains, phytic acid combined with calcium in the grain and prevented the calcium from being absorbed. Later research found when these grains were made into breads, the enzyme phytase became activated and liberated the bound up calcium from the phytic acid bonds during the rising of the bread. More recent research has found that over time, the body begins to produce its own phytase enzyme for breaking down the phytates. According to Bitar and Reinhold in *Biochemica et Biophysica Acta*, the phytase enzyme produced in our intestines releases the calcium from the phytate binding so that the calcium can be absorbed into the system.

The questions concerning the potential harmful effects of oxalates also require attention. Oxalic acid is found in many foods, such as spinach, caffeine products, sesame seeds, cola drinks, nuts, citrus fruit, tomatoes, asparagus, beets and beet tops, Swiss chard, dandelion greens, cranberries, and ascorbic acid supplements. Some researchers think that the oxalic acid combines with the calcium in these foods to form oxalates and then this calcium cannot be absorbed. My general observation, in examining the oxalate sediment in the urine of hundreds of people, is that oxalates from natural foods does not build up in the system if the fat metabolism and digestion are working well. Poor fat metabolism seems to be associated with a buildup of oxalate crystals. Dr. Loomis, in a personal communication, pointed out that if one eats lots of chocolate and takes more than 500 mg of vitamin C ascorbate, the oxalates will begin to build up and excess oxalate sediment will accumulate in the urine. Research does show, however, that with some plants, such as spinach and chard, the oxalates can bind with the calcium in a way that prevents some calcium absorption. However, Davidson, in *Human Nutrition and Dietetics,* points out that the chelating effect of oxalic acid on calcium and other minerals is most likely negligible. According to Dr. Ballentine, even the chelating effect of oxalic acid in spinach or chard can be nullified by eating them with rice. In this way, the high calcium present in spinach and chard can be assimilated into the system.

Organic oxalic acid, defined as that which occurs in nature in its raw form, can actually be beneficial to the system. Once foods containing oxalic acid are cooked, according to the dean of juice therapy and author of *Raw Vegetable Juices*, Dr. Norman Walker, the oxalic acid becomes a dead and irritating substance to the system. He feels that in its cooked form it binds irreversibly with the calcium and prevents calcium absorption. An excess of cooked oxalic acid may also form oxalic acid crystals in the kidney. In its live organic form, Dr. Walker feels oxalic acid stones and calcium blockage does not occur because the organic oxalic acid is able to be metabolized appropriately. According to Dr. Walker, oxalic acid in its raw form is one of the important minerals needed to maintain tone and peristalsis of the bowel.

Organic Calcium

On a Stage III diet it is possible to get plenty of organic calcium. Other excellent leafy green sources of calcium, which are also low in oxalates, are kale, collards, mustard greens, broccoli, and cabbage. According to the USDA publication *Nutritive Value of American Foods,* two thirds cup of collard greens has 91% of the calcium in a cup of milk. According to the *Composition of Foods Book* published by the USDA, other nondairy sources of calcium which are approximately equal to collard greens are almonds and kelp. Sesame seeds that have been hulled, sunflower seeds, and tofu have about one half as much calcium as collard greens. Kelp is extremely high in calcium, but should only be taken in moderate amounts because of its high iodine and salt content. By eating leafy greens, seeds, nuts, tofu, and dulse, vegetarians get more than enough calcium. Because they also eat a lot of fruit and vegetables which are high in boron (boron helps minimize loss of body calcium through the urine), the amount of calcium in the body stays high. As pointed out before, vegetarian men and women have considerably less osteoporosis than flesh-eating men and women.

One other significant factor in calcium absorption is the ratio of calcium to phosphorous in a particular food (see fig. 22). Too much phosphorous in a food causes a lowering of calcium in the blood and produces a tendency to lose calcium from the bones. This is what happens on a high flesh food diet because meat is high in phosphorous. The foods with the healthiest ratios are leafy greens, which have a ratio of between 2/1 and 6/1 times more calcium than phosphorous. Dairy is also good with 1.5/1 times more calcium than phosphorous. Foods like broccoli and green beans also have about 1.5/1 times more calcium than phosphorous. Fruits, such as apples, bananas, and pineapples, have slightly more phosphorous than calcium. Foods which have the worst ratios, which means they have much higher phosphorous than calcium, are meat, fish, and poultry at a ratio of calcium to phosphorous of 1/15. Yeast is 1/9. Grains and beans have more phosphorous than calcium, but only 1/2 to 1/5 times higher. The soft drinks on the market have enormously high phosphorous to calcium ratios and thus make a strong contribution to the creation of osteoporosis.

Think Zinc

The mineral input of a vegetarian diet is more than adequate. In a balanced, vegetarian diet, manganese intake is at least double that of an animal-based diet. Adding leafy greens, dulse, kelp, and herbs like thyme, ginger, and cloves, will increase the mineral content of any vegetarian dishes to adequate, and even what may be considered high, levels. The one possible exception to this is zinc, which may not be as plentiful on a vegetarian diet in relation to other minerals. In my own clinical practice, I have noticed that vegetarians and meat eaters alike tend to have zinc deficiencies. The study of Freeland and Graves on the zinc status of vegetarians published in the *Journal of American Dietetic Association* in 1980, suggests that vegetarians tend to have a marginal zinc status. Because only seventy-nine people were studied and there are few large studies on this subject, I feel these findings should not be considered definitive. As we have seen with the B_{12} work, the question remains to be answered what are actually low, and what are low but actually physiologically safe, levels of zinc for vegetarians? A diet high in grains, which are also high in zinc, may actually result in a lower zinc status because the phytates in the grain combine with the zinc to keep it from being absorbed. The phytase needed to release the zinc from the phytate turns out to be a zinc-dependent enzyme. This means that if you are already low in zinc at the time you switch to a vegetarian diet, you may not have enough zinc to make the zinc-freeing phytase enzyme work efficiently. Once there is enough phytase enzyme to release the zinc phytate bonding, then the cycle is broken and the zinc is able to be freed from the phytates. During the time of transition to vegetarianism one might want to check the zinc status and also eat more foods that are high in zinc, such as brewers yeast, wheat germ, and pumpkin seeds. Other foods

RATIOS of CALCIUM/PHOSPHOROUS

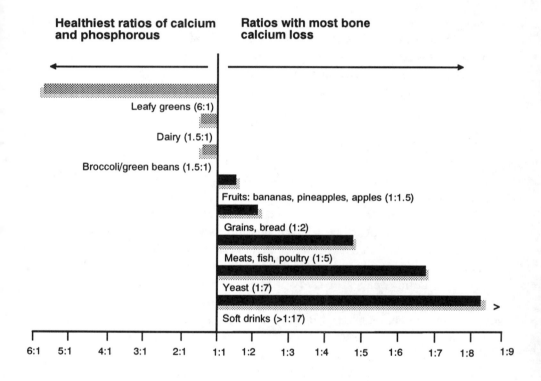

Fig. 22

that are high in zinc and do not have phytates are dairy products, tofu, beans, seeds, and nuts. Soaking and sprouting grains eliminates phytic acid and liberates zinc for absorption. People who are particularly at risk for zinc deficiencies are pregnant and nursing mothers, children, young males and females going through puberty, people undergoing physical and mental stress, those healing wounds, or those with a compromised immune system. Young men are more affected than young women since the male reproductive system requires ample amounts of zinc for its normal functioning and development. Increasing pumpkin seeds in the diet during stages of high zinc need helps to maintain a high zinc input.

Holy Cow!

When one establishes oneself as a vegetarian, questions may arise as to whether or not to include dairy in the diet. Throughout the world, the majority of people who do not eat flesh food are usually lactovegetarians. In many cultures, such as in India, dairy plays a role as a condiment and balancing element to the more spicy, fiery elements of the meal. In ancient India, where the cows were treated with much love and respect, dairy was seen as a sattvic, or pure, food. Today in the West the situation is much different. Cows are thought of as living, financial "stock" which produces a product called milk and later becomes another product called red meat that is eaten. Instead of specially respected animals, they are seen as objects to be exploited and milked of their life force. They become victims of our financial and flesh-food greed. Cows are victims in this exploitive system. One takes on their victim consciousness when one drinks their milk and eats their flesh. Because cows eat or graze on tremendous quantities of vegetable matter, when one drinks their milk, one takes on high concentrations of pesticides, herbicides, radioactive particles such as iodine 131, strontium 90, and cesium 134 and 137, antibiotics, and antibiotic-resistant microbes. One also becomes exposed to animal-borne diseases. Even when the milk is pasteurized, not all of the bacteria or viruses are killed. The acceptable standard for pasteurized milk is approximately 100,000 bacteria per teaspoon or 20,000 bacteria per milliliter. The January 1974 *Consumer Reports* found that one out of six milk samples bought from retail stores had a count of 130,000 bacteria per milliliter.

Another problem with pasteurization is that it destroys the live enzymes in the dairy. One of these enzymes is phosphatase, which is an enzyme that is important for the assimilation of minerals, including calcium, in the milk. The heating process, according to Dr. Morter, also alters the chemical bonds that hold the minerals together and the calcium becomes less available. The deleterious effect of pasteurization on the nutritive quality of milk is well-illustrated by the research of John Thomson of Edinburgh as reported by Dr. Bieler in his book, *Food Is Your Best Medicine*. John Thomson fed pasteurized milk to one calf of a twin and the other was allowed to continue to suckle. The calf that suckled grew strong. The calf that was fed only pasteurized milk died within sixty days. Unfortunately for the calves, these same results were found many times. Dr. Bieler asserts that milk must be raw and fresh if it's to have any nutritive effect on the body. His report that he has prescribed raw milk for 50 years without ever seeing a case of "undulant fever" casts some question on the necessity for pasteurization. Pasteurization also affects the acid-alkaline effect of the raw milk. Raw milk historically has a normally alkaline-producing effect in the body. Dr. Crowfoot, in a personal communication to me, reported that raw milk had an alkaline effect in the body as evidenced by alkaline urines that occurred after the ingestion of raw milk. After pasteurization it becomes acid-producing in the body. The acidity increases even more so if one chooses to boil the milk because one heats it to higher temperatures than pasteurization. Dr. Morter, in his book, *Your Health, Your Choice,* points out a new trend for raw milk. The dairy cows are being fed more protein because it increases milk production. The milk consequently has more protein in it. Because of the higher protein content, the acid-base balance of the milk has shifted and the total effect, of even the raw milk, is to add more acid to the body.

Problems Associated with Milk

There are other problems associated with milk once we get beyond infancy where mother's milk is the perfect nutrient food. One problem is that beginning between eighteen months and four years of age, humans lose the enzyme called lactase, necessary for digesting the lactose, which is the sugar in milk. Most adults have about five to ten percent of the lactase that they possessed as an infant. When there is a deficiency of lactase, the undigested milk sugar ends up in the intestine as the perfect culture media for bacteria to grow on. Depending on the degree of lactose intolerance and the amount of dairy eaten, lactose-intolerant people may get symptoms of bloating, intestinal pain, gas, and diarrhea. Black Americans and Japanese are more likely to have milk intolerance than Caucasians because they have not genetically adapted to the use of dairy as have those with a long history of consuming dairy. In the form of yogurt, the lactose is broken down by the healthy lactic acid bacteria, and therefore yogurt is easier to digest.

Milk, no matter if one has enough lactase to digest it, tends to produce mucous. This is especially true in adults who have already passed through the formative growth period of their life. Milk, with the exception of goat's milk, according to the Ayurvedic system, is a kapha food. If a kapha food is given to an adult, it will increase the tendency to gain weight as well as produce mucous. Cow's milk, as compared to mother's milk, has 300% more casein. Casein is a milk by-product that is used to make a tenacious type of glue for gluing wood together. The main ingredient in Elmer's glue is caesin. There may be so much kapha mucous that a cold develops in order to rid the body of this excess mucous.

Another problem with eating dairy is that many people have milk allergies. In children, I am always amazed how many have their chronic colds, sore throats, and earaches cleared up when I discover they are allergic to dairy and they stop eating dairy. Even without an allergy to dairy, the tendency to colds and flus is greatly decreased when dairy is eliminated.

There are also ecological concerns associated with the use of dairy products, such as the destruction of the rain forest and of the topsoil from cattle grazing, cruelty to animals, and excess methane gas from the bacteria in the cows gut which is belched out in tremendous quantities that significantly increases the greenhouse effect. If this sounds incredulous at first, it is a fact that the methane from the two billion cattle in the U.S. produces 16 million metric tons of methane per year. This is the third largest contributor to the greenhouse effect. The high fat in pasteurized dairy products is also associated with increased clogging of the arteries. Yogic traditions also teach that excess dairy clogs the subtle channels of energy flow in the body known as nadis.

The answer to the dairy question is that if one does not have milk intolerance, does not easily produce mucous, does not mind being exposed to increased concentrations of toxins, bacteria, and radioactive substances, does not have a milk allergy, does not care about taking on victim consciousness in every sip, clogging developing arteries and subtle energetic channels, does not mind increased weight gain, making your body more acid, or contributing to the destruction of the ecology, then dairy is acceptable, in moderation. For some, dairy can be an important supplement to their diet, but in any case, it should remain as a condiment rather than a major part of the dietary intake as it is for so many people today.

The Airola Diet

Paavo Airola, PhD., was one of the most knowledgeable natural doctors of modern times. The diet he recommends permits raw milk to be used as a condiment if one can tolerate it. The diet which he suggests is similar to the traditional way of natural eating characteristic of many cultures around the world who have good health and longevity. The Airola diet recommends a lot of seeds, nuts, and grains. Next in importance are vegetables and then fruits. These food groups may be supplemented by some raw dairy products from healthy cows or goats, preferably in cultured form such as yogurt. Although Airola doesn't recommend dairy products, he allows use of raw dairy as a condiment in a way similar to what one sees in India by lactovegetarians. Actually, in his own clinical healing practice, dairy would often be the first thing he would ask people to eliminate from their diet. He also points out that only those who are tolerant to milk might even consider using dairy as a supplement. In the conscious eating diet, **I suggest that if there is to be any use of dairy at all, it should be as a temporary transition step**. Airola strongly emphasizes eating approximately 80% of one's food in its live state in the warmer months and closer to 60% live food, if one feels the need for more cooked food, in the winter. He particularly emphasizes eating all the nuts and seeds raw, and sprouting much of one's nuts, seeds, and legumes. Airola also emphasizes some foods high in some source of high quality vegetable oils because they supply the essential fatty acids as well as vitamins E, F, and lecithin. He also recommends kelp as a source of minerals, trace minerals, and particularly for its high iodine content. It is a diet that can be adjusted to balance all three doshas.

The Macrobiotic Diet

Another major dietetic approach that many people use as their first entry into vegetarianism is called macrobiotics. The term macrobiotic did not start with George Ohsawa or even in Japan. It was coined one hundred fifty years ago by the German researcher and physician, Christopher Wilhelm Hufeland, in his book titled, *Macrobiotic, The Art of Prolonging Human Life.* This is not the macrobiotic approach to which I am referring when I use the term macrobiotic. George Ohsawa was the founder of modern day macrobiotics. The first and foremost student of his was Michio Kushi. Kushi brought macrobiotics to the West in the early 60s. In the 90s, several other macrobiotic leaders have emerged who have made minor alterations in its theory and practice. Although the most often-practiced macrobiotic diet includes white-meat fish 1-3 times per week, my use of a macrobiotic transition is a vegetarian version of macrobiotics.

The standard macrobiotic diet, as recommended by Michio Kushi, puts a high emphasis on cooked foods. In his basic diet, Kushi suggests that cooked grains be at least 50% of every meal. Vegetables are suggested to be 20-30% of the daily intake and are recommended at every meal with two thirds of them cooked. Cooked beans and sea vegetables, equal to 5-10% of the daily intake, are suggested. Soups made from sea vegetables, grains, or beans with seasonings from miso and tamari, are suggested to be 5-10% of the daily intake. The diet also strongly emphasizes cooking all fruit. There is no dairy in the diet.

Like the 80% live food diet and the Airola diet, the vegetarian version of macrobiotics is an organic, low-protein, and high-natural carbohydrate one; it is also a nondairy diet. I feel that the inclusion of sea vegetables in the diet is quite beneficial, as it adds minerals, iodine, and certain specific protectors from radioactive fallout particles. In the conscious eater's diet I suggest about 2-3 ounces of sea vegetables per week.

The other part of the macrobiotic approach which agrees with the *conscious eating approach* is their teaching that how and what we eat is part of a way of life. As I have pointed out earlier, what and how we eat is a reflection and cause of the awareness and harmony with which we lead our lives. As it has evolved, macrobiotics has included more room for individuality in the diet based on one's particular constitution. As a movement, macrobiotics has an effective and extensive public media outreach which makes it accessible and attractive for many to make the transition from the typical American diet. Because of all of the above factors, I applaud vegetarian macrobiotics as a fine transition diet to vegetarianism.

Part of the effectiveness of the macrobiotic diet is through the power of omission. Through the avoidance of high-protein flesh food, and high-pesticide dairy and junk food, it is a great support to general health. The power of omission in a diet should not be ignored or minimized because it allows the self-healing aspects of the body to be able to do their job. One of the most significant health-benefitting impacts of any vegetarian diet is that it is significantly lower in pesticides and herbicides than a flesh food diet. Stopping or lowering the intake of environmental toxins can't help but be a boon to our health.

Reservations About Macrobiotics

The generic macrobiotic approach emphasizes a fifty-fifty balance of yin and yang energies of the food in the diet as a major way to balance the yin and yang energies. The diet is complex and for most people requires some training in order to master the cooking and yin/yang balancing procedures. In the *conscious eating approach* the focus on the balancing of yin and yang energies uses the totality of one's life to create an overall yin/yang balance, rather than primarily through the diet. This is an important difference from macrobiotics because the conscious eating approach is primarily a live food diet, with a minimal amount of yang grains. The *conscious eating approach* is a powerful aid to spiritual life. It is easy to balance the yin effect of the conscious eating diet with other yang lifestyle activities. It is only fair to point out that although macrobiotics puts a high focus on a balance of yin and yang foods in the diet as a primary way to achieve this balance, it does not entirely ignore the existence of other lifestyle factors which balance the yin and yang of life. The more conscious one becomes, the easier it is to remain centered and grounded with yin foods as the main component of the diet. My observation, in working with many spiritually committed people, is that yin foods, especially a diet high in live foods, accelerates the consciousness process, and as consciousness increases, people are able to increase their percentage of yin live foods without becoming imbalanced. On a theoretical level, I hypothesize that God's Divine fire actually begins to add a yang element that balances the more yin foods.

Although certain key concepts of the theoretical orientation of macrobiotics are right on the mark, I feel the diet itself does not necessarily create a stable, long-term, high-energy, radiant health as compared to a properly implemented live food approach. The radiant energy of someone on live foods is easy to notice.

The standard macrobiotic approach is different in a major way from the guidelines of an eighty percent or more live food vegetarian diet recommended over the last hundred years by such nutritional lights as Dr. Airola, Dr. Ann Wigmore, Dr. Norman Walker, Viktoras Kulvinskas, M.S., Max Bircher-Brenner, M.D., Max Gerson, M.D., Herbert Shelton, Dr. Edmond Bordeaux Szekeley, Dr. Paul Bragg, and Dr. Patricia Bragg, who have found a primarily live food diet excellent for health and for healing severe degenerative diseases such as arthritis, heart disease, and cancer in hundreds of thousands of patients.

Macrobiotics does not address the scientific facts that show that cooking destroys self-digestive enzymes of the food, valuable antioxidant enzymes, and other living food factors. From this point of view, I particularly object to the roasting of the high life force foods, such as nuts and seeds, and insistence on cooking all fruits. This essentially total, cooked-food diet destructures the food with heat, resulting in a 50% protein loss, and approximately a 70-80% loss of the vitamins and minerals, including high losses of vitamin B_{12}. A high-grain diet also has a tendency to drive the body toward a more acid state, which for many people is not healthy. Cooked grains also have a tendency to produce excess mucous and destroy enzymes needed to enhance digestion and build the life force.

Although many of the principles of macrobiotics are drawn from age-old health wisdom of countries such as Japan and China, its present form, in actual practice on Westerners, is very new. Although there is some recent research showing it may be helpful in the healing of certain types of cancer, macrobiotics doesn't have extensive scientific, cultural, or health research in the western culture to show that it brings about optimal health on a large cultural scale over hundreds of years as the Airola and conscious eating approach of 80% live food does for the Western body. The use of sea salt, which is hard for the body to metabolize and can contribute to high blood pressure, is another potential health problem in the macrobiotic diet. With its high emphasis on salt and grains, and especially rice, from an Ayurvedic point of view, macrobiotics is particularly helpful for people who have a vata constitution and would be most imbalancing for those with a kapha constitution. Due to the above reasons, I am cautious to recommend it beyond the initial transition stage to vegetarianism. In any case, it has been a great service in helping people become vegetarians and making organic food items available in America. I have observed in my clients that both the vegetarian macrobiotic diet of Oshawa and Kushi, and Airola's diet, are supportive for spiritual life.

Fermented Live Foods

Fermented lactic acid foods, such as sauerkraut and fermented vegetables, are good ways to increase the amount of raw food in the diet and a convenient, viable way to store food during the winter. Dr. James Lind did the first scientific study of raw cultured vegetables, another name for sauerkraut, in the 1700s when he found that they prevented scurvy in Dutch seamen. The famous Russian scientist, Elie Metchenikoff, felt that one of the most important factors in the diet of the long-lived Russians he studied was a diet rich in lactic acid. Raw cultured vegetables have been used by the ancient Chinese, Romans, and even by the army of Genghis Khan.

Raw cultured vegetables are rich in the lactic acid bacteria lactobacillus plantarum and lactobacillus brevis. These bacteria, via enzymatic processes, convert the sugars and starches in the vegetables into lactic acid and acetic acid. This acid environment is excellent for a healthy colon where these same bacteria also grow. Because cultured vegetables are slightly acidic, they are a particularly good food for those people who tend to be alkaline.

When the conditions for a healthy colon environment are produced, the growth of healthy colon bacteria is stimulated and the overgrowth of candida yeast is prevented. In *The Complete Guide to Raw Cultured Vegetables* by Evan Richards there are many testimonials to the successful use of cultured vegetables to treat candida. Patricia Bragg, PhD., the daughter of the famous Paul Bragg, is quoted as saying that their "research and experiences have shown raw sauerkraut to help alleviate candida problems, digestive problems, ulcers, and in general, helps to rejuvenate and promote longevity." These claims only apply to raw, and not to canned or pasteurized, sauerkraut.

One of the most famous medical doctors who used the fermented vegetable approach was Dr. Johannes Kuhl. He regularly used cultured vegetables in his anticancer diet. He felt that the lactic acid produced by the lactobacteria helped to prevent chronic disease and cancer as well as promoted good health. One way that the cultured vegetables are so good for us is that they prevent the yeast, albicans candida, and pathogenic bacteria from taking over the colon and creating endotoxins which suppress the immune system. In essence, they create a micro-ecological balance in the colon that helps us maintain health. The vegetables mostly used in fermented cultures are cabbage, carrots, and beets. These are high in vitamins A and E. Cabbage is a cruciferous vegetable which is also high in vitamin C as well. The American Cancer society's epidemiological studies indicate that diets high in cruciferous vegetables have been associated with less cancer incidence.

The lactobacilli organisms found in fermented foods are very high in enzymes which add to our overall enzyme bank when they are taken into the system. These organisms help with the digestion and conversion of starches and sugars in the vegetables to lactic and acetic acid in our colon. This aid to our digestion further supports our overall enzymatic pool because now less enzymes have to be secreted by the pancreas for digestion. The friendly bacteria growing on the vegetables also digest the vegetables during the fermentation process so that vegetables become an easily assimilated, predigested food. The best and most inexpensive way to regularly have raw cultured vegetables in the diet is to make them in one's own home.

Nuances on the Stage III Diet

In Stage III, one's awareness of the acid-alkaline balance, food combining, low protein intake, and organic foods becomes more refined. As one begins to understand these issues, one then begins to increase sprouting skills and to understand the importance of using more of the rejuvenating foods, such as soaked or sprouted seeds, nuts, grains, and legumes. These types of foods are called biogenic because of their high life force energy. In the spectrum of the vegetarian diet one may find oneself shifting to 60–80% biogenic and bioactive foods and 20–40% cooked foods. Increased live food consumption may include soaked and sprouted nuts, seeds, vegetables, fruits, legumes and grains. In the later part of Stage III, biogenic foods may eventually reach 30% of the total dietary intake. About 30–40% of the diet is fruit. This is also the approximate percentage for vegetables, nuts, seeds, and grains. Over time, the fruits and vegetables become a larger part of the diet, and the grains, especially cooked grains, diminish in quantity. Soaked and sprouted seeds, nuts, grains, and grasses tend to stay about the same. Because the *conscious eating approach* is individualistically attuned to one's own constitutional needs, each person will adapt a little differently to the variations of the seasons and changes in one's lifestyle and environment. The percentages suggested are more to give a general sense of what this stage might resemble.

During the summer, one tends to eat more fruits and less grains. During the winter, the more heating foods, such as seeds, nuts, grains, and legumes, will often be increased. Vata people tend to do better with slightly more grains and soaked seeds. Kapha and pitta people tend to do better with slightly more fruits and vegetables and less oily nuts, seeds, and fruits, like avocados. The cooked foods that are usually part of the 80% raw, and 20% cooked, diet are usually potatoes, grains, and fibrous vegetables with much cellulose coating, such as broccoli and cauliflower.

As one progressively adapts to the Stage III way of eating, one may find oneself losing interest in dairy, even as a condiment, and eating closer to 80% raw, and 20% cooked, food cuisine. The main food groups in the end of Stage III are primarily nuts, seeds, grains, fruits, and vegetables. Dairy may be totally avoided or slipped into the diet occasionally as a condiment on special, rare occasions. The idea is not to be rigid about live food percentages or dairy on a daily basis, but look at an overall average of one's dietary pattern. **This general diet is one that will quite adequately support all one's nutritional needs and provide a gradual detoxification over the years, so one's body will progres-**

sively become healthier and be a better superconductor for the cosmic energy passing through. A general guideline of 80% raw, 20% cooked, and 33% biogenic diet will completely support all aspects of one's life, including the spiritual. Such a Stage III diet can be modified to be building or cleansing, acid- or alkaline-forming, warming or cooling, or more yin or yang. Stage III is also a diet that can still be comfortably adapted to social situations.

Eating or drinking dairy products contributes to iron deficiency because some factors in dairy products block iron uptake.

Dairy products, especially if pasteurized, create acidity and excess mucous.

Symptoms of dairy allergies and lactase intolerance are: gas, bloating, diarrhea, sinus congestion, earaches, chronic colds, rings under the eyes, headaches, and mental symptoms.

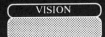

BLACKBOARD FACTS

Preview of Chapter 22
Stage Four: Olympic Vegetarian Diet

This is a diet that seems to accelerate the spiritualizing sensitivity and process in many people. It is a diet for spiritual athletes. The people who do best on it are those who have reached a certain amount of stability and harmony in their lives and are already experienced vegetarians. It is a 95% or more live food diet with about 50% biogenic food. Although this is a powerful diet for enhancing spiritual life, diet is still just an aid to receiving and holding God's Grace. This chapter describes how to apply the art of conscious eating in a refined way. Although you may not feel it is time to try a Stage IV diet, its principles are worth understanding and applying to your diet. Do you feel ready to apply conscious eating principles to your own diet?

I.   Becoming a spiritual athlete

II. One cannot eat one's way to God or personal happiness

III. Stage IV: high biogenic food diet

IV. Developing the intuitive art of conscious eating

Chapter 22

Stage IV: Olympic Vegetarian Diet

Stage IV marks the difference between a diet that simply aids health, well-being, and spiritual development and one that positively **accelerates** the process. Stage IV is ninety-five to one hundred percent live food with approximately fifty percent biogenic food, about fifty percent bioactive food, and zero to five percent cooked foods, like potatoes, or slightly cooked, fibrous vegetables. So far, I have not been able to detect a significant difference between one hundred percent raw and ninety-five percent raw in terms of day to day health or physical and spiritual energy. There may be a measurable difference in terms of longevity, however. My observation and hypothesis is that becoming in touch with just the right amount to eat rather than overeating, even of biogenic foods, plays a more critical role for health than whether it is a ninety-five or one hundred percent raw food diet. That five percent is important because it allows some social leeway, as well as avoids one getting stuck in a perfectionistic type thinking and eating.

Stage IV can be likened to the difference between a personal program of jogging, hiking, and aerobic exercises and a program actively training for the Olympics. Those who aspire for the "Olympic diet" in the context of a fully centered and balanced life, become spiritual athletes who often participate intensely in the shift of planetary consciousness. This in no way means that anyone who is not living on a Stage IV diet is not participating in the process of planetary transformation — we are all doing so in our own way, just by being alive on this earth at this time. So being on a Stage IV diet is not a prerequisite for being "on the team." There are many spiritually active people who are working very hard for the planetary shift in consciousness who are not even vegetarians. In time, for the reasons pointed out in this book, I feel that many of them will eventually make the shift to a vegetarian diet.

Those who choose to adopt a Stage IV level diet may find it hard to ignore the issues of planetary transformation, such as the ecology, peace, equal rights, and health concerns, et cetera. Their very lifestyle will impel them in life-positive, evolutionary directions where they will want to contribute to the greater good of humanity and all life.

A potential psycho-spiritual danger of the ninety-five to one hundred percent raw food diet is the tendency to follow it as some sort of obsessive, self-righteous, self-centered ritual in the hope of achieving happiness, purity, or God just from the diet alone.

One cannot eat one's way to God or even personal happiness. Happiness and God are never one's own. They are a state of awareness in which there is no "I" to claim ownership. God, when experienced as a state of noncausal happiness, is where the ego self or "I" is not. The "I" ceases to exist. It is a consciousness where polarities and distinctions of "I" and "Thou" end. **Diet is a most important aid to this process, but the stabilized peace and happiness of God-awareness requires far more than just a well-thought-out and executed Stage IV diet.** Intense focus on God with a clear heart and mind, supported by whatever psycho-spiritual tradition one chooses, has been the path for ages. Diet helps one walk more quickly and keep stabilized on that timeless path, but it is not "the path" in itself. I choose to eat at the Stage IV level because it is the diet which most powerfully enhances my communion with the Divine. I am grateful, but not at all surprised, that a diet that most enhances the communion with the One is also the most healthy and ecologically harmonious diet as well. It seems that everything that leads to the Divine inherently creates harmony.

Stage IV begins with a complete nondairy vegetarian cuisine of primarily live, soaked, or sprouted nuts, seeds, grains, grasses, vegetables, fruits, and sea vegetables. It is a fifty to sixty percent biogenic diet. As we progress in the process of the Stage IV diet, there is an increase in the amount of life-generating foods, such as all forms of soaked and sprouted nuts, seeds, grains, and grasses, including wheatgrass. There is a progressive decrease in cooked grains which are acid, mucous-producing, and devoid of life-force-filled enzymes. Eventually, there is very little cooked grains in the diet except on occasion as part of the cooked five percent. Depending on our constitutional type, one may vary the percentage of sprouted foods and fruits and vegetables. This diet also can be varied to balance acid-base ratio, the yin and yang balance, and heating and cooling elements. The Stage IV diet can be modified to have a cleansing, rebuilding, or maintenance effect, depending on how one organizes it based on one's individual requirements.

Because this diet is a "jet fuel," high-energy one, to successfully make it work in one's life requires more attention, knowledge, and spiritual maturity. We can no longer afford the luxury of a single theory or understanding guiding us at all times. It is necessary to become, as much as possible, in tune with the "holistic practitioner" within.

To do this requires a certain amount of trial and error experimentation with a variety of live food approaches with real attention to acid-base balance and Ayurvedic constitutional type. For example, one of my clients, who tested acidic, was primarily on live foods except for some grain each day. As soon as she stopped eating grains, her health improved considerably and her pH returned to the normal range. She also felt more balanced emotionally and spiritually. Theoretically one might claim that her new diet was incorrect because it was too yin, having eliminated the yang acid-forming grains, but the clinical results over time gave a total picture which goes beyond the limited theory of yin and yang balance in the diet as the only way to look at health.

My own diet is Stage IV with only occasional and incidental intake of raw or cooked grains. My personal and clinical experience is that grains slow down the movement of the spiritual energy in my body and dulls the sensitivity to this energy. This may not be true for everyone, but this is the way grains work for me and many people I have observed. Although my diet may be yin, I balance it with: the yang-generating heating energy of my physical activities of hatha yoga, fast walking, and running each day; the heating energy of some herbs, like ginger, black peppercorns, cardamom, and cayenne, especially during the winter months; the heating energy of the fire meditation; the yang fire of the sun each day; the grounding nature of my holistic health work; my garden work; and my full participation in my family life. The harmony I experience comes from the balance of the overall net dynamic of yin and yang energies in my total life rather than just the mere summation of the yin and yang energies of my food. This is what I call the wholeness approach.

Diet is an important part of the delicate creation of a total, balanced, harmonious life rather than being the focus of one's life in itself. The Stage IV diet of ninety-five percent living food is a powerful, purifying, energizing, and spiritualizing force in one's life. This diet can help to activate or awaken the spiritual energy. It accelerates the detoxification and healing process on a physical, emotional, and mental plane.

The root meaning of the Latin word "vegetarian" is vegetare, which means to "enliven." The Stage IV diet fulfills this definition to the utmost. It is so powerfully enlivening that to balance the energy created by the diet, one almost requires a life built on a spiritual foundation. Such a spiritual foundation may include some level of spiritual outlook or understanding, a supportive social, spiritual environment, a connection with nature, right livelihood, meditation, and love. Without these other supportive activities and structures in one's life, it is easy to get thrown off balance by the intense physical and psychological toxins that are initially released when one is on this diet. Whereas the Stage III, eighty percent raw, twenty percent cooked, vegetarian diet is generally easy to attain for most everyone who is ready and motivated, the Stage IV diet is more intense and more likely to be successful for those who are more mature and balanced in all areas of their lives. For most people, it requires several years of experience and self-experimentation to become balanced and grounded with the full life-force power of this diet.

In Stage IV, the practice of self-examination and observation is crucial. At this level of refinement our ability to absorb nutrients is continually improving. As already discussed, the 30-year research of the Wendts, a family of medical researchers, established that a high-protein diet clogs the basement membrane. As the excess protein is eliminated by eating less protein and no flesh food, the basement membrane becomes more and more porous. This allows the nutrients to be more easily absorbed. Using an electron microscope, photographs by the

Wendts showed that the basement membrane of babies were very porous. This may be why they can grow so fast on a breast milk diet that is only five percent protein. On a ninety-five percent live food diet, this process of clearing the basement membrane occurs more quickly than on other diets so that one can eat less and still absorb the same amount of nutrients. Eventually one discovers one does not need to eat three meals per day. In my own life, I have essentially eliminated the evening meal, except for occasional raw juices. It was fascinating and exciting for me to be able to comfortably make this switch and discover that my weight remained stable.

How Much Do We Need To Eat

Eating two, or perhaps even one, meal per day may be more closely aligned with what a healthy organism actually needs, although this will vary with one's constitution. As a baby, there is an intense growth phase with rapid gain in weight, brain and nervous system myelinization, and maturing of organs and enzyme systems. During this time, the baby feeds as much as every two hours. As children undergoing rapid growth and development, three meals per day and frequent snacks seem appropriate. In the teenage years there is another rapid maturational growth spurt in which the teenagers seem to always be eating. Sometime in the early twenties, physical growth of the organism is brought to a close and we shift over to more of a "repair and replacement" metabolism. Much less food is needed to sustain this phase of the life cycle. If one continues to eat like a teenager, the primary physical growth that occurs is sideways! With this overweight condition comes those unwanted "spare tires," but even more significant is that waste builds up in the tissues and the circulatory system. When physical growth has reached its peak in early adulthood, for many, two meals per day will be quite adequate to support the physical function of the body.

Although two meals a day may appear to be undereating, it actually isn't because one's rested digestive system is more efficient in absorbing more nutrients from what one eats. If one doesn't eat after 2:30 pm, until the next morning, the digestive system gets three-quarters of a day's rejuvenative rest every day. One of the ongoing issues in the Stage IV diet is eating too much based on one's increased ability to almost completely assimilate everything one eats. To clarify this concept, as the basement membrane becomes more porous, less and less food is needed to give the same amount of nutrients. To eat more than is needed to fulfill one's nutrient needs, even if one eats only one half as many calories as is recommended by government authorities, may still constitute overeating when one's basement membranes are clean.

Eating less is not a back door invitation to anorexia. It is easy to tell if one is undereating because there will be noticeable weight loss and a lack of vitality and health. My clinical observation of appropriate, healthy weight levels is similar to the 1959 weight standards for health set by Metropolitan Life Insurance Company and the weight chart for optimal longevity designed by Stuart Berge, M.D., in his book, *Forever Young*. Dr. Berge's chart reflects the approximate weights that longevity researcher and professor at UCLA Medical School, Roy Walford, M.D., suggests with his calorie-limiting diet approach to maximize a healthy longevity. It is approximately 20% less than what people normally think of as an acceptable body weight. In looking at Drs. Walford and Berge's data on longevity, I was delighted to find that my stabilized weight was precisely what they recommended. My focus, however, has never been on weight charts or calories. It has been on **developing the art of conscious eating, which is to eat just the right amount of food to be totally functional for every aspect of one's life and to enhance communion with the Divine.**

Another factor to consider on a live food diet is the improvement of the metabolic enzyme function as health improves. I have observed that some people initially need supplements, but after a while they need less and less. It seems that as health improves, enough life force is created to regenerate damaged and exhausted enzyme systems or even develop new enzyme systems. Dr. Kervan, in his classic book called *Biological Transmutation*, cites twenty-five years of research that shows how the body can make specific enzymes that can actually transmute one mineral into another. Biological transmutation is one explanation for how some people are able to live without food. They have created the prerequisite enzymes to biologically transmute the basic minerals and other substances to make what the body needs. Obviously, not everyone is able to do this at present, but everyone theoretically has the capability.

There are what seem to be several examples of people who have been observed to live on water alone. There is a Buddhist monk living in the Himalayas who was continually observed by medical researchers for forty-three months. During this time he only drank water. Theresa Neuman, a devoted Catholic peasant, is another individual who was observed to live just on water except for her once a week communion wafer. She too, was observed continuously by researchers who acknowledged the veracity of her ability to live without food. The Taoists in China also mention certain masters who have achieved this ability to live on just air and water. Although living on water is not a goal, it hints at our incredible potential as humans.

These stories are not told so that we should aspire to learn how to live on just water, especially since the water these days is not so reliable. The point is that our enzyme systems are constantly improving so one needs to eat less and less in order to assimilate the same amount of nutrients. Because of our different attachments on many levels to eating three meals including snacks, it is not necessarily so easy to give up these patterns. The secret to making these changes is to go slowly, patiently, and with a great gentleness on oneself. Make changes that one can comfortably make. Forcing changes in diet too quickly often results in reversals that are self-defeating.

On a living food diet, I have personally found that it is easier to experience an extraordinarily exquisite, gentle, eternal flow of the Divine energy coursing through the physical and subtle bodies. The more we experience this energy, the more we are filled with it. The more we experience ourselves permeated with this Divine energy, the more we experience the truth of our existence as "That," and know that this divine experience is our primary identity. This profound and continual experience is not the same, however, as awareness of the One, which is a totality beyond any experience of time, space, senses, and energy, and especially beyond words to describe the experience. The experience of Divine energy helps us feel connected and a part of the flow of the universe. It is the reflection of the One in the mirror of the human body. It is a constant reminder of our eternal nature, of our Divinity. To me, this is the great blessing and grace of a living food diet. **If we are to be in this body, why not live in a way that helps us feel connected to the Divine energy. Why not live in a way that has us experiencing the grace of God's touch?**

One cannot eat one's way to God or even to personal happiness!

Diet is a most important aid to spiritual life; the stabilized peace and happiness of God-awareness requires far more than just a well thought out and executed vegetarian diet.

It is aided by balanced lifestyle, healthy relationships, right livelihood, support from your spiritual friends, praying, meditation, grace, and devotion to God.

VISION

BLACKBOARD FOOD FOR THOUGHT

Preview of Chapter 23
Enzymes: A Secret of Health and Longevity

Enzymes are one of the most important health factors in our foods. The preservation of our enzymes is associated with better health, vitality, and longevity. In this chapter you will learn about food enzymes and how to preserve your own enzyme reserve. If you accept the importance of enzyme preservation, are you ready to change your dietary patterns to conserve them?

  I. Enzymes: a secret of health and longevity
   A. Enzymes are chemical protein complexes and bioenergy reservoirs
   B. Three main types of enzymes: metabolic, digestive, and food
 II. Importance of enzyme preservation
   A. Our bodies only secrete enough enzymes for each food we eat
   B. Enzyme energy is linked to SOEFs
   C. Enzymes decrease with age
   D. Animal research and enzymes
III. The role of food enzymes in digestion
 IV. Enzymes for health
  V. Enzyme-deficient is a hard way to start life
 VI. How do we preserve our enzymes?
   A. Eating raw foods
   B. Live enzyme supplements
   C. Fasting
VII. Not overeating:
   A. Animal life extended by underfeeding
   B. Not overeating results in optimal health
VIII. Enzyme supplementation: live plant digestive engymes
 IX. Persons to use enzymes
   A. Enzymes lost or destroyed in cooked foods
   B. Enzymes decrease with age
   C. Enzyme depletion during illness
   D. Digestive disturbances
   E. Enzymes help detoxify
  X. Food enzymes: a new perspective on food combining

Chapter 23

Enzymes: A Secret of Health and Longevity

As I explained with my new paradigm of nutrition, whenever we process foods in any way, we disorganize the SOEFs of the food, and hence, lower their life force. This manifests on the physical plane in a variety of ways. Enzyme destruction is one of the ways that SOEF disruption manifests. According to Dr. Howell, whom many consider the father of food enzyme research in this century, **enzymes are both chemical protein complexes and bioenergy reservoirs.** In the physical body, as bioenergy reservoirs, they are among the closest, analogously, in their patterning to SOEFs. I think of them as high-energy vortex points which step down the cosmic SOEF energy into the body. Dr. Robert G. Denkewalter, one of the first to synthesize an enzyme protein, says that enzymes are *"embarrassing because they can do at body temperatures and in simple solution what we organic chemists can do only with corrosive agents and at high temperatures and with laborious processes."* Dr. Troland, from Harvard University, who was one of the first scientists to put forth a living theory for enzymes, said *"Life is something which has been built up about the enzyme; it is corollary of enzyme activity."* Chemists concede that only the living organism makes active enzymes. Dr. Howell points out that **enzymes are not simple chemical catalysts, but have this vital life force that initiates biochemical interactions.** He also points out that the capacity of an organism to make active live enzymes depends on the available life force of the organism. The corollary to this is that the enzyme activity of an organism is a way to measure the life force of the organism. Ann Wigmore, the mother of the raw foods movement in America, feels that *"enzyme preservation is the secret to health."*

Two key concepts taught by Howell are: (1) that enzymes are living, biochemical factors that activate and carry out all the biological processes in the body, such as digestion, nerve impulses, the detoxification process, the functioning of RNA/DNA, repairing and healing the body, and even thinking; and (2) the capacity of an organism to make enzymes is exhaustible. Therefore, on the biological level, how we utilize and replenish our enzyme resources will be a measure of our overall health and longevity. By understanding how enzymes work, we will understand why it is best to eat a higher percentage of mother nature's offering "au naturelle."

There are three main types of enzymes: **metabolic**, which activates all our metabolic processes; **digestive**, for the digestion of food; and a relatively newly conceived category called **food enzymes**. Food enzymes are present in all live foods, and serve the function of specifically activating the digestion of those foods in which they occur. Live foods also contain a variety of metabolic enzymes as well, such as superoxide dismutase (S.O.D.).

There are over 1300 enzymes that have been identified today in the human body. Each organ has its own set of enzymes. Of the 1300-plus enzymes, about 24 of them are digestive enzymes. The three main types of digestive enzymes are proteases, which digest proteins; amylases, which digest carbohydrates; and lipases, which digest fats. Mother Nature works in conjunction with us by adding what we will now call from our human-centered point of view, "food enzymes," to each living element of nature. These food enzymes contained in the food have the exact ratio of proteases, amylases, and lipases that are required to begin the digestion of the food for the body.

Importance of Enzyme Preservation

The relevance of this gift of Mother Nature becomes more obvious when we explore what Dr. Howell called the Law of Adaptive Secretion of Digestive Enzymes. Based on research at Northwestern University and confirmed by many other researchers, the law of adaptive secretion proposes that **the living organism will secrete no more enzymes than are needed for digestion of a particular food.** This means that if a food from Mother Nature comes into our system in its live form, filled with exactly the right proportion of food enzymes to begin digestion, then it will result in less digestive enzymes being secreted by our organism for the digestive process. Researchers have found that when dogs are given cooked foods, after a week the enzyme content of the saliva greatly increases in order to digest the cooked foods. When the dogs were put back on their normal diet of raw foods, within a week, the enzyme content of the saliva went back to its normally low content. The implication of these studies is that since the raw food contained the self-digesting food enzymes, the dogs did not have to use up its own enzyme reserves to digest the food as it did with the cooked food.

Human research as far back as 1907 has shown that the type of enzymes secreted in the human system also depended on the type of diet. Simon, in 1907, showed that the starch-digesting enzyme, amylase, in human saliva increased with a high-starch diet and decreased with a high-protein, low-starch diet. In 1927, Goldstein showed that the content of fat-digesting lipase, protein-digesting trypsin, and starch-digesting amylase in the pancreatic secretions of humans varied in direct relation to the amount of fats, protein, or complex carbohydrates in the diet. The implication of this and the dog research is that by taking in foods high in live enzymes, less of our own digestive enzymes need to be used, so we are able to conserve enzyme energy. Enzyme energy is linked to our vital force and therefore the energy of our SOEFs. The higher our vital force, or SOEFs, the better is our health.

The significance of enzymes preservation and the Law of Adaptive Secretion becomes even clearer when we see how much our enzymes level is linked to chronological age and disease. For example, Dr. Meyer and his associates at

Chicago's Michael Reese Hospital, found that the amylase in the saliva of young adults was thirty times greater than in people with a chronological age of 69. Dr. Eckardt in Germany found that young people had 25 units of amylase in their urine as compared to 14 in older people. Other researchers have found that the amount of S.O.D. in an 80-year-old person is 57% of that of a newborn and 61% of that of a 10-year-old child. In a 40-year-old person, the S.O.D. was found to be 84% of a newborn and 87% of a 10-year-old child. Individuals of 27 years of age have been found to have twice the amount of lipase than that of 77-year-old people. A lower enzyme content is also found in people with chronic diseases. In 111 Japanese patients with tuberculosis, 82% had lower enzyme contents than normal. In 40 patients with liver diseases, all had lower levels of amylase. In diabetes, it has been found that 86% are lower in amylase. Researchers have also found a lowered lipase level in people with obesity, arteriosclerosis, and high blood pressure. Directly and indirectly, we can see how important enzyme preservation and harmonious utilization is to health and vitality.

This same sort of enzyme decrease with chronological age happens in the animal kingdom. Researchers have found the enzyme content of younger Daphnia insects, potato beetles, grasshoppers, fruit flies, fire flies, and rats to be significantly greater than for their older counterparts.

The above findings may be quite connected with the research of Dr. Kollath of the Karolinska Hospital in Stockholm, who found that when he put animals on a diet of cooked and processed foods similar to the regular Western diet, they initially appeared to be as healthy as animals on live foods. As the animals reached adulthood, those on the cooked and processed foods began to age more quickly. They also developed chronic, degenerative disease processes at an earlier age. The animal's degenerative diseases resembled the very human diseases that are common in the western industrialized world, such as osteoarthritis, osteoporosis, and constipation, et cetera. He called the state of health of these animals, meso-health, a sort of half-health. Those animals raised on raw foods did not suffer from these problems. The good news was that the meso-health of these animals could be reversed. It couldn't be done with megadoses of vitamin or mineral supplementation, however. The only thing which worked to reverse the aging process and bring the animals back to a normal state of health was to give the animals raw foods. Dr. Kollath called these heat-sensitive, unknown factors in the raw food "auxones." Most likely what he termed auxones were enzymes. There are many other factors in raw foods that also support health, but the enzymes are probably the most significant.

Similar animal research was done over a ten-year period by Frances Pottenger, M.D., using 900 cats. He gave half of the cats raw milk and raw meat and the other half were given pasteurized milk and cooked meat. In the first generation, the cats on the cooked food developed a pattern of degenerative disease similar to what we see in humans. In the second and third generations of

THREE STAGES OF DIGESTION

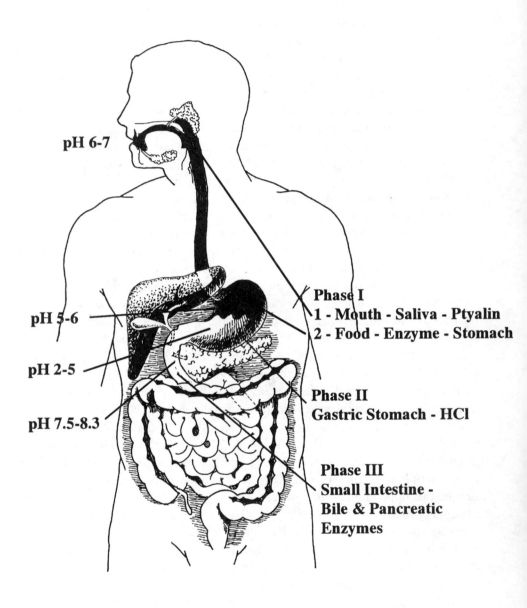

pH 6-7

pH 5-6

pH 2-5

pH 7.5-8.3

Phase I
1 - Mouth - Saliva - Ptyalin
2 - Food - Enzyme - Stomach

Phase II
Gastric Stomach - HCl

Phase III
Small Intestine -
Bile & Pancreatic
Enzymes

Fig. 23

cooked-food-eating cats, he observed the onset of congenital bone deformities, hyperactivity, and sterility. The cats became so dysfunctional that plants would not even grow on their manure. The conclusion he made was that some critical, heat-sensitive factor was missing from the cooked food. The main factors known to be completely destroyed by heat—are enzymes.

According to Dr. Howell, temperatures of 118° F applied for one half hour will destroy all the food enzymes in a particular food. This is a temperature that is sensed as warm to the hand. One can see that any kind of cooking, boiling, baking, or frying destroys essentially 100% of the enzymes as does canning, food irradiation, and microwave cooking. Dr. Howell points out that even boiling food for three minutes will kill all the enzymes. His research shows that even at 145° F, the temperature for pasteurization, 80-95% of the enzymes are destroyed after one half hour.

The Role of Food Enzymes in Digestion

To develop an overview, we need to dissolve some false concepts about the process of digestion and understand how food enzymes work in our total organism. Contrary to the myth that our stomach is simply one big container for the digestion of protein, researchers have conclusively shown that there are two distinctly different digestive sections of the stomach. There is an upper part of the stomach which retains food for 30-60 minutes. There is no peristaltic action in this part of the stomach and there are no enzymes secreted from its walls. The second part of the stomach is the lower part, called the pyloric stomach. This is where the hydrochloric acid and pepsin are secreted and considerably more protein digestion is carried on. During the first 30-60 minutes in the upper stomach, digestion takes place primarily by the food enzymes released from the raw foods. The digestive process actually starts in the mouth where the ptyalin in the saliva begins to digest the carbohydrates. In the process of chewing, the cell walls of the plant food are broken down and the food enzymes begin to get released also. Most green foods are covered by a thin layer of cellulose for which humans have no digestive enzymes. For this reason, it is important to chew our food well because when the cell walls of the plant are opened up by the action of chewing they release cellulase in the food itself, which helps to digest this cellulose. It is my impression that some of the green plants that are more difficult to digest in their raw form, such as broccoli, have a thicker layer of cellulose, and the problem is that we do not chew it well enough to break open the cell walls and release the plant cellulase (see fig. 23).

Given this new perspective on the upper part of the stomach, which is anatomically known as the cardiac area, we will now call this upper part of the stomach the 'food enzyme stomach.' A food enzyme stomach is found in many animals. Cattle, sheep, whales, dolphins, and chickens all have them, although often called by different names, such as the rumen in cows and crop in chickens. Support for this idea of two parts of the stomach is also found in one of the medical school anatomical classics, *Gray's Anatomy*. It states that the stomach consists of two anatomically distinct parts. The first part is called the upper, or cardiac portion, where salivary digestion continues and in which there is no peristalsis. The lower part is called the pylorus. Pepsin and hydrochloric acid are secreted in the pylorus. This lower section has a pH of 1.6-2.4. The upper stomach has a pH that ranges from 5 to 6. This is important because the food enzymes are still active in this 5 to 6 pH range. They are temporarily inactivated in the 2.4 or lower range. A number of researchers show that the food enzymes again become active in the alkaline pH of the small intestine where they complete their work.

Although this seems like a new concept, research by a variety of people shows digestion does occur in the food enzyme stomach. Dr. Beazell reported in the *Journal of Laboratory and Clinical Medicine* that 20% of starch was digested in the stomach, and only 3% of protein, in this first hour of digestion. Olaf Berglim, a professor of physiology at the Illinois College of Medicine, found that 45 minutes after giving his subjects mashed potatoes and bread that 76% of the starch in the mashed potatoes, and 59% in the bread, was digested. Other researchers have found similar results. This research was most likely done with cooked foods and so probably only the ptyalin (amylase) from the saliva was active in the food enzyme stomach. Dr. Howard Loomis, who is considered to be Dr. Howell's successor, estimates that **an average of 60% of starches, 30% of protein, and 10% of fat are digested in the food enzyme stomach.** We can only assume that considerably more would be digested if it were raw food because the raw food would have its own digestive enzymes that would be released for self-digestion. The point is, as with the rest of nature's animals, the food enzyme stomach is where all the food enzymes in the raw foods are engaged in active digestion along with our own ptyalin and amylase secretions from our own saliva.

The result of this food enzyme digestion in the food enzyme stomach is that the pancreas is not forced to work so hard to secrete so many enzymes. This conserves the body's enzymes for use toward nondigestive, metabolic purposes such as detoxification, repair, and the health and proper functioning of the endocrine glands and other vital organs. Because eating raw foods liberates enzymes for use in other parts of the body, the importance of making a high percentage of our diet biogenic and bioactive is obvious.

Evidence compiled by Dr. Howell strongly suggests that eating of foods that have become devoid of enzymes by way of cooking, food irradiation, and microwaving causes an enlargement of the pancreas and also stresses out other associated endocrine glands, such as the adrenals, pituitary, ovary, and testes. In all of nature, the human pancreas is three times larger, as compared to total body weight, than that of any other animal. What is interesting is that when mice are fed cooked foods, the ratio of their pancreas weight to total body weight becomes approximately that of a human's. When they are switched back to a raw food diet, their pancreas shrinks back to normal size. The most obvious conclusion is that the pancreas becomes hypertrophied, or enlarged, because it is forced to keep up a high digestive enzyme output.

A great deal of the body energy goes into the process of digestion. Sometimes so much energy is needed for digestion that we tend to become sleepy after a meal. This increased amount of energy implies a large input of enzymes are used up in the digestive process. In order to keep this enzyme production up, some theorize that the pancreas has to draw enzymes from other bodily glands. This forces these other glands to overwork and eventually enlarge to compensate for the demand. This hypertrophy primarily starts with the endocrine glands. Hypertrophy of a gland eventually leads to its early exhaustion.

Perhaps associated with the phenomena of increased enzyme secretion by the pancreas due to cooked food eating is the startling findings mentioned earlier of a Swiss physician, Paul Kanchaukoff. In 1930, he showed that the eating of cooked foods caused leucocytosis which is an increase in white blood cells in the blood. This even occurred when water was heated above 191°F. There are two hypothesis that explain this. One is that the white blood cells, which have a similar lipase, protease, and amylase ratio as the pancreas, are actually taking enzymes to the pancreas to boost its supply. The second explanation is that when the food is cooked and the water is boiled the body recognizes them as a foreign body and has an immune response to it. Both explanations may be true simultaneously. In any case, the repeated leucocytosis with every meal certainly puts a strain on the immune system. Kanchaukoff also found that when subjects started a meal with raw foods which equaled more than half of the meal, they were able to have some cooked foods and not produce a leucocytosis. When people ate biocidic, highly processed, or junk foods, not only did they get leukocytosis, but the normal white blood cell ratios became deranged to the extent that they resembled the pattern one sees with blood poisoning from contaminated meat. From the point of view of the SOEFs, one can see how eating biogenic and bioactive foods brings SOEF and enzyme energy into the system, and eating biostatic (cooked foods) or biocidic foods requires SOEF and enzyme energy to complete the digestion, and therefore depletes the SOEFs and enzyme reserves.

Enzymes for Health

In order to understand the importance of enzymes for our health, it would be useful to understand how they specifically affect our health. For example, a medical doctor at Tufts Medical School found that in 100% of the cases of obesity he studied, all had lipase deficiencies. The implication was that they had a decreased ability to assimilate fat properly. The fat ended up being stored as fatty tissue rather than being broken down.

Cooked food also seems to stimulate the craving for food because the organs are not getting the nutrients they would normally get in uncooked food. The body naturally craves more nutrients, which may translate into an uncontrollable appetite and lack of willpower. Farmers have known for awhile that if you give raw potatoes to hogs they will not gain weight, but if you give them cooked potatoes they gain weight. In my clinical practice, I often will see people lose weight readily when they go on a raw food diet. Many times this is all that is needed to help people lose weight.

As pointed out in an earlier chapter, cooked fats are missing lipase and have significantly less biologically active cis fatty acids. The difference in the digestive pattern of the raw versus cooked fat may also be important. The raw fat begins its digestion with its own lipase in the food enzyme stomach under slightly acid conditions. The cooked fat, without its own lipase, doesn't begin a significant digestive transformation until it is in the highly alkaline pH of the small intestine. When they both reach the small intestine, the predigested raw fats or oils are already beginning the next step in the digestion, while the undigested cooked fats are just starting their digestion. This may result in a slight shift in how it is metabolized and could cause some altering of the cholesterol. This interference with the fat digestion sequence may be another reason a high, cooked, fat intake is so deleterious to our health. The other reason is that eating cooked fats or oils causes an eventual lipase deficiency in the system. It could be that lipase is in some manner involved with fat and cholesterol metabolism. For these reasons, a deficiency of lipase may have a profound metabolic effect on both obesity and cholesterol disorders. It will be interesting to see what the researchers will discover in the next few years about this important health question.

Enzyme Deficient is a Hard Way to Start Life

For babies who are not breast fed, they are immediately forced to deal with a lipase and amylase deficiency in their food because they get almost no enzymes at all in pasteurized milk. In a study of over 20,000 babies, the rate of illness was compared between completely breast-fed babies and bottle-fed babies. Pasteurized milk-fed babies had a mortality rate 56 times greater than breast milk-fed babies. The general rate of sickness was nearly double for the pasteurized milk fed babies. Although there are other factors involved with breast feeding that make it desirable for health, it is very important to realize that babies who are not fed with breast milk are being short changed by the enzyme-deficient foods they are being fed. This is probably true for the majority of our children in America who have become addicted to enzymeless junk and fast foods. We are paying the

346

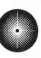
price for altering the way Mother Nature presents us with Her gifts. By cooking food we contribute to the loss of our health at an earlier age.

For diabetics and hypoglycemics, it seems that whether the food is cooked or raw is very important for their well-being. In research at George Washington University Hospital, when 50 grams of raw starch were administered to patients, the blood sugar only rose 1 mg in one half hour before it began to decrease. With the cooked starch there was a dramatic average increase of 56 mg in one half hour and then a 51 mg average drop by one hour. This is quite a significant shift in blood glucose. The major difference between the raw and cooked is the raw starch came with its own amylase and so was able to be predigested in the food enzyme stomach. Raw food and low-fat diets, with the use of added food enzymes, have been found to be a very effective treatment of adult onset diabetes. On such a diet, if properly managed by a physician, adult onset diabetics can actually stop needing insulin injections or oral medications.

How Do We Preserve Our Enzymes?

Eating raw foods is the number one activity which preserves enzymes and maximizes health. It is the diet of choice of all the rest of Mother Nature's children that dwell on this planet. Animals which live in the wild do not suffer from chronic degenerative diseases as does the human race and domesticated animals. It is a striking fact that all other species, without exception, eat their foods raw, whereas the overwhelming majority of humans do not. When these same animals are fed cooked foods, they too, begin to suffer chronic degenerative diseases.

The foods with the highest amount of live enzymes are biogenic, predigested, and fermented foods. Seeds that have the highest enzyme content are those with a 1/4 inch sprout. Some have estimated that the enzyme content is ten times greater at this 1/4 inch sprouting stage. In Asia, the idea of fermenting soybeans by exposing them to the enzymatic action of fungal plants has been practiced for thousands of years. The fungal plants not only add enzymes to the food, but predigest the protein, carbohydrates, and oils. Miso, a fermented soy bean product, and tempeh, a soy product with a cultured fungus, are examples of this. One can also make enzyme-rich, fermented, raw seed and nut cheeses through a fermentation process (see recipes section).

Although all live foods are high in enzymes, there can be a tendency for some people on a live food diet to become too thin if they just eat vegetables, fruits, and sprouts. Through self-experimentation, I found that on a vegan diet of 99% live fruits, vegetables, seeds, and sprouts, with occasional sprouted or cooked grains, I am able to maintain my weight. By adding certain foods that not only are high in enzymes, but also high in carbohydrates, or lipids, I am able to increase my weight at will. These foods primarily are: bananas, avocados, and soaked or sprouted raw seeds and nuts. Other foods that are high in enzymes, as well as calories, are: grapes, mangos, dates, raw honey, raw butter, and unpasteurized milk. Though raw dairy products are high in enzymes, I do not necessarily endorse their consumption.

Fasting is another powerful way to conserve and redirect enzyme potential. During a fast, we stop producing digestive enzymes and the enzyme energy is diverted to the metabolic sphere of operations, which include an increased rate of autolysis (breakdown of old cells), as well as a breakdown and elimination of fatty deposits, incomplete proteins, and other toxic material in the system. The enzymes become a rejuvenating power for us. Raw food expert and author of *Survival into the 21st Century*, Victoras Kulvinskas, suggests that during a fast, our natural, body bacteria have an opportunity to add a great deal more of their enzymes to our system and thus increase our total enzyme force. My observation in guiding many individual fasts and running several spiritual fasting retreats per year is that fasting is an incredible way to rejuvenate our total life force and SOEFs. When we fast on water or juices, we are giving a substantial rest to our digestive enzymes systems, and this takes the burden off our enzyme pool.

Not overeating: The Secret to Health, Longevity, and Enzyme Preservation

Not overeating raw foods is itself another way to conserve enzymes. It is different than an obsessive undereating which can result in a physical and mental deprivation syndrome. **Not overeating is what I call the art of conscious eating. It is learning to take just the right amount of food and drink to support our individual needs on every level of our spiritual and worldly functioning.** Researchers have shown that not overeating increases longevity. World-famous nutritionist, Paavo Airola, Ph.D., has proclaimed that undereating is the most important health and longevity secret. He felt that overeating of even health foods was one of the main causes of ill health.

Jesus, in the *Essene Gospel of Peace, Book One (p. 31)*, said,

"And when you eat, never eat unto fullness."

Moses Maimonides (1135-1204), one of the most celebrated of all Jewish healers and spiritual teachers taught:

"Overeating is like a deadly poison to any constitution and is the principle cause of all disease."

Animal research by Dr. Clive Mckay of Cornell University showed that when their food intake was halved, the life span of rats was doubled and they were healthier. The rat's life span increased to the equivalent of approximately 170 human years. At Brown University, 158 animals were overfed and another group was put on a near starvation diet. Those on the sparse diet lived 40% longer. For those who might be concerned that they have been irreversibly overeating to the detriment of their health, research by Roy Walford and Richard Weindruch showed that one could extend the life of even middle-aged animals by underfeeding them. Some of their mice lived 40% longer, and fish lived three times longer, on a sparse diet. They also noticed that degenerative diseases, such as cancer, and heart and kidney disease, occurred less frequently and the onset of these diseases occurred at a later age in the underfed mice. These researchers even discovered that the mice's immune systems were rejuvenated. For example, underfed mice had only 13% spontaneous cancer as compared to 50% for mice on the same type of foods, but with no limits on the food intake. Kidney disease was 25% in underfed mice verses 100% in the mice with an unlimited diet. There was 26% heart disease for the underfed mice verses 96% with heart disease for the overfed. Other animal research has now confirmed their findings. The underfed animals stayed physiologically younger for a longer time. Animal research in both America and Germany has also shown that rats fed once per day had higher enzyme activities in the pancreas and fat cells and a 17% increased life span over that of the frequent eaters. It seems that if the enzymes are only secreted once per day, there will not be as many of them used up as with frequent meals. **The evidence of the effects of not overeating is that it is actually a method for life and vitality extension as well as prevention of degenerative disease**.

Research suggests that excessive eating causes oxidative stress to the system which results in free radical damage to the tissues and an increase in cross-linking of the active protein in the tissues and cells so that they do not function properly any more. Free radicals are harmful molecules that can be generated by poor nutrition, emotional stress, environmental pollution, surgery, radiation, food irradiation, physical stress, bacterial and viral illnesses, and the aging process in general. These free radicals have a free electron that disrupts the integrity of cell membranes. They are quenched and neutralized by molecules called antioxidants.

Eating a dietary program which is low in protein and total calories helps the body fully assimilate what is eaten. This way of eating creates a minimum of metabolic by-products such as free radicals. Protein cross-linking in the tissues is a sign of aging and has been found to be connected to free radical formation. Eating less food and increasing the quality of food is something everyone can do if they put their awareness on this aspect of a balanced life. Not only will this approach cut down on the rate of aging, but unlike most medical approaches, this way of living will actually save money by not having medical problems to begin with.

Not overeating results in optimal health and not malnutrition. **Not overeating in our society is eating what we need rather than what we desire or that to which we are addicted.** This is not so easy for most of us. We live in an environment of excessive stimulation from empty calories and negative thoughts. We are undernourished from not getting enough from all our processed foods and overfed with junk in order to compensate for not getting enough real nourishment. Not overeating is a part of conscious eating. It means eating what is appropriate to our health, vitality, longevity, and what will bring us into harmony with our body and the planetary body. This understanding of the importance of not overeating has inspired me to switch in my own life to two meals instead of three meals per day.

Historical and Cultural Evidence for the Benefit of Not Overeating

Cultural evidence supports this not overeating approach also. The cultures in which people have been found to live long and healthy lives, such as in the Vilcabamban region of Ecuador, the Hunzukuts of West Pakistan, the Tarahumara Indians of Mexico, and the Abkhazians of Russia, all consume a low-protein, high, natural carbohydrate diet that have about one half to one third the calories and the amount of protein that the average American eats.

Historically, there have been several cases of longevity associated with eating less. Saint Paul the Anchorite lived to be 113 on dates and water. Thomas Carn, born in London in 1588, lived to be 207 on two vegetarian meals per day. This health wisdom as been with us for thousands of years, but few really put it into practice. On a 5000 year old Egyptian pyramid an inscription of this wisdom was found, "man lives on one quarter of what he eats, on the other three quarters, his doctor lives."

One of the most famous of the "non-overeaters" was Luigi Cornaro, a Venetian nobleman who lived from 1464 to 1566. By his late 40s, he had become deathly sick from overeating. A doctor, Father Benedict, who had been trained in the Essene health philosophy, explained to him about eating less. He simplified his diet to 12 ounces of solid, and 14 ounces of liquid, food per day and recovered to live to be 102. Luigi went on to teach many people about this Essene way of health, including the Pope. His writings on not overeating are summed up in two statements:

"The less I ate, the better I felt." and " Not to satiate oneself with food is the science of health."

From what we now know about the importance of enzyme preservation, not overeating, especially of raw foods, less frequent meals, no snacking between meals, and fasting are effective ways to conserve enzymes and thus build and maintain a high quality of vitality and healthy longevity. The idea of not overeating may be threatening in America where we have over 80 million people who are considered overweight. We are a country of overabundance in which overeating has become a major way of avoiding unwanted feelings, such as intimacy, sex, feelings of loneliness, feeling unloved, and anger. It can also be a form of self-sabotage and self-abuse, as well as a slow form of suicide. Overeating food has become one of America's most serious drug habits.

Enzyme Supplementation

In addition to eating live food, and not overeating, the use of exogenous enzyme supplementation is another way to build up enzyme reserve. Since 1949, enough research has thoroughly documented that these enzymes are not only active in the digestive system but will increase in concentration in the blood after taken orally. For example, researchers who fed raw soybean lipase to rabbits demonstrated that the blood serum lipase was elevated in response to the administration of lipase orally. Work by Peter Rothchild, M.D., PhD., has found that in a double blind study using the antioxidant enzymes from a wheat sprout matrix that there was a 70-90% increase in blood levels of serum glutathione peroxidase after giving these oral wheat sprout concentrates. In another similar wheat sprout enzyme study, he found a 40% increase in SOD and a 60% increase in serum catalase. The fact that we can absorb these enzymes through our digestive tract is important because it means we have a way of correcting some of these enzyme deficiencies. Of course, it is a lot easier and less expensive if we do not create the deficiencies by not eating cooked foods in the first place.

Live plant digestive enzymes may be the best source of enzyme supplementation. They seem to be active at a much fuller pH range than animal enzymes. These plant enzymes show some activity in the stomach, especially the enzyme stomach, and become immediately active in the small intestine. One study, reported in the *Journal of Clinical Nutrition,* found that 70% of plant amylase is active in the small intestine after it was ingested orally. Because of these facts, I recommend that people consider using plant digestive enzymes for their digestive supplementation. They are actually concentrated food enzymes from nature. This is welcome news to those who feel they need digestive enzymes, but who do not like to eat animal pancreas products taken from animal slaughterhouses.

Animal enzymes, such as pepsin, only work in a moderately strong acid environment, such as the stomach. Trypsin only works in a slightly alkaline environment, such as in the small intestine where it is secreted. Because of the versatility of their activity, plant digestive enzyme supplementation can take the stress off the entire digestive enzyme system. Some pancreatic animal enzyme tablets have an enteric coating which protects them from inactivation in the stomach. These enzymes require the pancreas to secrete enough enzymes to digest their enteric coating before they start to operate. Thus, they do not give the pancreas a chance to conserve its digestive enzyme power for uses in other places in the body like the plant enzymes do.

Another form of enzyme supplementation is produced by growing and harvesting wheat berries which are specifically cultured to be high in antioxidant enzymes. These antioxidant enzymes neutralize free radicals throughout the system at the cellular level. In addition to the medical use of these enzymes, we live in such a toxic environment that most everyone needs to maintain proper antioxidant enzyme levels as a critical protection barrier. Some of the preliminary research has suggested that once optimal blood levels of these antioxidant enzymes are obtained, they do not go any higher by increasing the dosage. This suggests the possibility that some of these live enzymes might be converted to other types of metabolic enzymes in the system. Thus, the use of these enzymes affords an opportunity to protect against free radicals as well as increase general enzyme reserves.

Reasons to Use Enzymes

1. Anyone eating cooked, microwaved, or irradiated food should take food enzyme supplements to compensate for the lost and destroyed, naturally occurring food enzymes that were previously in the food. This approach is still not the same as eating the food in its active, live state. Even if a person eats 90% live food, if they still have imbalances in their health, they would do well to take enzyme supplements.
2. Since age correlates with a decreasing enzyme reserve, enzyme supplementation should theoretically slow down the aging process by building up the enzymes and quenching free radicals.
3. During acute and chronic illnesses, there is often an enzyme depletion that can be alleviated by enzyme supplementation. In my clinical observations as well as those of others, enzyme supplementation seems to increase the rate of recovery.
4. I have found that people with digestive disturbances, endocrine gland imbalances, blood sugar imbalances, diabetes, obesity, cholesterol excesses, stress-related problems, and arthritic inflammations all seem to benefit from enzyme supplementation. Dr. W.W. Oelgoetz has shown that partially digested fats, protein, and carbohydrate molecules get into the blood system when the blood enzymes become too low. He observed that when he gives clients oral supplements of amylase, lipase, and proteases, the allergies which seem to be associated with these incompletely digested molecules subside. Thus, enzyme supplementation can be a support to the immune system.
5. Enzymes help the detoxification process because they free up more metabolic enzyme energy for this work.

Those who probably do not need food enzyme supplementation are people who are healthy, eating at least 80% live foods, and are living the holistic awareness of the Essene Tree of Life.

Food Enzymes: A New Perspective on the Theory of Food Combining

The generally held theory of food combining in certain sectors of the vegetarian community is that certain combinations of foods will disrupt digestion and cause putrefaction, fermentation, toxic acids, and heartburn. The combining at the same time of certain foods is said to disrupt digestion, for example: fruits and vegetables; fruits and starches; fruits and protein; starches and proteins; simple sugars, complex carbohydrates, and proteins; fats and protein; acid fruits and proteins; acid fruits and starches; two different types of concentrated starches; two different types of concentrated proteins; and dairy or melons with any other food. These poor combinations are said to take longer to digest and use up a great deal of enzyme energy. Many find these "rules" to be obsessively overwhelming The idea of food combining is not new; it is historically recorded in Exodus 16:8 which says, "And Moses said...the Lord shall give you in the evening flesh to eat, and in the morning bread to the full." This can be interpreted to mean that we should not combine starches and proteins. Another Kosher food-combining law from the Torah is not to combine flesh and dairy at the same meal.

The general theoretical principle behind food combining is that the different food classes require different enzyme secretions and digestive pHs for their digestion. They also have different rates of digestion. For example, food-combining advocates claim that fruit digestion requires an alkaline solution that neutralizes the acid medium needed for the protein digestion and, therefore, fruit and proteins are a bad combination. Also, fruit has a faster digestive rate than protein and if the fruits are held up for the slower protein digestion, they will begin to ferment. This is also why fruits and starches should not be combined. Fruits and vegetables are said to be incompatible because the enzymes required for their digestion neutralize each other and block digestion.

From a live food perspective, there are some major incongruities in the orthodox food combining approach that need to be considered. The first is the scientific evidence that live foods bring with them their own active digestive enzymes which digest a considerable amount of the food in the enzyme, or upper, stomach. Therefore, the concept of different bodily enzyme secretions for the different foods cancelling each other is much less an issue, especially in the food enzyme stomach where no enzymes other than saliva and those released by the living foods themselves are activated. It is a proven scientific fact that each raw food comes complete with its own set of specifically combined enzymes to digest that specific food. For example, seeds are made up of primarily oils and protein, so Mother Nature has packaged in the seeds sufficient amounts of lipase for the oils and proteases for the protein. In seeds there is not much amylase present because they do not contain much starch.

Another scientific fact that needs to be considered is that there are two distinctly different digestive stomachs. There is the pyloric, or primarily protein-digesting, stomach, and the food enzyme stomach, in which all the raw food starches, protein, sugars, and lipids are self-digested. We do not have just one stomach in which competing enzymes are poured as if into a bag, cancelling each other out. In the food enzyme stomach, the pH is between 5 and 6, which is a range in which all of the plant food enzymes for all the different classes of food are active. No enzyme of any class of food is neutralized by any other food enzymes in the food enzyme stomach.

A third point is a set of foods which are called the predigested foods. This predigestion process happens primarily by soaking or sprouting the seeds, nuts, and grains. In this process, the enzymes inhibitors, phytates, and oxalates are deactivated and almost entirely washed away after 6-24 hours of soaking. During soaking, complex carbohydrates are broken down to simple sugars, oils are broken down into free fatty acids, and proteins are broken down into free amino acids. In these predigested forms, these foods are much easier to digest and assimilate. Some examples of these highly assimilable predigested foods are: raw, soaked, and sprouted seeds; nuts, grains, and legumes; bee pollen; raw nut and seed ferments; nut and seed cheeses and yogurts; and other fermented products, such as sauerkraut, tempeh, and miso. Most of these foods, except the tempeh and miso, which are cooked, can be digested easily with all classes of foods, including fruits.

The ability to comfortably combine predigested protein and fruits is particularly important for people with hypoglycemia. I have found a great deal of my patients who have hypoglycemia become imbalanced by just eating fruit by itself in the morning. By adding the predigested seeds and nuts either directly to the fruit, or blending them into seed sauces, hypoglycemics have stabilized well and improved with this approach. I have also had good results using these predigested proteins for people with digestive disorders or other forms of malnutrition.

The fourth consideration is food enzymes are not destroyed in the very acid, protein-digestive part of the stomach. They again resume active digestive capacities in the more alkaline-digestive part of the small intestine. They are also not neutralized by either the acid secretions or the alkaline pancreatic secretions of the small intestines and so they keep their digestive powers to a lesser or greater extent throughout the full digestive process.

I do not intend to negate the orthodox theory of food combining. It is, however, put into a less significant and proper perspective if one eats primarily live or predigested foods. By presenting this more liberal view, I will be very happy if just one less person doesn't become obsessive about food combining; or if one less person stops breaking down in frustration and stops becoming

Food Combining Self-Experiment

Eat only a single combination at a meal and observe

What I Ate

- Grain & Vegetables
- Bean & Vegetables
- Fruit & Beans
- Fruit & Vegetables
- Fruit & Grain
- Grain & Dairy
- Melons & Fruit
- Melons & Anything Else
- Dairy & Fish

When
Breakfast / Lunch / Dinner

How Much
Little / Moderate / Too Much

SYMPTOM

What I Ate

	Gas	Bloating	Headache	Feel Full	Feel Hunger	Indigestion	Food is a Lump	Feel Fine
Grain & Vegetables	1hr☐ 2hr☐ 3hr☐	1hr☐ 2hr☐ 3hr☐	1hr☐ 2hr☐ 3hr☐	1hr☐ 2hr☐ 3hr☐	1hr☐ 2hr☐ 3hr☐	1hr☐ 2hr☐ 3hr☐	1hr☐ 2hr☐ 3hr☐	1hr☐ 2hr☐ 3hr☐
Bean & Vegetables	1hr☐ 2hr☐ 3hr☐	1hr☐ 2hr☐ 3hr☐	1hr☐ 2hr☐ 3hr☐	1hr☐ 2hr☐ 3hr☐	1hr☐ 2hr☐ 3hr☐	1hr☐ 2hr☐ 3hr☐	1hr☐ 2hr☐ 3hr☐	1hr☐ 2hr☐ 3hr☐
Fruit & Beans	1hr☐ 2hr☐ 3hr☐	1hr☐ 2hr☐ 3hr☐	1hr☐ 2hr☐ 3hr☐	1hr☐ 2hr☐ 3hr☐	1hr☐ 2hr☐ 3hr☐	1hr☐ 2hr☐ 3hr☐	1hr☐ 2hr☐ 3hr☐	1hr☐ 2hr☐ 3hr☐
Fruit & Vegetables	1hr☐ 2hr☐ 3hr☐	1hr☐ 2hr☐ 3hr☐	1hr☐ 2hr☐ 3hr☐	1hr☐ 2hr☐ 3hr☐	1hr☐ 2hr☐ 3hr☐	1hr☐ 2hr☐ 3hr☐	1hr☐ 2hr☐ 3hr☐	1hr☐ 2hr☐ 3hr☐
Fruit & Grain	1hr☐ 2hr☐ 3hr☐	1hr☐ 2hr☐ 3hr☐	1hr☐ 2hr☐ 3hr☐	1hr☐ 2hr☐ 3hr☐	1hr☐ 2hr☐ 3hr☐	1hr☐ 2hr☐ 3hr☐	1hr☐ 2hr☐ 3hr☐	1hr☐ 2hr☐ 3hr☐
Grain & Dairy	1hr☐ 2hr☐ 3hr☐	1hr☐ 2hr☐ 3hr☐	1hr☐ 2hr☐ 3hr☐	1hr☐ 2hr☐ 3hr☐	1hr☐ 2hr☐ 3hr☐	1hr☐ 2hr☐ 3hr☐	1hr☐ 2hr☐ 3hr☐	1hr☐ 2hr☐ 3hr☐
Melons & Fruit	1hr☐ 2hr☐ 3hr☐	1hr☐ 2hr☐ 3hr☐	1hr☐ 2hr☐ 3hr☐	1hr☐ 2hr☐ 3hr☐	1hr☐ 2hr☐ 3hr☐	1hr☐ 2hr☐ 3hr☐	1hr☐ 2hr☐ 3hr☐	1hr☐ 2hr☐ 3hr☐
Melons & Anything Else	1hr☐ 2hr☐ 3hr☐	1hr☐ 2hr☐ 3hr☐	1hr☐ 2hr☐ 3hr☐	1hr☐ 2hr☐ 3hr☐	1hr☐ 2hr☐ 3hr☐	1hr☐ 2hr☐ 3hr☐	1hr☐ 2hr☐ 3hr☐	1hr☐ 2hr☐ 3hr☐
Dairy & Fish	1hr☐ 2hr☐ 3hr☐	1hr☐ 2hr☐ 3hr☐	1hr☐ 2hr☐ 3hr☐	1hr☐ 2hr☐ 3hr☐	1hr☐ 2hr☐ 3hr☐	1hr☐ 2hr☐ 3hr☐	1hr☐ 2hr☐ 3hr☐	1hr☐ 2hr☐ 3hr☐

alienated from Mother Nature and his or her own intuition because of not knowing what to eat out of intellectual fear of combining the wrong foods. I will be happy if one more person is not psychologically and gastronomically blocked by all the food-combining concepts. Human beings are extremely capable of creating what they believe and expect is supposed to happen. The more we can put orthodox, food-combining theory into perspective, the easier it will be to establish our own harmony with the gifts that Mother Nature offers us.

Honor Your Food Combining Needs

The simplest rule of food combining is to eat a food, or combinations of foods, that in our direct experience are easiest for us to digest and maintain our life energy and enzyme reserve. If we are eating a primarily live- and predigested-food diet, the food combining rules are considerably less applicable. If we have a mono diet, but eat too much of that one food, we will still have digestive difficulties because overeating of any food, no matter how well-combined or raw, is still a stress on the digestive system. Overeating is a primary cause of digestive difficulties.

When I was in India, I lived on very little food. Often in the morning, about four hours after getting up, I would have raw tahini mixed with banana on a chapati (a piece of flat bread). Theoretically, this was the worst of three combinations: fruit, protein, and starch. I never had digestive difficulties from this simple meal because I ate so little of it and so little food altogether. If, however, we eat when we are emotionally upset, or are rushed, we will tend to cause digestive difficulties. Some people, especially pittas, have very strong digestive constitutions and so are less affected by their food combinations. Others have delicate digestive constitutions and need to pay more attention to their harmony with nature. It behooves us to become our own scientists and experiment to discover what are the best food combinations for us. The food combining ideas can serve as a rough guideline for this.

Now that we have taken a new look at orthodox food-combining rules, we can appropriately consider some ideas of food combining. Whether or not the food-combining rules are based on accurate explanations for why people have digestive troubles when eating certain combinations, there are some combinations of foods, particularly if cooked, that are more likely to create fermentation or putrefaction than others: milk and meat, protein and starches, fruit and vegetables, and melons with any other foods. Eating too many different types of foods, even of the same food class, can also result in disrupted digestion.

Papaya and lemons seem to go well with any type of food. Avocados can also go with fruits or vegetables. A few easy-to-digest combinations are predigested proteins with vegetables or sweet and subacid fruits, sprouted grains with vegetables, or protein with vegetables.

The timing of eating plays a role in digestion too. A little water at meals if one is thirsty is acceptable, but drinking many glasses of liquid at a meal dilutes the digestive enzymes and therefore tends to impair digestion. A good time to drink liquids is 20 or more minutes before meals. If one must have dessert, it is a good idea to eat a fruit dessert one or two hours after a nonfruit dinner. Paavo Airola used to teach that if one is eating a salad and a protein, it is better to eat the salad either with the protein or afterwards. The roughage of the salad may tend to block the hydrochloric acid secretion from reaching the protein if it is eaten beforehand.

The best way to tell if our food combinations and volume of food intake are good for us is through the results. If we get gas, constipation, bloating, nausea, or exhaustion after eating, these are distinct signs that our combinations can be improved and the amount decreased.

In a quote from the Essene Jesus in the *Essene Gospel of Peace Book One (p. 38)*, the concepts for proper food combining are nicely described:

> "Take heed, therefore, and defile not with all kinds of abominations the temple of your bodies. Be content with two or three sorts of food, which you will always find upon the table of our Earthly Mother. And desire not to devour all things which you see round about you. For I tell you truly, if you mix together all sorts of food in your body, then the peace of your body will cease, and endless war will rage in you."

It is more difficult to enjoy the flow of the cosmic energies and the peace of meditation when gas warfare is raging inside the bowels. In the U.S., Tagamet, a drug for digestive disorders, is the number-one-selling drug. This suggests people have not yet begun to pay attention to what, how much, and how they are eating. Part of the reason is that the traditional, "home economics, basic-four-food-groups-at-each-meal" concept is still being taught in our schools. It is hard to overcome old food thoughtforms, no matter how unscientific they may be. In general, however, if we eat live food with some degree of awareness of food combining, eating the appropriate combinations will no longer be a big issue and we will not need Tagamet for dessert. The more we become attuned to the laws of nature, the simpler our meals become, with fewer combinations at each meal. Please trust in your own experience and use some artful intelligence.

You and Your Family Deserve Fresh Food

1. Shop for organic life in your foods.

2. Smell and touch foods to feel aliveness

3. As you eat these foods, the memory of soggy, frozen, overcooked cheesy, goopy vegetables will fade.

Preview of Chapter 24
Live Food Nutrition, a Gift of Nature

The essence of this chapter is—if it is not broken, don't fix it. Raw foods are the original creation and nutrition gift of God. Do we really think we can improve on them? In the process of trying to "fix" live foods to appease our taste buds, we destroy their SOEFs, deplete and disrupt their bioelectrical energy, disrupt their immune-protecting factors, destroy a high percentage of nutrients, destroy the living enzyme force, and destroy many known and unknown heat-sensitive health factors of the living food. As with the rain forest, there is much we don't even know we are destroying. In this chapter you will also learn about the ancient and modern history of living food cuisine and health practices, an energy system for classifying foods, and potentially harmful natural factors in foods. For many, increasing the living foods in the diet means letting go of culturally programmed habits of cooking and taste. Are you ready to begin eating more foods for health and begin learning new tastes?

    I. Live food nutrition, a gift of nature

        A. Raw foods as healers

        B. Energy categories of food

   II. Bioelectric energy of live food

  III. Biophysics of live foods

  IV. Raw food boosts immunity

   V. Cooked foods are damaged goods

        A. Cooking is a risky business and can transform certain fungicides into cancer-causing agents

        B. Browned or burn sections of food are mutagenic

  VI. Lesser-known health factors in live foods

        A. Wholeness of raw foods is health-producing

 VII. Potentially harmful factors in food

        A. Oxalates and phytates

        B. Estrogens in vegetables

Chapter 24

Live Food Nutrition, a Gift of Nature

The necessary, life-supporting process of nutrition starts with suckling at our mother's breast and continues as we suck our life force from the all-giving breast of Mother Nature. Live foods, because of their high, energetic structural integrity, give us the healthiest, physical, food-sourced nurturance on the physical plane. Raw foods contribute the most to the energy of our SOEFs. Extensively processed fast foods give the least energy, and may actually serve to disrupt our own SOEFs. In order for us to absorb the processed food, energy from our own SOEFs is needed to reorganize the disrupted SOEFs of the processed food before we are able to assimilate it. This means assimilating processed foods indirectly depletes our SOEFs and accelerates the aging process.

History of Live Foods for Health

The use of live foods for creating health has had a strong foundation of medical support in the last 100 years. One of the first clinics to adapt a raw food for health approach was the Bircher-Benner clinic started in 1897 in Zurich, Switzerland. Its founder, the world famous Max Bircher-Benner, M.D., discovered the power of raw foods when he experimented upon himself for his own healing. He found that live foods healed his jaundice and inability to eat. Later, he had a patient who was unable to digest anything, including cooked foods, and who was slowly degenerating in his health. In his studies, Dr. Bircher-Benner discovered that the wise teacher, Pythagoras, who lived in 500 B.C., had used raw foods to heal people with poor digestion. He applied Pythagoras' cure to the patient and he recovered. This is significant because there was, and still is, in some circles, a current myth that live foods are difficult to digest. What makes the raw foods easier to digest is that they have their own digestive enzymes that do most of the digesting. In my own practice, I often start people with severe digestive disorders on blended raw foods. This approach is very successful, and again confirms that properly prepared raw foods are effective for digestive disorders where cooked, enzymeless foods have failed. Bircher-Benner began to investigate the properties of live foods and found that regardless of the seriousness of the disease, the living food treatment was a powerful healing approach. Based on these principles, his clinic became one of the most respected healing centers in the world. He understood the causative role cooked and processed foods play in the epidemic of degenerative diseases. The tremendous increase in disease that we in the West are today witnessing is not something that has to be. Bircher-Benner wrote:

"We are oppressed by an overwhelming burden of incurable disease which hangs over our lives like a dark cloud. It is a burden that will not disappear until men become aware of the basic laws of life."

One of the basic laws of life is to eat our foods whole, organic, and in their natural, raw state.

In the early part of this century another great physician, Max Gerson, M.D., also discovered the healing power of live foods. First for the healing of his own migraines, and then later for the supposedly incurable disease called lupus. He then applied this approach to every sort of medical disease, from clogged arteries to mental disorders. He believed that a live food and a live juice diet was more than just a specific cure for certain diseases. He said that eating raw foods was a way of eating which restored the diseased body and mind's ability to heal itself. Dr. Gerson recognized raw foods as a way to rebuild the vital regenerative force of the total organism. In 1928, he was even able to cure Albert Schweitzer's wife of tuberculosis with this diet. Later, he put Albert Schweitzer on a raw food diet for his diabetes. As a result of this, Schweitzer was cured of diabetes and was able to stop using insulin.

Dr. Gerson also found that a live food diet high in potassium would restore the potassium-sodium balance and improve cellular respiration as well as enhance the immune system. He began to apply this principle to the treatment of cancer with great success. This work was highlighted by his extensively documented book, *A Cancer Therapy, Results of Fifty Cases,* which he published in 1958. His successful cancer clinic, using these live food principles, is successfully under the direction of his daughter, Charlotte Gerson, in Mexico.

Many of the great European healers and clinics advocate the use of live foods for healing and for maintaining high-level wellness. The internationally re-spected Dr. Paavo Airola, whom I studied with over a period of seven years, recommended a 100% raw food diet for regaining health and an 80% raw food diet for maintenance and prevention. During the winter, he recommended a little less raw foods. My personal and clinical experience with raw foods is that after about two years on an 80% live food diet, the immune system seems consider-ably stronger and people essentially stop getting colds and the virulent flus that prey on most of the population.

At first, in my transition, I felt colder on raw foods, but by the second or third year, I felt comfortably warm. Now I even go outside many mornings before the sunrise, barefoot in the frost, as part of my way of communing with the earthly and heavenly forces. I just would not have been able to comfortably do that before beginning a raw food diet. My personal experience was validated by a workshop on spiritual nutrition I gave in Anchorage, Alaska. As I mentioned earlier, I met a wonderful group of people who operated a live food restaurant called the *Enzyme Express*. All the folks connected with the restaurant have discovered the same thing: that after a few years on a raw-food diet, they actually feel warmer during the cold Alaska winters and generally have a better tolerance for the cold. They shared with me that they also went through a transition where they felt colder in the beginning of their raw-food experience.

My hypothesis for this increased health and vitality is that during the initial beginning of the 80-95% raw-food diet there is sometimes mild healing crises. In this stage, one may become more vulnerable and sensitive to the environment since the body's innate intelligence directs its energies inward to cleanse and rebuild the system. Once one passes through this stage, there is a building up of the vital force and the immune system. Once this force has become strong again, no matter what one's body type, one becomes more resistant to all adverse forces, including the cold weather. I find that I am now able to go out without a jacket while it is still in the high thirty degree Fahrenheit range. My ability to do this is a dramatic contrast to what it used to be like before I switched to primarily live foods back in 1983.

Other physician pioneers have had their own positive healing experiences with raw foods. The Danish physician, Kristine Nolfi, switched to raw foods to heal herself of breast cancer. Based on her positive experiences with herself and her patients, she started the successful Humlegaarden Sanatorium in Denmark. While doing workshops in Sweden, I had a personal interview with Dr. Aly, who runs a famous clinic in Sweden. He has been highly successful with the use of fasting and live foods as a way to restore health.

In America, Ann Wigmore has been an active and successful proponent of live foods for over thirty years. Blossoming out of her work have been a variety of live-food centers sprouting up all over the country. Victor Kulvinskas, who began his work with Ann, is another well-known proponent of live foods for healing.

Dr. Paul Bragg was one of the original American pioneers of raw foods and natural living in accordance with the laws of nature. His work has reached millions of people in this country. Until he passed away in an unfortunate swimming accident at age 96, Bragg was in vigorous health in large part because of his 80% raw food, "fresh is best" diet and regular fasting as a way of life.

Dr. Norman Walker, who lived to age 108, and ate primarily raw foods and juices, is another famous raw-food pioneer in the United States with thousands of clinical successes.

One of the greatest pioneers of live foods for maintenance of optimal health, as well as for the treatment of disease, was Dr. Szekely, who translated the *Essene Gospel of Peace Books I-IV*, and brought the Essene teachings into the awareness of the 20th century. Over a period of 33 years, from 1937 to 1970, at his clinic at Rancho La Puerta, Mexico, he established one of the greatest modern human experiments using live foods. He saw over 123,600 people (approximately 17% of them came with the diagnosis of medical "incurables") with over

90% of them regaining their full health. His translation of the Essene healing methods into his clinical work highlights that live foods for optimal health and for the treatment of disease is not a new discovery but has been part of the Western and Judaic-Christian tradition for over two thousand years. The Essenes, who lived in communities for 200-300 years before the time of Jesus, were said to eat primarily live foods and were reported by historians to live an average of 120 years.

Based on his study of the Essenes and his own clinical experience, Dr. Szekely developed a useful way to categorize foods based on their energetic and physiological effects rather than their biochemical makeup of calories, protein, carbohydrates, and fats.

To briefly review, foods that had a high degree of life force and, in turn, enhanced the human life force (SOEFs), Dr. Szekely called biogenic. **Biogenic foods increase the SOEF organization on every level. They help to reverse entropy and the aging process. These are high-enzyme, raw foods that have the capacity to revitalize and regenerate the human organism.**

The second category of foods are called bioactive. These are foods which are capable of sustaining and enhancing an already healthy life force. They add to our SOEFs. **Bioactive foods include fresh, raw fruits and vegetables.** They have less enzymes and inherent life force than biogenic foods but are still very beneficial to the system.

Biostatic is the name of the third category. It includes fresh foods that have been cooked. These foods can be slightly life-sustaining in the short-term, but are gradually life force depleting in the long-term because they require the human organism to give of its SOEFs to reactivate the SOEFs of the cooked foods so they can be absorbed. The end result is a slow depletion of the human SOEFs. Biostatic foods are cooked or minimally processed foods, as well as foods which are raw, but no longer fresh.

The fourth category of foods are called biocidic. These are life-destroying foods — foods which without question disrupt and deplete the SOEFs. Biocidic foods have gone through much processing and are full of additives and preservatives. They are the plastic, fast, "convenience foods." Biocidic foods also include all cooked flesh foods because of their rapid putrefication, unless they have been freshly killed and eaten.

Mother Nature has given us a wide variety of food choices. Hopefully we will choose foods which reverse the effects of entropy on our system. To reverse entropy is to help to reverse aging and enhance health. These are the biogenic and bioactive foods. Unfortunately, despite all the information available, most of our population still chooses foods which increase our entropy and accelerate the aging process. These choices are difficult because so many of us are so addicted to satisfying our taste buds and are attached to fixed eating habits and cultural concepts.

Paavo Airola often pointed out that in making the transition to live foods it is important to be sensitive to the type of foods traditionally eaten by the individual's family of origin, their ancestors, along with considering the genetic background. Sometimes the question is raised as to whether certain ethnic groups without a major, live-food tradition, such as the East Indian, Chinese, and Japanese, can, or should, make the transition. In these cultures people had to, and still do, cook their food in order to kill parasites, virulent bacteria, and amoebas. This may be one of the main reasons for cooking food in these cultures, but it does not mean that these individuals cannot make an intelligent and careful transition.

In India, there has always been a tradition of vegetarianism. There is also a history of those who ate very little, or only raw foods, as part of their spiritual development. One of the most famous of these was Shivapuri Baba who lived to be 137 years old. At the age of 50, after living in the forest on just roots and tubers for 30 years, he went on a 35-year, world walking tour. He spent time with different spiritual, cultural, and political leaders, including four years with Queen Victoria in England. Born in 1826, he left his body in 1963. It was said that he ate raw foods up until a few years before his death, when he began to accept the cooked food of his visitors. It was said, that after this that he began to lose some of his vitality and began to noticeably age. He was, however, quite alert and clear until the time he left his body.

Satya Sai Baba, one of the few Indian spiritual teachers who has transcended his culture's food traditions, gets to the core issue of the resistance to live foods:

> "Out of all the species...Man alone tries to cook and change his food. A seed when planted will sprout into life...but when cooked, the life is destroyed...it is man alone who is subject to the most health trouble....The reason is that man does not like to partake of food as God created it. He is the victim of his tongue, which he wants to be satisfied in terms of taste, and so his own likes and dislikes come in the way of what he should eat. Man seeks to change the foods available in nature to suit his tastes, thereby putting an end to the very essence of life contained in them. Because he is exterminating the life-giving forces in the food available to him, he is increasingly subjecting himself to disease. So, it follows, again, that if man were to eat foods in their natural states, he certainly would not be subject to disease."

Cooked Foods are Damaged Goods

A variety of research has shown that a good percentage of nutrients are destroyed in cooking. Viktoras Kulvinskas estimates that the overall nutrient destruction is around 80%. Although there is some variation in research findings, most agree that over 50% of the B vitamins are destroyed by cooking. Thiamine

(B-1) losses have been recorded up to 96%, folic acid losses up to 97%, and biotin losses up to 72%. Vitamin C losses are up to 70-80%. The Max Plank Institute for Nutritional Research in Germany has found that there is only 50% bio-availabilty in protein that has been cooked. Cooking alters protein into substances which disrupt cellular function and speed up the aging and disease process. In general, it can be said that cooking also coagulates the bioactive mineral/protein complexes and therefore disrupts mineral absorption, such as calcium in pasteurized milk. Cooking foods disrupts RNA and DNA structure, and, as already discussed, destroys most of the nutritive value of fats, creates carcinogenic and mutagenic structures in the fats, and produces free radicals in fats. According to Dr. William Neusome of Canada's Department of Health and Welfare Food Research Division, cooking transforms certain fungicides into cancer-causing compounds. We can assume that with all the potent pesticides, herbicides, and additives that have been added to our foods, that cooking will also transform a certain percentage of these into more carcinogenic or mutagenic (producing changes in gene patterns) compounds. Cooking is risky business.

Other research has uncovered the fact that even when cooking organic foods, there is a burned or browned section of the food after cooking which is highly mutagenic. This comes primarily from the heated protein. Some of these chemicals in the cooked protein have been isolated and fed to animals and they appear to be cancer-causing. The browning that comes from the interaction of carmelizing sugars and amino acids, such as the brown crusts on bread and toast, have also been found to be mutagenic substances.

There is an old saying, **"If it's not broken, don't fix it."** I believe this applies to the way Mother Nature has presented us with Her food, in an "unbroken" way. Nevertheless, humans insist on virtually unrestricted use of cooked foods. The message of Jesus in the *Essene Gospel of Peace Book I* (p. 36) rings as true today as it did then:

> **"For I tell you truly, live only by the fire of life, and prepare not your foods with the fire of death, which kills your foods, your bodies, and your souls also."**

The Bioelectricity of Live Foods

The electrical potential of our tissues and cells is a direct reflection of the aliveness of our cells. Live foods enhance the electrical potential of the cells by maximizing the electrical potential in cells, between cells, and the interface of cells with the micro-capillary electrical charge. The proper micro-electrical potential gives the cells the power to rid themselves of toxins and maintain the selective capacity to bring in the appropriate nutrients and oxygen supplies. In *Spiritual Nutrition and The Rainbow Diet*, I describe a model for how this selection process works on the electromagnetic level. Researchers have discovered that with disease there is a decrease in selective capacity of the cells to absorb and excrete. This results in a buildup of toxins in the cells and a decrease in efficiency of cell metabolism. There is also a weakening of cell membranes of tissue cells and blood capillary cells through which nutrients and oxygen are selectively filtered in, and toxins are filtered out.

I am particularly interested in this lowering of electrical potential effect because many of the people I see are just not feeling well, but all the lab tests they have had with other doctors show that they are not overtly, clinically diseased. The drop in the electrical potential is the first step in the disease process. These are the people who are in a state of meso-health, or subclinical "dis-ease."

Professor Hans Eppinger, chief medical doctor at the First Medical Clinic of the University of Vienna, found that a live-food diet specifically raises the microelectrical potentials throughout the body. He found that a raw-food diet increases selective capacity of the cells by increasing the electrical potential between the tissue cells and the capillary cells. They found that the raw foods significantly improved the intra/extra-cellular excretion of toxins and absorption of nutrients. Dr. Eppinger and his co-workers found that **live foods were the only type of food that could restore the microelectrical potential of the tissues once their electrical potential and the ensuing subtle cellular degeneration had begun to occur.** This correlates with the research by Dr. Kollath that raw foods alone, and distinctly not vitamins and mineral supplements alone, were able to restore his animals back to health from the half-health condition of meso-health. Their research findings that live foods have a regenerative power and ability to restore orderly functioning of the cells on the cellular and electromagnetic level of the organism supports my own clinical observations over the last 19 years. In essence, we can say that **by restoring the electrical potential of the cells, raw foods rejuvenate the life force and health of the organism.** A live-food cuisine is a powerful, natural, healing force which gradually restores the microelectrical potential and overall cell functioning in every cell in our body. Eating primarily raw foods is a gentle, delicious, nature-orientated and gradual way to restore health. Eating live foods means that one is paying attention to Mother Nature and accepting Her gifts the way She gives them to us. It is a specific and daily way to commune with Mother Earth.

Kirlian photography has been a useful tool to validate our understanding of the bioelectric affect of live foods on the health of the human organism. Kirlian photographs by Harry Oldfield and Roger Coghill, in their book, *The Dark Side of the Brain,* reveal electroluminescent fields (natural radiation field) surrounding living organisms that take the form of a coronal discharge. It is thought that what is seen in the photographs is the electrical conductivity of the skin cells as they are influenced by the cellular radiations of the rest of the cells of the body. From the point of view of the SOEF theory, the strength of these fields indicate the SOEF strength of the cells. Oldfield and Coghill feel these actual electrical fields maintain the integrity of the biological system. According to them, if these fields have more energy, they better maintain the physical structure and function. If their fields are depleted, they are less able to maintain both structure and function. In their theory, they hypothesize, as I do, that human beings and all living organisms are ultimately made up of patterns of resonant energy. This energy is reflected in the functioning of each cell. The actual molecular structure of the cells is guided by DNA, which acts as a resonant receiver of the different resonant frequencies of the body and also as a transmitter of a specific resonant frequency. The stronger the resonant frequency of the cell, the stronger the natural radiation field. **In other words, the electroluminescence is a measure of the life force of the cell.** The stronger the life force of each cell, the stronger the electroluminescence is of the total Kirlian photographic field, which is the sum of the electrical potential of each cell.

By using this system, they were able to understand how the life force of people and foods are affected by various conditions. One of their photographs shows a person when they had been on junk food for 24 hours. It shows an absence of any electroluminescence energy. This picture is typical of 12 subjects who were put on junk food. They then showed a picture of the electroluminescence of a man who had been on whole foods for 40 years. There is a dramatic difference between his highly charged field and the junk food absence of any field. Another photographic comparison they made was that of the electroluminescence of the same cabbage live, and then cooked in a pressure cooker for ten minutes. The live food cabbage had a significantly brighter and larger electroluminesent field than the cooked cabbage.

They also applied this technology to assessing storage techniques and effect of different processing methods on foods. They found that the natural radiation of the processed food varied corresponding to the cooking method. The results of food processing, in order of highest natural radiation, were:

1. raw
2. wok cooking
3. steaming
4. microwave cooking
5. pressure cooking and prolonged boiling
6. deep frying
7. barbecue and grilling
8. oven baking

The results with food storage, in order of highest natural radiation, were:

1. Fresh raw food had significantly the most energy
2. Raw stored in the refrigerator for four hours was the next highest
3. Freeze-drying showed 75% of the original energy
4. Freezing showed 30% of the original energy
5. Gamma radiation leaves almost no natural radiation left, and in the case of avocado, it was totally obliterated by the gamma radiation

Biophysics of Living Foods

The new scientific models developed by the brilliant minds in submolecular biology and quantum physics have made it possible to develop corresponding scientific models in the biophysics of nutrition. This broadened, conceptual understanding helps us better understand the importance of living foods, the rainbow diet, and an expanded comprehension of multi-energetic, nonmaterial aspects of nutrition. In the future, the bioelectric energy of food may become one of the most important considerations in the field of nutrition.

Nobel laureate Szent-Gyorgyi describes the essential life process as a little electrical current sent to us by sunshine. He is referring to highly charged single electrons that are involved in transferring their energy to our own sub-molecular patterns without changing our molecular structure. These wandering sunlight electrons belong to the electron clouds of the sub-molecular world described by quantum mechanics. These quantum physics models begin to validate our more intuitive model of vegetarian food as condensed sunlight energy which is then transferred to our human organism.

Another little piece of the biophysics of live foods is the theory of John Douglass, M.D., Ph.D., who feels that live foods have a higher energy ability to awaken relatively inert molecules in our system by either taking an electron or giving them one. This high-energy, electron transfer ability is described as the "high redox potential" of a particular molecule. Vitamin C has this property of a high redox potential, as do raw foods. Dr. Douglas believes the high redox potential of raw foods, which is destroyed by cooking, is an important factor in their healing power.

There is some interesting original work by the German fatty acid and light researcher, Dr. Johanna Budwig, with what she calls the sun-electron or biotron. Dr. Budwig feels that the biotron "guides" the Krebs cycle, one of the bio-electron cycles involved in the production of cellular energy. The biotron is also thought to be directly absorbed into our brain from the sun. Some theorists feel the biotron supplies up to one third of our energy directly into our system from the sun. Dr. Budwig feels that several tablespoons of flax seed oil per day will enhance this biotron energy absorption. The concept of the biotron is a very beginning stage of exploration, but worth contemplating.

367

The sunlight energy, when transferred to us indirectly through our food, is almost completely lost to us if the transfer of the vegetarian nutrients is second-hand through animal foods. The Kirlian photography studies suggest the sunlight energy in vegetarian food is also significantly lost if the bioelectric, resonant energy patterns are disrupted by cooking or processing our foods. Another message, then, which comes through when we think of food and the human body in terms of bioelectric energy, is that **foods in their live state pass on the bioelectrical energy from the sun directly and maximally to us**. The plants store it for us in the process of photosynthesis. Then, as I have suggested before in a more metaphoric way, they release their stored light into us. One ramification of this is the plants transfer their bioelectrical energy into our cells in a way which increases the individual, electrical potential of each cell, and therefore enhances the health and bioelectrical energy of our whole living organism. This is one of the secret stories of live foods and even the rainbow diet. **Our biological lives and health are dependent on the electric radiation of the sunlight. This bioelectric radiation stored in the plants, as nature's gift to us, is lost or greatly diminished when live foods are cooked, irradiated, or even stored for more than a few days. By increasing this bioelectrical energy in our cells, we increase our health, vitality, and longevity.**

Live Food Boosts Immunity

As described earlier, research by Paul Kouchakoff, M.D., in 1930 showed that every time we eat cooked foods, we get an increase of white blood cells in our blood stream. Dr. Howard Loomis has regularly repeated some of Dr. Kouchakoff's results in his clinical work with hundreds of patients. This finding is a potentially significant discovery for helping us learn how to protect and maintain our immune system. Overstimulation of the immune system three or four times a day by ingestion of cooked food is definitely an ongoing stress on the system. Specific immune factors in the raw foods, such as the gibberellins and abscisic acid (found in avocados, lemons, cabbage, and potatoes), also help support the immune system. The other major way raw food helps boost the immune system is that it keeps us healthy by its total detox, 'anti-' free radical enzymes, cleansing properties, and physical and energetic enhancement of our total biological organism. When we are healthy, the immune system naturally follows suit. Research at the Linus Pauling Institute found that a raw-food diet in mice had the same cancer-preventing properties as high doses of vitamin C. In general, I have observed that my clients who have been on an 80% or more live-food diet for six months to two years have a significantly stronger immune system than the general population and get significantly less colds and flus than they did previously.

Lesser-known Health Factors in Live Foods

Raw plants have an incredible variety of health-promoting factors, such as plant hormones, that help our metabolism, and paciferans, which are antibiotic substances. They are loaded with a variety of bioflavonoids, such as rutin, hesperidin, vitamin P, flavons, flavonals, and methoxylated bioflavonoids, including nobelitin and tangeretin. Nobelitin and tangeretin have more cortisone activity per weight than injectable cortisone. These two bioflavonoids have been found to remove heavy metals, drugs, and hydrocarbons from our bodies. They also have been found to decrease red blood cell clumping. In one experiment, three to four oranges or five tangerines decreased blood viscosity by 6%. In beet roots there are anthocyans which have been shown to be helpful in treating cancer and leukemia. There are also a variety of plant fibers that completely fulfill our need for fiber in the diet. Some plants have bitters which help our digestive secretions. Plants contain essential oils, saponins, and also chlorophyll, which is so important for our health.

Researchers have also found that some factors in raw foods stimulate the production of the healthy bacteria flora. This is significant because healthy colon bacteria protect against candida overgrowths, the growth of numerous pathogenic bacteria, constipation, and colon, blood, and tissue toxicity.

These myriad of health-restoring components contained in the unbroken wholeness of raw foods are partially or completely destroyed by cooking. Trying to list them all is like trying to list all the known and unknown herbal medicines in the rain forest. I want to expand on the concept that the wholeness of a food is crucially important. **On this level, it is the wholeness of raw foods which is health-producing and nonreproducible by science.** We do not fully understand why a raw-food diet is so effective, but it is clear that the whole is greater than the sum of the parts. **Cooking or other forms of processing destroy qualities and components of our food of which the significance is not yet, or perhaps never will be, known in its totality.**

We do know that live foods have been used as a powerful healing treatment primarily in Europe, but now also here in the U.S. A live-food diet has been used with great success to heal arthritis, high blood pressure, menstrual difficulties, obesity, allergies, diabetes, ulcers, heart and other circulatory diseases, hormone disturbances, diverticulosis, anemia, weak immune system, and other degenerative diseases or poor states of health. Many have found a live food diet an excellent aid for improving the brain/mind function. The research on animals, as well as longevity studies in cultures around the world, all suggest that a high, live-food diet plays an important part in creating a healthful longevity.

Some Food Factors with Bad Reputations

Within almost all foods there are also some factors which may be toxic in high concentrations. According to research compiled by the Food and Nutrition Board of the National Academy of Science National Research Council, these factors are not significant if taken in moderate amounts and one's general health is good. Research into the question of the goitrogenic (antithyroid) effect of eating raw cabbage and other members of the brassicae family and their seeds, peaches, pears, strawberries, spinach, carrots, soybeans, and peanuts, has found that, according to the Food and Nutrition Board of the National Academy of Science, "The goitrogenic effects in man of edible portions of Brassicae other than rutabaga and white turnips are not regarded as firmly established." The research has found that most of the goitrogenic factors of the Brassicae family was in the seeds rather than the edible portions. It has also been suggested that some of the goitrogenic factors from the rutabaga or white turnips could be transferred through cow's milk. It is generally thought that even these effects can be offset by increasing one's intake of high-iodine foods, such as kelp or dulse.

Another concern is the effect of naturally occurring oxalates in spinach and rhubarb. Many researcher's believe that it would take eating almost nine pounds of rhubarb to get any acute poisoning and that the oxalate content of vegetables has no significance in causing acute poisoning. The research on problems of chronic oxalate intake suggest it would be impossible, with an adequate calcium intake, to have a problem of calcium deficiency from a normal oxalate intake from vegetables. One two-year study on rats showed that with a diet of 0.1% to 1.2 % oxalates there were no abnormalities. In one extensive study on children put on a high-spinach diet and other high-oxalate foods, no evidence of any alteration of calcium, vitamin D, or phosphorous metabolism was found. It is possible, however, if a person has a low calcium intake or poor calcium metabolism, a high-oxalate diet could cause a calcium deficiency. One way to avoid the oxalate issue in nuts and seeds, such as sesame seeds and sunflower seeds, is to soak them overnight and rinse several times in the morning. By this process much of the oxalates are washed out and therefore do not pose a problem. **In general, unless one has a low calcium problem, one need not be too concerned about a moderate intake of oxalate foods.**

Phytates are another natural substance in some foods, especially grains such as wheat, rye, and oatmeal. They also occur in some nuts and seeds as well. They form a complex with calcium that keeps the calcium from being absorbed. Fortunately, a normally functioning intestinal tract produces an enzyme called phytase which releases calcium from its phytate-bound complex when it is transiting through the intestinal tract. The calcium is freed up to be absorbed. Unless we take an excess amount of phytates into the system, there is usually enough phytase to keep the phytates from having any effect on our calcium absorption. By soaking and rinsing the nuts and seeds we also wash out the phytates. **The way the body eliminates phytates seems to mirror the general way the body handles most of these naturally occurring, seemingly adverse factors in our food. If they are taken into the system in small enough quantities, our bodies usually have the enzymatic systems that will protect us from their potential negative effects.**

We should also be aware there are naturally occurring estrogens in carrots, soybeans, wheat, rice, oats, barley, potatoes, apples, cherries, plums, garlic, sage, parsley, licorice root, wheat bran, wheat germ, rice bran, and rice polishings. Estrogens are also found in edible oils such as cottonseed, safflower, wheatgerm, corn, linseed, peanut, olive, soybean, and coconut oil. Researchers in the publication put out by the Food and Nutrition Board of the National Academy of Science have concluded that:

> "...the consumption of any food product in a quantity sufficient to cause a physiologic effect due to estrogens it contains seems remote."

On the other hand, someone with an estrogen-sensitive cancer should be aware of these naturally occurring estrogens.

There are a variety of toxins in some of our naturally occurring foods. In some aged cheeses there are high concentrations of histamine, tyramine, and tryptamine which are normally detoxified by an enzyme in our system called monoamine oxidase. Some people under psychiatric treatment are given drugs that are monoamine oxidase inhibitors. If these people eat these cheeses, they may get severe cases of acute high blood pressure. These substances are not a problem, however, as long as the body biochemistry is functioning in a normal manner and we are not taking any antidepressive drugs.

In nutmeg and mace there are high concentrations of a toxin called myristicin. Carrots, parsley, celery, and dill have a little myristicin also. In small amounts myristicin has been noted to be helpful for toothaches, dysentery, diarrhea, rheumatism, and skin problems. **In large doses, such as one ounce of nutmeg or two whole nutmeg nuts, it may cause shock, stupor, acidosis, and/or intoxicating symptoms with euphoria for up to 24 hours after ingestion.** As in most cases, a little is okay, and a lot may be dangerous.

Another poison is thujone, an oil of wormwood; it is mentioned in the Bible nine times. It is the primary flavoring of the liquor called absinthe. In high doses it may produce convulsions. A muscle weakness and paralysis of the lower legs, called lathyrism, can occur when eating various types of vetch. Some people can develop favism, an anemia in which the red blood cells break down from eating uncooked fava beans. It occurs primarily in Mediterranean cultures and is transmitted by a sex-linked gene of moderate dominance. In brown mustard, horse radish, broccoli, cabbage, and arugula, there is an irritant called isothiocyanate which acts as a mucous membrane irritant.

Some **beans, such as raw soybeans, lentils, black-eyed peas, partridge peas, and mung beans, as well as peanuts and vetch, have trypsin inhibitors which block this class of digestive enzymes.** The trypsin inhibitors cause poor protein digestion and result in putrefaction and gas. Research on raw soybeans shows that their trypsin inhibitors decreased growth in chickens. Researchers have also specifically found that the trypsin inhibitors are a major cause of the poor utilization of raw soybeans. Kidney, soy, and lima beans are the highest in trypsin inhibitors and have the best improvement of digestibility after heating which destroys this inhibitory enzyme. The other beans and peas do not show such a dramatic improvement in digestibility after heating. Trypsin inhibitors were found in 23 of 26 pulses in India and also in wheat and guar gum. They are also found in egg whites, but research shows that dogs are more affected by it than humans. Much of these trypsin inhibitors are found in the seeds and are not present before the seeds develop. No research was available on the effect of sprouting on trypsin inhibitors. My observations and reports from other observers is that there is some improvement with sprouting, but that even sprouted beans and peas are still not so easy to digest even if sprouted. **I do not recommend more than occasional use of even sprouted beans or peas for those on a live food diet because of this research and my personal observations. This is especially true for those with a vata constitution.**

Raw soy beans, kidney beans, and other legumes, such as peanuts, groundnuts, jack beans, sword beans, horse beans, sweet peas, lentils, common vetch, and mung, green, Lima , navy, kidney, pinto, French, black, white, casto, and horse beans, also have factors called hemagluttins. When 1% of the diet is raw soybeans or .5% of the diet is raw kidney beans, growth in rats is suppressed. The theory is that the hemagluttins line the intestine and block fat and protein uptake. **All edible legumes which contain hemagluttins are poorly absorbed unless they are cooked thoroughly until the hemagluttins are destroyed.**

Sprouts are a wonderful, healthy, biogenic food; yet even alfalfa sprouts eaten in excess and harvested before they are mature contain a small percentage of an amino acid analog called canavanine, which has been reported in several cases to cause a worsening of symptoms of people who are suffering from systemic lupus erythematosus (SLE). The canavanine concentration is highest in the alfalfa seeds and decreases in concentration after the third day of sprouting. Because canavanine is water soluble, rinsing the sprouts each day also decreases the concentration. Alfalfa sprouts are best to eat when they are fully mature. This mature stage is their nutritional peak and they will have become a rich green in color and have their first leaf division. This is usually around day seven. For several years, I have advised my SLE clients and others with rheumatoid-like diseases about these considerations when using alfalfa sprouts. As yet, no one following this advice of selecting mature alfalfa greens and not eating them in excess has suffered an exacerbation of their symptoms.

372

Buckwheat sprouts require some moderation also. I have found two people who developed what seems to be cold sensitivity, allergic symptoms and painful skin nerve sensitivity worse with sunlight, after eating the super nutritious buckwheat sprouts in amounts equal to 20% of their dietary intake for six months. Prior to this extended excessive intake, these two people had eaten buckwheat in moderation without developing any symptoms. Their symptoms almost all went away when stopping this excessive amount of buckwheat sprouts. I have heard several secondhand reports of similar symptoms in others who have eaten an excess of buckwheat sprouts. Again, all the symptoms immediately went away on the cessation of excessive intake of buckwheat sprouts. The message is that almost any food, no matter how biogenic and healthy, may have small amounts of hidden toxins that may cause symptoms if eaten in excess for a long enough period of time.

Another enzyme found in plants are cholinesterase inhibitors. Cholinesterases are enzymes that play an important role in nerve impulses. Raw potatoes had the highest concentration of these inhibitors of 17 vegetables studied. The fruit of eggplants has some of these cholinesterase inhibitors, as well as roots and leaves of tomatoes. There is a small amount in asparagus, Valencia oranges, turnips, radishes, celery and even carrots. In potatoes exposed to sunlight, there is a buildup of cholinesterase inhibitors called solanine alkaloids, particularly in the eyes, skin, and sprouts of the potato. This alkaloid buildup can be toxic. A potato in which these alkaloids have accumulated will have a green tint to it. The way to prevent this sunlight-activated alkaloid buildup is to store potatoes away from the sunlight. Putting potatoes in a brown paper bag is one way to shield it from light. Researchers have not detected any harmful effects from any other vegetables because the cholinesterase inhibitors occur in such low amounts. These **green potatoes with solanin are still poisonous even when cooked.** One way to protect yourself and others is to tell produce markets and health food stores about the danger of potatoes exposed to sunlight. The potatoes can be stored in a covered bin.

Although it is useful to be aware of the little-known potential toxins in fruits and vegetables, it is important to maintain the larger perspective that sprouts and other live foods contain many anti-oxidants, anticarcinogens, live enzymes, electromagnetic energies, a high zeta potential, and high levels of minerals, vitamins, nucleic acids, paciferans (plant antibiotics), auxones (beneficial plant hormones), and other factors, which health benefits far outweigh the potential dangers of naturally occurring toxins. A healthy body has a sufficient defense to metabolically detoxify the naturally occurring toxins as long as we are not eating them in excess. Although excess is hard to define, I eat two to four ounces of mature alfalfa sprouts almost every day as part of my sprout salad. I consider this a moderate amount. Part of being a conscious eater is to have a holistic perspective about these issues and to eat in a moderate way using a variety of sprouts and live foods in the diet. In this way, Mother Nature's gifts of food can be eaten with love and not fear.

Preview of Chapter 25
Traveling in the Raw

Travelling in the United States and many countries around the world is not always easy for an inexperienced vegetarian. One of the main challenges is that most of the world is not vegetarian and may have some difficulty understanding your needs. If it's your family who is not vegetarian, they may even feel a little threatened by your new change. This chapter addresses the challenge by explaining how you can tactfully and gracefully maintain dietary and health patterns almost anywhere. The real challenge is whether you are willing to make the extra effort to make it happen. Are you?

I. Traveling in the raw

    A. Bring along whatever your need to restaurants or on trips

    B. Use the Yellow Pages to find health food restaurants and stores

II. Dinner invitations

III. Camping

Chapter 25

Traveling in the Raw

People frequently ask me how they can best eat vegetarian, and particularly raw, foods while travelling. There are a few tips I would like to share from my own travels that may be helpful. The first point to remember is that when one travels, one might face social pressures to conform, as well as be subtly ridiculed for "being different." In these situations, one should remember that one eats vegetarian or live food not to please others but because it is the healthiest diet for our species. Once outside the home, overcoming shyness about eating differently is an important challenge to face. On some level, many people intuitively know a vegetarian and/or a live-food diet is healthier than the standard American diet. Despite this unconscious inner knowing in some folks, they still consciously might feel threatened by it. By being firm about one's dietary needs, without adopting a "holier than thou" or a "self-righteous crusader" attitude, one can travel almost anywhere and manage to get one's dietary needs met.

One of the best ways to get one's culinary needs fulfilled is to take care of them for oneself. For example, when going to a potluck, don't depend on someone else to make something that one can eat. To play safe, bring one dish that supports your own dietary needs. If one is going out for a meal with a group of friends and one doesn't know much about the menu or have much say in selecting the restaurant, when arriving at the restaurant order a small salad but bring one's own supplemental sprouts, avocado, sunflower seeds, or whatever else one might want on a salad. Since most salad dressings in restaurants have a lot of pesticides, preservatives, and cooked oils in them, it is a good idea to also bring a homemade salad dressing.

More and more restaurants nowadays will prepare a vegetarian plate or salad if they are specifically asked, so bringing extra backup foods isn't always necessary. While traveling on the road, there is usually a salad bar somewhere which will have enough healthy items to eat. One might still want to bring one's own salad dressing because the salad bar dressings are often high in synthetic or regular dairy, fats, preservatives, additives, and color dyes. The foods of choice to eat in a salad bar are sprouts, and dark green vegetables like spinach and sunflower seeds. Avoid the white-colored head lettuce since it is a nutritional waste of time (and stomach space).

Eat the simple, fresh foods and avoid the foods with lots of sauces. Sometimes these sauces sit around for a long enough time that bacteria begin to grow in them. It is also a good idea to ask if any items have monosodium glutamate (MSG), a harmful additive that causes a violent reaction in some people. Salad bar items are sometimes also sprayed with sulfites to help preserve the appearance of the displayed foods.

The best policy when taking car trips of a few days is being prepared. Our family often takes an ice chest filled with several days' foods when we go traveling. We periodically get ice refills along the way to keep the food cold, as well as stock up, whenever we need food, from local health food stores that we pass. Looking in the Yellow Pages under the category "Health Foods" is a good way to find out if there is a health food store in the area.

It is relatively easy to find health food stores or health food restaurants in large cities to supply vegetarian needs while travelling in the United States or Europe. A thorough examination of even a standard restaurant may yield something. For example, our relatives in England took us to a fancy traditional restaurant in London. Sitting next to the roast beef was one of the best salad buffets I've ever experienced in a restaurant anywhere. In travelling throughout Mexico, Canada, Europe, Eastern Europe, India, and the U.S., I have always seemed to get by with little difficulty finding vegetarian and primarily live foods.

One compromise that I've found in my travels is that I have not always been able to find organically grown foods. Admittedly, unless there is a health food store with organic produce or someone's organic garden that one stumbles upon, organically grown foods are harder to find. However, eating a limited amount of nonorganic foods for a short while is not going to hurt one's health unless one's immune system and general health is already very run down. In places like India or Mexico, plenty of raw foods are available if one likes fruits with a hard outer covering, such as bananas or papayas. The covering gives protection against parasites.

It is possible to maintain a live-food diet while traveling if one carries one's own extra supplies. For example, sunflower seeds, almonds, pumpkin seeds, alfalfa seeds, dried fruit, and dried vegetables work well. Taking along a light-weight, portable water filter to purify drinking water and for soaking the dry foods overnight is a must. With the purified water one can even have sprouted seeds the next day. Fresh fruits and vegetables are usually available in most countries during the summer.

There are two excellent foods to take when traveling. One is spirulina and the other is a new product called Juice Plus. If I had a choice of one food to bring with me on a desert island, it would be spirulina. Gram for gram, spirulina could be the most nutritious and well-rounded food on the planet, which stores almost indefinitely. It is about 70% assimilable protein. The following properties make spirulina a number one food choice: it has all the essential amino acids in correct proportion; it contains the needed omega 3 and omega 6 fatty acids; it has 14 times the daily dose of human-active B_{12} (per 100 grams); it contains glycolipids, sulfonolipids, vitamins, 17 different beta-carotenoids, and over 2,000 enzymes; and it contains a full spectrum of well-assimilated minerals, especially iron and magnesium. Spirulina is the only substance that contains phycocyanins and it is second only to mother's milk in concentration of natural gamma linolenic acid (GLA). Spirulina is 0.5% glycogen, which is a ready-made glucose energy in a stored energy form. It contains 9% rhamnose, which is a biologically active and unique sugar important for transporting essential substances across the brain barrier as brain food.

Unlike other algaes, the cell wall of spirulina has high concentrations of mucopolysaccharides, which are easily digestive and form glycoprotein complexes that are important in the formation of protein and building of cell membranes. Primitive foods such as spirulina contain the highest food energy, the highest nutrient value, and use up the least amount of the planet's resources. Spirulina is also a powerful alkalinizing and healing food. It is an excellent support for the healing of hypoglycemia, diabetes, chronic fatigue, anemia, ulcers, and for boosting the immune system. It has been shown to repair free radical damage. Researchers have found it to contain a tumor necrosis factor. The anti-cancer power of spirulina is significant enough that at Harvard Medical School they found extracts of spirulina were extremely effective in treating cancer in hamsters. In my preliminary personal and clinical research, I have found spirulina and Phycotene Cream (a skin cream produced by Light Force, Inc. and made of the phycotene extract of spirulina) effective in preventing sunburn, while actually helping to absorb the sun's solar photon energy.

In 1977, I, my family, and others who were on prolonged stays in India, began to use spirulina. It was my impression that those who took one tablespoon of spirulina a day maintained their health better in India than those who did not use it.

A second excellent food is Juice Plus, which is a flash-dried concentrate which comes either as a vegetable combination or a fruit combination. In addition, it contains some grains, soluble and insoluble fiber, and enzymes. These elements are synergistically combined to provide a whole variety of nutrients and subtle energies designed to balance all the body subtle systems and organs. Two capsules have the equivalent nutrition of one glass of live juice. Although not the same vitality as a fresh glass of juice, it comes close and supplies the healing and detoxifying power of live juice. Juice Plus is also a convenient short cut for people on a fresh juice diet for detoxification, weight loss, or for those people who do not have time to prepare fresh juices. For those who do not believe they have the time to eat fruits and vegetables every day, it serves as an entry point into live foods. A high-quality spirulina and Juice Plus can be obtained by calling 602-394-2520.

Part of the adventures of traveling can be exploring the open markets or health food stores in a town or city. This becomes an interesting way to learn about a culture. I once was attending a seven-day program where there was no health food store produce available. However, I was able to procure fruit, avocados and sprouts at the local market and was able to pick fresh, organic vegetables from someone's garden. I completely enjoyed my meals that week despite the initial paucity of health food outlets.

I don't want to make it sound too easy; I'd be the first one to admit in this society eating vegetarian, and particularly live food, on the road is not always easy, but with a little creativity and effort one can make it work. While one is traveling there is no need to give in to the momentary conveniences that are always tempting us away from a healthy diet.

Dinner Invitations

Dinner invitations are sometimes trickier. It is advisable to tactfully ask the host what might be served ahead of time. If nothing the host mentions is considered healthy for the stage of diet that one is in, confide in the host that one is a vegetarian. Sometimes they will be very glad to make a little side dish on one's behalf. If your host still somehow doesn't get it or is unreceptive to one's hints, remember that the main purpose of the gathering is to socialize and not to eat. With close friends it is often possible to be so informal as to bring a salad or some "special dish" that just has to be shared as part of the meal for everyone to enjoy.

If one is visiting relatives, volunteering to help prepare the food is both a nice offering and a way to help steer the meal toward including at least something live. Sometimes one can have fun preparing the whole meal. Preparing food in a fun way allows relatives to enjoy the special offering. If they don't want the type of food one offers to prepare, then take everyone out to dinner. If nothing works, the art of delicately and lovingly making one's boundaries clear, without confrontation, is sometimes necessary. The bottom line for a successful friendship or family relationship is love. While it is important to be loving, it is also important to be truthful and to maintain one's integrity. Just because a relative thinks one should eat meat doesn't mean one has to please them by eating flesh foods. This is more likely to create a resentment that ruins the digestion of the whole meal, as well as alter the relationship with the relative.

Recreational Camping

Camping trips require a different sort of creativity. Although I do not generally recommend dehydrated food as a regular part of one's diet (because its SOEF energy is depleted as compared to fresh foods), dehydrated foods are very handy on camping trips. Dehydrated foods are also good to take traveling in cars and airline trips. Dehydrated foods at 118° F are the closest to live foods in energy. Once these foods are exposed to water, the enzymes are often reactivated with a minimal loss. In the recipe section, there is a variety of soups, snacks, crackers, and cookie preparations of organic foods that are dehydrated in a way which maximally preserves the enzymes. Dehydrated food is also the best way to store food with the minimum amount of enzyme and energy loss.

On a camping trip, a good water filter that is able to filter out bacteria is important. No commercially available filter works for viruses. If one is concerned about hepatitis and other viruses in the water, there are oxidative preparations, such as stabilized oxygen solution by the brand name of Aerobic 07 and its associated product called Floc, which interact with the oxidized viruses so they clump and can be filtered out. The makers of Aerobic 07 claim this combination completely sterilizes and purifies the water. Boiling the water for twenty minutes and reactivating it with the product, Crystal Energy, is also a good way to have safe drinking water.

If while traveling one is unable to find acceptable food to eat, one can either decide not to eat or remember that eating some nonorganic food for a short period of time will not cause great harm. The biggest problem I often see with traveling is not the food people eat while traveling, but how to return and successfully reestablish a nonsugar or sweets program, or a newly started, live-food or vegetarian program. If one is not careful, it is easy to slip back into old patterns and start feeling bad about oneself. What helps this tendency is to understand that this is just a temporary situation and not take it as if it is the end of all of one's good progress. This is the time to get some positive social support and maybe fast for a couple of days to clean out and then start again on one's health program. Sometimes reexperiencing how poorly one felt on one's old diet is a blessing in disguise and may reinforce the desire and fortitude of how to proceed to make the necessary future dietary changes. The usual process to a healthy diet and lifestyle is an up and down "sine wave" rather than a straight line graph going upward to a "perfect" diet. By not holding oneself to unrealistic standards, a failure and discouragement syndrome is avoided. At all times during the transition to a healthier dietary practice, be gentle on oneself.

New eating habits thrive best in the company of friends who understand and appreciate your motive for change.

Find a supportive friend or group with which to discuss your ideas and with whom you can share food.

BLACKBOARD FOOD FOR THOUGHT

Preview of Chapter 26
How Diet Can Protect You
From the Dangers of Radiation

One of the most alarming and pernicious threats to our health is radiation. Everyone is exposed to it. In this chapter you will understand the sources of radiation to which we are exposed, the ways in which these sources of radiation exposure are dangerous to us, general dietary adaptions that can be made to help protect you and your family, and specific nutrients and herbs that offer protection. The good news of this chapter is the general conscious eater's diet I recommend is basically the best diet to eat for radiation protection. Isn't it interesting that a conscious vegetarian diet is good for preserving health in so many different ways. Do you think the source of the Divine inspiration for dietary blueprint given in Genesis 1:29 knew about this potential use?

   I.   Major sources of radiation exposure

  II.   A nuclear blast is not the most serious radiation threat unless it lands on your head

 III.   Yes, something can be done—four principles of protection

       A. Selective uptake

       B. Chelation

       C. Antioxidant nutrients and enzymes

       D. Certain foods and special herbs

 IV.   Summary of the conscious eater's radiation protection diet

       A. A low-fat, high-natural carbohydrate, high-fiber, high-sea vegetable, 80%-live, vegetarian cuisine optimizes radiation protection.

Chapter 26

How Diet Can Protect You From the Dangers of Radiation

Major Sources of Radiation Exposure

Excessive radiation exposure comes from: 1) radioactive fallout from nuclear testing; 2) major nuclear power plant accidents, such as from Three Mile Island and Chernobyl; 3) accidents at sterilization and food irradiation facilities; 4) unreported minor radioactive leakage from smaller mishaps at other nuclear plants; 5) routine leaks and emissions from common devices and products that use nuclear technology; 6) radiation from medical radiation techniques such as X-rays, fluoroscopy, mammography and C.A.T. scans; 7) military nuclear activity, such as nuclear weapons plant site accidents, storage difficulties, and nuclear submarine accidents; 8) radon gas; and 9) cigarette smoking.

Accidents at nuclear plants occur more frequently than one would ever expect. The *Radiation Protection Manual* points out that there were 2,974 reported mishaps at nuclear plants filed in the records of the Nuclear Regulatory Committee in 1985 alone. According to the September 1985 report released by the U.S. General Accounting Office, there were **151 "significant nuclear safety incidents between 1971 and 1984 in fourteen Western countries."**

The lack of civilian regulation of military nuclear facilities adds an additional danger. The General Electric contract-managed Hanford facility in Washington State is a good example of a health threat stemming from a military-run operation. In the 1940s and '50s the Hanford weapons plant exposed people to the radiation equivalent of 3000 chest X-rays per year, without reporting it, or warning the one quarter of a million people who were exposed. Regularly occurring nuclear submarine accidents are also a hazard.

Radon gas is another source of radiation exposure. Radon is a radioactive by-product of naturally occurring uranium decay which is often found in granite deposits, shale or phosphate rock, concrete made with uranium-containing phosphates, gypsum, or brick. The radon gas is released from these sources and seeps up from the ground where it may accumulate in unventilated basements and in other rooms of the home. According to Dr. Steven Schechter, the author of *Fighting Radiation and Chemical Pollutants With Foods, Herbs, and Vitamins—Documented Natural Remedies that Boost Your Immunity and Detoxify*, the National Cancer Institute officials now say that radon gas may be responsible for at least 30,000 lung cancer deaths each year. According to 1988 Environmental Protection Agency (EPA) estimates, approximately 20% of all homes in the U.S. contain potentially toxic levels of radon gas. Good ventilation and sealing off the cracks in the basement floor can help protect against radon gas seepage through the floor.

Although it may be a surprise, cigarette smoking is another significant source of radiation. Dr. Schechter points out that with the inhaling of cigarette smoking comes two radioactive particles: polonium-210 and lead-210. These are breakdown products of radium-226. Radium-226 is found in the phosphate fertilizers used in commercial tobacco farming. Cigarette smoke has also been found to contain radioactive radium-226 and potassium-40. In an article published in the *American Scientist* entitled *"Tobacco, Radioactivity, and Cancer in Smokers,"* Dr. Edward Martell points out that when tobacco smoke is inhaled, these radioactive elements create an alpha radiation exposure that is hundreds of times greater than naturally occurring background radiation. He also points out that large amounts of polonium and lead-210 are found in the lung tumors of smokers and in their adjacent lymph nodes.

A Nuclear Blast Is Not The Most Serious Radiation Threat

Contrary to popular belief, the most serious threat of radiation exposure is not the big nuclear blast of ionizing radiation which occurs with a nuclear explosion. **Low-level radiation over a long period of time causes the most radiation damage to the cellular structures.** This low-level radiation comes from small amounts of chronic radiation exposures that arise from eating the airborne radioactive particles that have fallen on food, or from the water and soil radiation incorporated in the cellular structure inside of the food. The end result of low-level radiation over a long period of time is the production of a great deal of free radicals. This free radical production causes lethal radiation sickness and contributes to high rates of cancer.

A free radical is created when one molecule which possesses a highly reactive electron "robs" electrons from other atoms. Free radicals can be thought of as molecules that are out of electron balance. The way they rebalance themselves is to steal a molecule from another molecule which subsequently unbalances the next molecule in a chain reaction type fashion. When the electrons are stolen from atoms in biological structures, the structure and function of those biological tissues are disrupted. Free radicals can destroy lipids, enzymes, and proteins and cause cells to die. An especially negative effect of free radicals is the disruption of the function of the cell membrane and the membranes of the intracellular structures. DNA/RNA structure and function is also disrupted, as well as protein synthesis and cell metabolism in general.

Free radicals may also cause cross-linking among tissue proteins. The cross-linking phenomenon involves the shape of protein structures which results in these protein strands getting entangled in each other. When this happens they can no longer perform their normal function and this can contribute to the aging process.

Free radicals can cause inflammations, damage lung cells and blood vessels, produce mutations, and cause degenerative diseases, including cancer. Free radicals disrupt and deplete the immune system. Ultimately, it can even be said that free radicals disrupt and deplete the SOEFs of the organism. Many researchers in the field of aging hypothesize that free radical destruction is the basis of aging, or at least always accompanies the aging process.

The danger of chronic, low-level radiation exposure was discovered in 1972 by Dr. Abram Petkau, a Canadian physician. He found that the cell membranes were considerably more damaged by long-term, low-level exposure to radiation than by a brief, but high-level exposure to radiation of the same total equivalent dose. He discovered that the main damage of low-level radiation was not from direct ionizing radiation bombardment of our genes and causing mutations, but from the production of free radicals. According to Ernest Sternglass, professor Emeritus of Radiological Physics at the University of Pittsburg School of Medicine, **Dr. Petkau found the free radical effect from chronic low radiation exposure was one thousand times greater than from a single large exposure.**

Dr. Petkau's finding represents a significant shift in understanding. Until 1972, the "permissible safe exposure" from nuclear plants, atomic fallouts, and nuclear arms plants were estimated on the basis of experience with brief and intense radiation exposures, such as from a nuclear blast. The implication was that regular and chronic, low-dose radiation exposure was relatively "safe." In physiological reality, the low level radiation is actually a thousand or more times more damaging to our health than estimated. At low levels of radiation, the free radical process becomes more efficient. According to Dr. Petkau's observation, the more protracted the radiation dose, the lower the dose needed to break the cell membrane. This helps to explain why leukemia and other cancers are occurring 100 to 1000 times more than the initially predicted rate at Hiroshima. With this finding, one begins to understand that **there is no "safe" dose of radiation since radiation is cumulative.** According to the nuclear physicist, John Gofman Ph.D., M.D., in *Radiation and Human Health:*

> "Harm in the form of excess human cancer, occurs at all doses
> of ionizing radiation, down to the lowest conceivable dose and
> dose rate."

Dr. Karl Z. Morgan, after 30 years as director of the Health Physics Division of Oak Ridge National Laboratory, wrote in the *September 1978 Bulletin of Atomic Scientist* that,

> "There is no safe level of exposure and there is no dose of
> radiation so low that the risk of malignancy is zero...the genetic

risks, and especially those associated with recessive mutations, may be as harmful and debilitating to the human race as the increases of cancer."

According to Lita Lee, PhD., in her book *Radiation Protection Manual,* the latest estimate for the yearly radiation dose received by Americans has increased from 170 to 360 millirems. The permissible maximum allowable radiation for the general public is 500 millirems. This dose is not related to safety or health, but "what those in power can get away with." We are constantly being exposed to radiation. The more serious exposures are often for those living near nuclear plants. For example, the July 12, 1990 edition of the *San Jose Mercury* reported that Department of Energy (DOE) Secretary James Watson admitted that a study financed by his agency found large radiation releases in the 1940s and 1950s from the Hanford nuclear plant. It is possible that the thyroids and other organs of infants living downwind from Hanford nuclear reactor in Washington State could have received radiation doses of iodine-131 as high as 2,500 rads. This is five times greater than the yearly permissible dose.

Physician and physicist John Gofman was hired by the Atomic Energy Commission (AEC) to investigate the impact of radiation on human beings; **he concluded that radiation exposure produces a direct linear correlation in the increase of cancer incidence.** Gofman's findings indicated the permissible dose of radiation allowable from nuclear plants, 170 millirems at that time, would result in an additional 16,000-32,000 cancer deaths per year. In *Killing our Own: the Disaster of America's Experience with Atomic Radiation,* authored by Harvey Wasserman, it is reported that following the Three Mile Island nuclear reactor accident the cancer rate of those living near the nuclear reactor increased sevenfold and that 58% of the births had complications.

An airplane flight from coast to coast will expose the flyer to several hundred millirads. The average radiation dose for medical X-rays is 300-500 millirads for pelvic X-rays, 10-500 millirads for chest X-rays, and 100 to 1000 millirads to the face for a full set of dental X-rays. Dr. Gofman, in his book *X-rays Health Effects of Common Examinations,* estimates that more than 45,000 fatal cancers are induced yearly by X-rays. The data is overwhelming that nuclear energy plants, nuclear arms production, irradiation plants for medical instruments and food, and the excessive use of X-rays is a tremendous threat to the health and safety of the human population.

Radiation is far more toxic than chemicals or pesticides. Radioactive isotopes which concentrate in specific organs are very damaging because, according to Dr. Sternglass, each electron emitted by a radioactive nucleus has several million electron volts of energy which is enough energy to disrupt millions of molecules in the living cell. These radioactive isotopes emit radiation as they decay. This means that when certain isotopes, such as I-131, concentrate in the thyroid, they give off radiation that causes cellular membrane damage, inactivates enzymes, alters cell metabolism, and may create abnormal cell division. Accumulation of radioactive isotopes in vital organs creates the worst damage because it results in long-term exposure to a particular tissue.

Another problem with radioactive isotopes is they stay around for a long time. Strontium-90 has a radioactive lifetime of 560 years, plutonium-239 has a full radioactive life of 500,000 years, cesium-137 has a radioactive lifetime of 600 years, and I-131 is radioactive for 160 days.

Dr. Sternglass points out that epidemiological studies showed mortality rates have started to rise again in population centers near nuclear plants just as they did at the height of the nuclear testing in our atmosphere. In those states where there are no large nuclear reactors, no nuclear bomb facilities, and no nuclear test sites, Dr. Sternglass finds the total mortality rate is dropping.

Englishwoman Dr. Alice Stewart, a recognized world authority on nuclear epidemiology, discovered that women exposed to diagnostic X-rays during pregnancy had children who developed twice as much leukemia as children who had not been exposed in utero. It seems that just a small dose of radiation, approximately the equivalent of a single year of background radiation from the environment, doubled the rate of cancer for in utero babies. She also found that the risk of children developing childhood leukemia was twelve times greater if their exposure to X-ray diagnosis was in the first three months of pregnancy rather than at the end of pregnancy.

Dr. Sternglass points out that this discovery of a one thousandfold radiation sensitivity in the early human embryo could explain his findings of increased infant mortality due to all causes following an exposure to nuclear fallout from bomb testing or nuclear plant explosions like Chernobyl. Sternglass feels that when the fetus or infant is exposed to radioactive elements, such as strontium-90, the radioactive particles accumulate in the bone marrow, where the cells of the immune system are developing, and disrupt their functioning.

Iodine-131, which is absorbed in utero or through the milk of the mother or cow, disrupts the thyroid gland. A poorly functioning thyroid gland affects growth and metabolism of infants. Radioactive decay of strontium-90 creates yttrium-90 which goes on to disrupt the function of the thymus gland. The thymus gland is extremely important for immune function. The yttrium-90 also accumulates in the pituitary and gonads and disrupts the critical secretory and regulatory functions of the these glands. All these vital glandular organs affect the birth process and the onset of labor. Their disruption from radioactive particles from fallout may explain the increasing epidemic of spontaneous miscarriages and premature deliveries associated with the onset of nuclear atmospheric testing in general, and the Chernobyl accident in particular.

According to Dr. Sternglass, the iodine-131 is concentrated one hundred times more in the thyroid of a fetus than in an adult. Since this radioactive poisoning of the thyroid affects the growth and development of all organs,

Sternglass feels this helps to explain the epidemic of underweight babies and is also associated with the reported increased incidence of brain damage and dyslexia that began during the time of nuclear testing. In other follow-up research on radiation-related brain damage, Dr. Sternglass has noticed a correlation between prenatal radiation exposure and an 18 year follow-up that showed a drop in SAT scores in those who were exposed by living in areas of nuclear testing. According to Dr. Sternglass, as long as unborn children are exposed en masse to radiation, there is a possibility of widespread intellectual decline.

The post-Chernobyl statistics in the United States, compiled by Dr. Sternglass and presented at the First Global Radiation Victims Conference in New York in September 1987, impressively conveys the seriousness of the radiation problem. The infant mortality rate following the arrival of the Chernobyl fallout in early May of 1986 showed a 54% increase in June 1986 in the Pacific region of the United States. Washington State had the highest rate in the region with a 245% increase in deaths per thousand live births. California was next highest with a 48% increase in infant mortality as compared to June of the year before. These high rates lasted for July and August. Massachusetts lead the nation in post-Chernobyl rate increase of infant mortality with an infant mortality increase of 900% per thousand live births! Massachusetts had a decline of 70% of live births. The rate of live births also decreased throughout the country in response to the Chernobyl fallout. The U.S. fertility rate decreased 8.3% in July and August to the lowest level ever observed in United States history. In the eight months following the accident, there was a total drop of 60,000 live births in the United States. This was followed by a return to the approximated rate of live births in September. This suggests that the sharp decrease in live births in July and August 1986, following the arrival of radioactive particles from the Chernobyl fallout, probably accounts for the sudden increase in miscarriages, fetal deaths, and still-births observed. We are profoundly affected by accidents of our nuclear technology. It is time to move out of government-supported denial and do something about it and at least protect ourselves with diet.

In his paper, Dr. Sternglass suggests that this rapid rise in perinatal mortality and decrease in live births was associated with an increase of radioactive iodine in the rain water in New England, which was the highest in the country at the time. At this time, I covered my organic garden with plastic for the first several rains after the fallout from Chernobyl came to California. The rise in Iodine-131 in the water correlates with rise of radioactive Iodine-131 in milk. The rapid rise and fall of these statistics suggest that it had to be associated with a short-lived, radioactive agent, such as Iodine-131, which has a half life of eight days and a radioactive release life of 160 days. Although the developing fetus and infants are the most sensitive to radioactive fallout for the reasons already explained, the post-Chernobyl fallout was associated with an overall rise in mortality for all ages. Massachusetts was the highest, with an increase in total deaths of 43%, and

California and Washington State were next, with an increase in total mortality rates of 39% and 40%. The statistics show 35,000 more deaths in the U.S. in the eight months following the arrival of Chernobyl radioactivity than would be expected based on the normal rates for this time in the previous years. Dr. Sternglass feels that his Chernobyl accident observations can explain the unexpectedly large increases of infant and total mortality rates in areas located near nuclear reactors. Sternglass further points out that the:

> "...effect of the radioactivity appears to have been similar to that of the intense (radioactive), air pollution episodes of the 1950s and 1960s during the period of large-scale, atmospheric testing of nuclear weapons."

According to *Diet for the Atomic Age* by Sara Shannon, as of 1980, about thirty million Americans live within thirty miles of a nuclear power or weapons plant. Those living within thirty miles receive a higher dose of radiation than those living farther away.

Something Can Be Done

I share this information to alert people to a situation which the government of the United States apparently wants to ignore or minimize. **On the positive side, there is a lot we can do to minimize the negative effects of radiation.** In addition to the general prescription to live as healthful a lifestyle as is possible, **there is a specific radiation protection diet that maximizes the preservation of health and specifically neutralizes the effects of radiation.**

Decreasing one's susceptibility by improving one's overall health is one place to begin. A person's susceptibility usually is not included in calculating risk factors among radiation workers and those exposed to radioactive fallout by the medical profession who used nuclear medicine (including X-rays). Taking the average dose does not allow for the increased danger for those who are not in optimal health or who fall into the more susceptible age groups. This point was driven home by Dr. Stewart's study entitled, *"Delayed Effects of A-Bomb Radiation: A review of Recent Mortality Rates and Risk Estimates for Five Year Survivors,"* published in the *Journal of Epidemiology and Community Health* in 1982. She established the fact that **those who were the healthiest were the ones with the best survival rates.** Dr. Irwin Bross, in his article published in the *New England Journal of Medicine* in July 1972, was able to select which children would be twenty-five times more likely to develop leukemia from X-ray exposure. His work reinforces the point that one cannot determine "safe levels of radiation exposure" based on an "average exposure" of "average individuals." This fallacious concept of an "average," safe exposure limit does not provide an exposure limit that protects the most susceptible groups. **There is no such thing as an average or safe dose of radiation.**

Principles of Dietary Protection from Radiation

The population groups that are most susceptible to radiation poisoning are those in poor health, fetuses, infants, young children, and older people. The older people are more affected because their immune systems are often weaker and because of an already preexisting accumulation of radiation exposure throughout their lives. Whether one is in a susceptible group or even in optimal health, the ability to minimize the affects of radiation can be greatly enhanced by a healthy diet and lifestyle and the inclusion of special foods in the diet known to maximize protection from all forms of nuclear radiation. We have already extensively discussed the meaning of a healthy diet, so now we will explore the use of foods and herbs which specifically minimize the effect of radiation.

The antiradiation diet is built on four principles. The first is the **principle of selective uptake,** which essentially means that if one has enough minerals in the system, the cells become saturated with minerals. Once cellular mineral saturation occurs, there is less opportunity for the radioactive minerals to be absorbed into the system. For example, with such minerals as calcium or iodine, if there is sufficient natural calcium or iodine in the system, the body will not tend to absorb additional strontium-90, which is a close equivalent to calcium or iodine-131. If the normal mineral levels are low, then strontium-90 and iodine-131 will be more easily absorbed. When any of these radioactive minerals are absorbed into a particular tissue, they immediately begin to irradiate the surrounding cells and tissues. Each element is attracted to the organs in which it is normally utilized. The main radioactive minerals and the organs which they specifically target, and therefore, irradiate, can be seen on the chart on page 392. Also listed are the healthy minerals which inhibit this radioactive uptake by the principle of selective uptake.

The second main concept in protection against radiation exposure is that of chelation. This means there are certain foods which will actively draw the radioactive materials to them and pull them out of the body via the bowel excretion process.

The third concept is to keep the body high in antioxidant nutrients and enzymes which will nullify the free radicals that are created by the radiation exposure.

The fourth concept is that there are certain foods and herbs that specifically protect against the overall effects of radiation or radiation treatments.

There are also other ways to protect against radiation exposure. Research published in the *International Journal of Radiation Biology* in 1980 indicated that the pH of the cellular fluid could influence the cell's response to radiation. *Diet for the Atomic Age,* by Sara Shannon, says that many studies have suggested a slightly alkaline to middle range of body pH enhances the resistance to radiation.

Stopping smoking is an immediate way to reduce self-induced radiation exposure. Dr. Schechter, in his book, *Fighting Radiation and Chemical Pollutants with Foods, Herbs, and Vitamins,* estimates that the pack-a-day smoker exposes themselves to the equivalent of 300 chest X-rays per year. Avoiding living near nuclear plants and avoiding unnecessary diagnostic X-ray procedures are other ways.

Radiation Protection from Selective Uptake

The principle of selective uptake gives us specific ways to minimize the dangerous effects of radiation exposure. As pointed out in the Chernobyl studies, one of the main causes of radiation sickness and death was radioactive Iodine-131. In a November 1987 *East-West Journal* article, Dr. Schechter points out that Dr. Russel Morgan, who served as the chief radiologist of Johns Hopkins University, reported that **one milligram of iodine for children, and five milligrams for adults, per day would reduce the amount of radioactive iodine accumulated in the thyroid by 80% from direct I-131 exposure.** This is the equivalent of five to ten tablets of kelp per day or one to two teaspoons of kelp granules. **For preventative purposes one needs closer to one milligram per day for an adult, which is about one half an ounce of dulse or other sea vegetables per day.** Other high-iodine foods are swiss chard, turnip greens, wild garlic and onions, watercress, squash, mustard greens, spinach, asparagus, kale, citrus, watermelon, and pineapple. These vegetables may be lower in iodine in the Great Lakes area and the Pacific Northwest of the United States due to a low iodine in the soil (see fig. 24).

Too much iodine may cause an over stimulation of the thyroid. If one is being treated for thyroid disease, hyperactivity, or cardiovascular disease, it is important to consult your physician or health practitioner before adding high-iodine tablets or lots of sea vegetables to your diet.

An additional approach to radiation exposure is to avoid eating foods high on the food chain (animal foods) which dramatically concentrate these radioactive minerals. Radioactive particles can originate in the air, such as in fallout, or through water contamination, as has happened with the leakage of cesium 137 at the Georgia radiation sterilizer plant. Statistics adapted from the *Radiological Assessment of the Wyhl Nuclear Power Plant* by the Department of Environmental Protection of the University of Heidlberg, Germany in 1978, showed that by air exposure, cow's milk is about 15 times more concentrated with radioactive materials, and beef is more than thirty times more concentrated, than are leafy vegetables. Root vegetables are about four more times concentrated than leafy vegetables and about three times more concentrated in radioactive material than grains. In the area of radiation exposure from water, fish were the most concentrated on the food chain. They contained about 15 times more radioactivity than leafy green vegetables. It is also important to note that the concentration of radioactive nucleotides in freshwater fish is considerably higher than saltwater fish because saltwater fish have more minerals, and therefore are better protected.

In general, however, foods lower on the food chain have less radiation contamination than those higher on the food chain, such as milk and flesh foods. Milk is the main carrier for strontium-90 and also is a major carrier for iodine-131 to enter the system. One interesting point about the food chain is that it does not necessarily mean the concentration of radioactive materials dissipates the farther away one is from the contaminating source. Aside from wind currents, that in the Chernobyl accident carried contaminants in high concentrations to such places as Massachusetts, the concentration of radioactivity up the food chain definitely makes the problem worse. Therefore, **eating low on the food chain is the best way of minimizing dietary-sourced radioactivity.**

Chelation Protection

Another important way of neutralizing radioactive buildup is that of chelation. The best chelator for pulling radioactive material out of the system is sodium alginate. According to studies by Yukio Tanaka and other researchers at the Gastrointestinal Research Laboratory at McGill University in Canada, sodium alginate reduces the amount of strontium-90 absorbed by the bone by 53-80%. The sea vegetables that have the most sodium alginate are in the kelp family which includes: kelp, arame, wakame, kombu, and hijiki. Other research reported by Dr. Schechter suggests that sodium alginate not only protects us from absorbing strontium-90, but also helps pull out the existing strontium-90 from our bones. What is especially interesting is that sodium alginate does not seem to interfere with normal calcium uptake. Work by J. F. Sara at the Environmental Toxicology laboratory of the EPA, and A. Huag, that was reported in the *Composition and Properties of Alginates, Report no. 30,* showed that the alginate binds other metal pollutants, such as excess barium, lead, plutonium, cesium, and cadmium. Research by Tanaka showed that the alginate decreased the uptake of strontium-90, strontium-85, barium, and radium by a factor of twelve. These radioactive elements are then transformed into harmless salts and excreted by the system. Schechter points out that the different sea vegetables seem to be selective in regard to which radioactive element they tend to bind the most. Brown sea vegetables bind excess strontium and iron. Red sea vegetables, such as dulse, are best for binding plutonium. The green algaes bind cesium-137 most effectively.

The United States Atomic Energy Commission, which has recognized the effectiveness of the sea vegetables for minimizing the intake of radioactive minerals, recommends a minimum dosage of two to three ounces of sea vegetables per week, or ten grams (two tablespoons) per day of sodium alginate supplements. Dr. Schechter, in his optimum, antiradiation diet, also recommends three ounces per week of sea vegetables. During an actual acute radioactive exposure, Dr. Schechter feels the dosage should be increased to two full tablespoons of alginate four times per day, or six ounces per week of sea vegetables (see fig. 25).

Fortunately, sea vegetables are great-tasting foods as well as being our antiradiation friends. Sea vegetables have all the 56 minerals and trace elements our bodies require. This is about 20 more minerals than land vegetables have. They have the highest amounts of magnesium, iron, iodine, and sodium and rank second in calcium and phosphorous. For example, four ounces of hijiki contain 1,400 mg of calcium. Dulse ranks first in potassium of any plant food.

Sea vegetables are high in vitamin A, chlorophyll, enzymes, all the Bs, some vitamin E and D, and vitamin C content equal to that of green vegetables. They are an excellent source of human-active B_{12}. They have about 25% protein, 2% fat, and are very high in fiber. Laver nori, for example, has approximately twice as much protein as tofu per weight and more insoluble and soluble fiber than oat bran. Because sea vegetables often come with sea salt still on them, I recommend soaking them before using to rinse off the salt.

Another chelating agent which protects the body from absorbing radioactive materials is zybicolin, a fiber that is especially good for drawing out radioactive materials and that is found in miso. Other fiber foods with high chelation properties include the fiber found in whole grains, nuts, seeds, and beans. Fiber found in pectin, which is a soluble fiber found in fruits and seeds, especially sunflower seeds, also has high chelation properties. Phytates, found in grains and beans, and sulfur-containing amino acids, found particularly in the cabbage family, are also good chelators. Not only do these have a chelating affect, but the sulfur-containing amino acid vegetables prevent the uptake of sulfur-135.

Special Foods Which Protect Against Radiation Exposure

Miso is a food that has been acclaimed as a general protector against radiation sickness and chronic disease. Miso is an alkaline-forming, fermented paste made from soybeans which may also be mixed with rice or barley. Unpasteurized miso, which is the only type to eat, has many healthy bacteria and enzymes which help digestion and keep the bowels healthy. Its B_{12} protects against the absorption of cobalt-60. Miso has many other minerals which protect against the uptake of other radioactive minerals (see fig. 26).

The anecdotal evidence that has made miso famous as an antiradiation food was the story of Dr. Akizuki of the St. Francis clinic in Nagasaki during World

PRINCIPLES OF SELECTIVE UPTAKE

HEALTHY MINERALS	RADIOACTIVE MINERALS	ORGANS PROTECTED
Calcuim	Strontium$_{90}$, Strontium$_{85}$, Barium$_{140}$, Radium	Bone
Potassium	Cesium$_{137, 134}$ and Potassium$_{42, 40}$	Muscle, Kidney, Liver Reproductive Organs
Iodine	Iodine$_{131}$	Thyroid and Gonads
Iron	Plutonium$_{238, 239}$ and Iron$_{238, 239}$	Lungs, Liver, and Gonads
Zinc	Zinc$_{65}$	Bones, Gonads
Vitamin B$_{12}$	Cobalt$_{60}$	Liver, Reproductive Organs
Sulfur	Sulfur$_{135}$	Skin

Fig. 24

CHELATION NUTRIENTS

CHELATION AGENTS

Sodium Alginate
- Kelp - best chelates $Strontium_{90}$, $Strontium_{85}$, $Barium_{140,}$ Radium
- Dulse - best chelates Plutonium
- Blue-Green - best chelates $Cesium_{137}$
- Other Sea Vegetables

Pectin — Soy, apple, sunflower seeds

Zybicolin — Miso

Phytates — Grains, beans, peas

Cellulose & Lignin — Nondissolvable food fibres

Fig. 25

War II. Dr. Akizuki's clinic was one mile from the bomb blast when the atomic bomb went off in Nagasaki. Dr. Akizuki and his staff, who took miso regularly, did not suffer radiation sickness as they cared for the victims of the atomic blast in the weeks and years afterward the blast. Unfortunately, according to Dr. Schechter in a personal communication, when scientists such as himself tried to validate this great story, they were not able to find any proof of its veracity or any documentary research.

In *Macrobiotics for Personal and Planetary Health,* autumn/winter 1990, there is one article that supports the antiradiation power of miso. Scientists in Japan found that laboratory mice who were fed miso daily were five times more resistant to radiation than mice who were not eating miso. One consideration about miso is its high sea salt content. Those with high blood pressure or heart disease should monitor their intake carefully.

Beets are another special food. Not only are they known as a liver and blood detoxifier, but they protect the nervous system and also help to treat anemia. Radiation may cause difficulties in all these areas. Beets are high in iron, which protects against absorption of: plutonium-238 and 239, iron-55, and iron-59. The most startling study done on beets was reported in the *Journal of Dental Research* by J. Wolsieffer in 1973. Rats fed a diet of 20% beet pulp had 97-100% less cesium-137 absorption than rats exposed to the same radiation, but which were not given the beet pulp. Work by Dr. Siegmund Schmidt, reported in *Raw Energy* by Susan and Leslie Kenton, indicated that raw beet juice has been successfully used to prevent and cure radiation-induced cancers. The beet juice is particularly high in a specific anthocyan which is active against cancer and leukemia. It must be mentioned that if one lives in an area where the ground-water might be contaminated with radioactivity, beets, since they are below-ground vegetables, may be more exposed to the radioactive water than above-ground types of vegetables.

Bee pollen is another potent antiradiation food as well as a general health enhancer. Bee pollen helps to support the immune system and protects both red and white blood cells against their usual depletion from radiation. Bee pollen is also high in vitamins A, B, C, and E, nucleic acids, lecithin, cysteine, and vital minerals such as selenium, calcium, and magnesium. All of these nutrients contribute in their own way in helping to protect against radiation.

One study, reported in *Fighting Radiation and Chemical Pollutants With Foods, Herbs, and Vitamins,* conducted by Dr. Peter Hernuss at the University of Vienna Women's Clinic, showed that bee pollen significantly reduced the usual side effects of both radium and cobalt-60 radiotherapy in twenty-five women treated for inoperable uterine cancer. As compared to the women who did not receive bee pollen, the bee pollen women had one half as much nausea, 80% less loss of appetite, 50% less sleep, urinary, and rectal disorders, and 30% less general malaise and weakness after the treatment. They were given approximately two tablespoons of bee pollen three times per day. Other clinical research has shown similar results. Researchers at Stanford Research Institute found that bee pollen also protected mice against X-ray treatments.

Bee pollen has 15% lecithin, which helps to protect the nervous system and brain against radiation. Lecithin is useful in protecting against strontium-90, X-rays, iodine-131, krypton-85, ruthenium-106, zinc-65, barium-140, potassium-42, and cesium-137. Bee pollen specifically protects the gonads against the accumulation of iodine-131 and plutonium-239. It also gives some protection against environmental contaminants such as lead, mercury, aluminum, DDT, nitrates, and nitrites. Bee pollen is also high in nucleic acids, which a variety of research has shown to increase survival of mice against radiation. One Soviet study showed a 40% survival rate increase in rats after they received nucleic acids before radiation exposure.

Bee pollen is much more than simply a radiation protection food. It, along with sea vegetables, is a food I recommend to take regularly as part of the *conscious eaters approach* whether or not you are concerned with radiation protection. **Bee pollen is the procreative life force of the plant world.**

> "Pollen is the finest food and best medicine ever discovered. Pollen contains the richest source yet revealed of vitamins, minerals, proteins, amino acids, hormones, enzymes, and fats. Pollen also contains other substances which so far defy identification."

This is the opinion of Dr. G. J. Binding, M.B.E., F.R.H.S., a British scientist, author, and world-famous expert on nutrition. Dr. Binding feels that the honeybee pollen has a powerful life force that:

> "...not only builds up strength and energy in the tired body, but acts as a tonic. People have more vigor, vitality, and increased resistance to infection....Honeybee pollen has shown itself to be a complete nourishment in every sense of the word."

The high life force in the pollen comes from the millions of living plant forces contained in the pollen. Each pollen granule contains four million pollen grains. One teaspoon contains about two and one half billion to ten billion pollen grains. Each of these grains is the male semen, seed, or germ cell of the plant kingdom. Every pollen grain has the power to fertilize and create a fruit, a grain, a vegetable, a flower, or a tree. **Pollen is the ultimate biogenic food.** It is filled with life force of the entire plant kingdom.

The Bible mentions bee pollen 68 times. The Talmud, the Koran, ancient Chinese scriptures, and Roman and Greek civilizations, as well as the Russian and Slavic people, have all praised bee pollen and honey as a source of rejuvenation and health. Many Greek philosophers claimed that bee pollen held the secret to eternal youth. The original, Greek, Olympic athletes used pollen-rich honey as part of their training diets.

Pollen is said to contain all the elements necessary for the sustenance of human life. The San Francisco Medical Research Foundation estimates that pollen has more than 5000 different enzymes and co-enzymes, which is more than any other food in existence. The high amount of enzymes, such as catalase, and amylase, and pectin-splitting enzymes, make it an aid to digestion. Some research suggests that pollen is absorbed directly from the stomach into the blood stream. Pollen is a vegetarian source of human-active B_{12}, most of the B vitamins, vitamins A, C, D, and E, rutin, all the essential amino acids, the essential fatty acid called linoleic acid, fats, complex carbohydrates, simple sugars, RNA and DNA, steroid hormone substances, a plant hormone similar to the human pituitary called gonadotropin, 15% lecithin, and many other unknown factors. According to research by doctors from France, Italy, and the USSR, pollen is the richest source of protein in nature. Gram for gram, pollen contains an estimated 5-7 times more protein than meat, eggs, or cheese. The protein in pollen is in a predigested form and therefore is easy to assimilate. Pollen is also abundant in minerals and trace minerals, such as calcium, phosphorous, magnesium, iron, manganese, potassium, copper, silicon, sulfur choline, titanium, and sodium. These minerals are highly assimilable because they are bound organically from plant metabolism.

According to Dr. Airola, research in Russia and Sweden has found that bee pollen is both rejuvenating and life-prolonging. Bee pollen seems to improve general health, prevent disease, boost the immune system, and stimulate and rejuvenate the glandular system. M. Esperrois, M.D., of the French Institute of Chemistry, concluded from his experiments that pollen contains potent antibiotics and also reverses the aging of the skin. Research reported by Dr. Airola has found that bee pollen is good for prostate difficulties, hemorrhoids, asthma, allergies, digestive disorders, curing intestinal putrefaction, chronic bronchitis, multiple sclerosis, gastric ulcers, arthritis, hay fever, and possesses antiaging properties. According to Dr. Alain Caillais, in *"Le Pollen,"* 35 grams of bee pollen per day would satisfy the total nutritional needs of the average person. That is about three and one half tablespoons per day. Dr. Airola feels that it fulfills Hippocrates requirement of the ideal food:

"Let your food be your medicine...let your medicine be your food."

Pollen is harvested by the female worker bee when she brushes up against anthers of the flower. The pollen sticks to her legs. When she returns to the hive, she passes through a screen that rubs off some of the pollen pellets. Like fruit, the pollen does not require the killing of the plant. Some beekeepers feel that pollen turns rancid in as short a time as one week, even in the hive, if the harvesting is done less than weekly and the weather is hot. Dried pollen is also said to become easily rancid. The best technique for eating pollen, given these possibilities, is to get it from a local beekeeper within a week of harvest and put it in the freezer and not the refrigerator. Curiously enough, it doesn't seem to freeze in most freezers. This may be because pollen is only 3-4% water. In the freezer, it goes rancid a lot slower than out in the open or in the refrigerator. Other beekeepers do not seem to think it is necessary to freeze or even refrigerate it. The final test is—does it have a bitter, rancid taste. If it does, do not buy it. Research of Haydak, et al., reported by the San Francisco Medical Research Foundation, suggests that one-year-old bee pollen loses 76% of its effectiveness when not refrigerated. The San Francisco Medical Research Foundation estimates that after five months bee pollen loses up to 50% of its potency. The implications of these diverse opinions lead me to suggest that one should try to get bee pollen that has been at least refrigerated as soon as possible after harvest. The best way to do this is to make a connection with a local beekeeper and get it directly from the beekeeper. Depending on one's health, taste, and sensitivities, a good supplemental amount is one teaspoon to one tablespoon per day.

Yeast is another antiradiation food. It is particularly high in selenium, all the B vitamins, including B_{12} and nucleic acids, all of which give protection against the side effects of radiation. A study done at Montefiore Hospital in New York, in which three tablespoons of yeast were given daily for one week before cancer patients received radiation treatments, showed that these patients did not develop any side effects to the administered radiation. The control patients, who were not given yeast, developed severe vomiting and anemia. Although initially there was some confusion about avoiding all yeasts if people had candida infections, it has now become clear that the yeast that causes candida infections is Candida Albicans, and not saccharomyces cerevisiae, which is primary grown yeast and a genus and species different than candida. Unless a person's immune system is so deranged that it begins to cross-react against all yeast in the system, there is no major problem taking yeast. The dosage for radiation treatments is one tablespoon three times per day. Yeast and lecithin are high in phosphorous, so taking a calcium supplement or eating high-calcium foods is a good way to balance the phosphorous excess.

Garlic is another specific antiradiation food. Although garlic has many different, health-producing qualities, the properties which may be most active against radiation are amino acid cysteine, the high-quality organic sulfur, and an unidentified substance named vitamin X by the Soviets, which both prevents the absorption of radioactive isotopes and helps to draw them out of the body. Wild

ANTIRADIATION FOOD, HERBS, AND SUPPLEMENTS

FOODS

Miso	High Minerals, Zybicolin, 5% Ethyl esters (anticancer elements)
Sea Vegetables, Kelp	Iron, Potassium, Iodine, and the rest of the 56 land/sea minerals, Sodium Alginate
Sunflower Seeds, Apple and Soy	Pectin
Cereals, Fruit, Vegetables	Fiber, Phytates
Raw Food	Alkalinizes the system and has a general detox effect
Sulfur Vegetables (Broccoli, Cabbage, Cauliflower & Radish)	Sulfer, cysteine
Bee Pollen	B_6, B_{12}, Inositol, Folic Acid, RNA, DNA, and improves survival from X-ray treatment by 40%; contains 15% lecithin which protects nerve, brain, and gonads from radiation
Chlorophyll-containing Foods	Reduces radiation side effects by 50%
Beets	97-100% protection against $Cesium_{137}$
Garlic, Ginseng and Onion	Protects against mutagenisis, high selenium, anti-oxidative effect
Blue-green Algae	Protects against $Krypton_{85}$, $Cesium_{137}$, improves cellular immutability; high in chlorophyll

HERBS

Siberian Ginseng	Adaptogenic, doubles postradiation life span of rats
Chaparral	Potent anti-oxidant NGRA

SUPPLEMENTS

Germanium	Anti-oxidant
Cysteine	Removes free radicals, protects against X-ray, $Cobalt_{60}$, $sulfur_{35}$
Vitamin C with Rutin	Reduces radiation side effects by 50%, supports blood vessels
Vitamin A/D	Removes $Strontium_{90}$ from bone
Vitamin E	Protects fetus from $Cesium_{137}$, boosts immune system, anti-cancer effect, protects from free radicals
Detox baths	1lb. sea salt + 1 lb. Bicarbonate of Soda

Wash and peel produce in Clorox - Removes 100% of immediate, radioactive fallout

Fig. 26

onions and wild ginseng also seem to have this vitamin X. The sulfur, which is high in all the cabbage family, prevents the uptake of sulfur-135.

Cysteine may be the most active factor in garlic, however. Cysteine is an antioxidant which helps to quench free radical production. Cysteine also binds with, and deactivates, cobalt-60. It also protects against X-rays. Dr. Schechter points out that the Japanese first reported the protective effects of cysteine in 1972 when they found that mice fed cysteine were able to survive 600 rads of radiation when 70% of the mice who did not receive cysteine did not survive the radiation. This finding of cysteine's protection against cobalt-60 radiation has been confirmed by several researchers.

Foods containing **chlorophyll** have long been known to protect against radiation. Generally speaking, any green foods have chlorophyll. From 1959 to 1961, the Chief of the U.S. Army Nutrition Branch in Chicago found that high-chlorophyll foods reduced the effects of radiation on guinea pigs by 50%. This includes all chlorophyll foods: cabbage, leafy green vegetables, spirulina, chlorella, wheatgrass, any sprouts, and the blue green algae from Lake Klamath called Alphanizomenon-on-Flos-aqua (AFA). This variety of blue green algae is an excellent antiradiation food because of its high cellular immutability and high regenerative energy, as well as its high chlorophyll content. It should be taken in a dose of four capsules (one gram) four times per day for one week before, and several weeks after, radiation exposure.

One gram of the freeze-dried AFA, taken directly from Klamath Lake and prepared for regular consumption, also contains 0.279 milligrams of the active form of vitamin B_{12} for humans. Much of the B_{12} found in other algae, like spirulina, or even the various marine algae, are primarily in analog form. An analog form means that it is close to B_{12} in chemical structure but that it is not utilizable in the same way by humans, and actually might compete for receptor sites on the cellular level with the real B_{12}. The implication of all this is that one gram of AFA supplies the minimum daily need of B_{12} as established by researchers.

AFA also seems to help balance blood sugar and the mood swings associated with glucose fluctuations found in hypoglycemia. In conjunction with a well-designed diet for hypoglycemia, AFA has been a helpful adjunct. It is important to note my clinical findings on hypoglycemia and for other medical conditions have not been tested by strict research procedures. Further formal research studies need to be done to corroborate my limited clinical findings before a definitive statement can be made.

The most unique property of AFA, however, is its effect on the mind-brain function. In my work with AFA, I have observed with myself and with my clients that it has an extremely high SOEF that seems to regenerate mind and body energy. I use two forms of AFA. One is a unique, concentrated liquid, which is live and unprocessed until just before put into the bottle. This fresh, liquid preparation is the only one of its kind available today. The other form is freeze-dried and is available either in powder or capsules.

I find that the liquid works synergistically with the freeze-dried form. The freeze-dried form is about one hundred times more concentrated than the liquid, live form. The liquid form seems to have more of a pure energetic mind-brain effect. The freeze-dried form adds the energized neurotransmitters, sulfonolipids, and B_{12}.

As I point out in my book, *Spiritual Nutrition and the Rainbow Diet,* AFA seems to activate mind-brain function in about 70-80% of those who use it. It has been a blessing for those who do much mental work. It is also excellent for those doing a lot of high-stress work or for students taking exams. Of course, I do not recommend it as a substitute for healthy living habits or adequate sleep.

I have found that AFA also enhances one's ability to sustain concentration while taking or giving workshops. In my spiritual nutrition workshops, I teach nonstop from 7:30 am to 10:00 pm at night. I find AFA to be a tremendously helpful adjunct that helps me sustain my energy and mental concentration. It seems to create a subtle clarity of mind that potentiates both creative thinking and deep meditations.

Because of the brain-enhancing qualities I observed with this algae, I became interested in exploring its effect on Alzheimer's disease. In my preliminary research, which was published in the *Journal of the Orthomolecular Society* in the 1985 Winter/Spring issue, I reported two cases of people who had been diagnosed as having Alzheimer's disease at two highly respected university medical centers. In one person, the course of Alzheimer's was partially reversed; in the other, a rapidly moving senility was halted.

Along with bee pollen and sea vegetables, I recommend AFA as a whole food supplement for regular use in one's diet.

Antioxidant enzymes from wheat sprouts not only protect against all types of radiation exposure, but protect against the dangerous level of air, water, and food pollution, which also increases our exposure to free radicals. Mental stress and severe viral infections can also greatly increase the amount of free radicals in the system. As explained in detail in *Spiritual Nutrition and The Rainbow Diet,* free radicals are intimately connected with speeding up the aging process.

These live enzymes are specially formulated, organic, whole food supplements which are designed to neutralize free radicals. The entire dehydrated sprout is used in their product so it remains essentially a whole, live food when taken as a supplement. Nowadays, many antioxidant nutrients are offered in a variety of multivitamins. These work to some extent but these are usually synthetic vitamins and thus they lack a wholeness and integrity that is only found in whole foods and whole food supplements. These wheat sprouts are genetically selected and grown in a way that produces a high concentration of antioxidant enzymes, such as superoxide dismutases, methionine reductases, glutathione peroxidases, and catalases.

The two main enzyme companies that produce these wheat sprout antioxidants are *Bioguard* and *Biotech*. According to Dr. Steven Levine and Parris Kidd, in their book, *Antioxidant Adaption: Its Role in Free Radical Pathology*, antioxidant enzymes are described as the first line of defense against free radical stress. I also recommend them to protect against radiation exposure in my jet lag program.

These enzymes also adequately support the antioxidant systems in the body that protect us from free radicals. It is also important to note that the free radicals are most commonly active at the cellular level, but none of the ordinary vitamin-based antioxidants act as free radical scavengers at the cellular level. The vitamin antioxidants, such as C, A, and E, act primarily as free radical scavengers in their free form in the blood. The antioxidant enzymes, on the other hand, act as free radical "quenchers" at the cellular level.

The number of wheatgrass antioxidant enzyme tablets one takes varies and depends upon one's body weight and the amount of free radical exposure to which one is subjected. The maximum number of tablets per day from either of the two main companies presently manufacturing the wheat sprout product is about twelve tablets per day. For maximum free radical stress, three tablets taken four times a day at least one half hour before eating food is an optimal way to take them. The documented research suggests that as one increases the tablets up to a certain level per day, the enzyme activity in the blood increases. After a certain amount per day, the enzyme activity does not seem to increase in the blood and taking any more is redundant. Those who lead more toxic lifestyles, or who live in more toxic environments, should take close to the maximum suggested per day.

Herbs that Protect Against Radiation

Siberian ginseng, also known as Eleuthero, or Eleuthrococcus senticosus, despite its name, is not the ginseng we usually associate with the name ginseng. Siberian ginseng comes from an entirely different herbal family and originates in Russia and China. It comes from a bush, unlike ginseng panax, which is a root. Most of the research on it has been done by the Soviets.

Siberian ginseng is referred to as an adaptogen because it produces a generalized rebalancing and healing effect on the body from all types of physiological, emotional, and environmental stressors, including radiation. In the book *Fighting Radiation and Chemical Pollution With Foods, Herbs, and Vitamins,* many Soviet research articles are quoted which essentially show that Siberian ginseng is one of the best herbs for minimizing the effects of radiation. It has been used successfully in situations of acute or chronic radiation sickness, which include the conditions of hemorrhaging, severe anemia, dizziness, nausea, vomiting, and headaches due to X-rays. Siberian ginseng has been shown to lengthen survival time after exposure as well.

In one study, Siberian ginseng given one hour before radiation treatments improved the patient's general state, appetite, sleep, and normalized unhealthy shifts in the vital signs. Soviet medical researchers found that the best post-radiation treatment results were observed when the Siberian ginseng was started two to four days before the X-ray treatment. When two milliliters of the herbal extract was used per day, patients showed almost no usual reaction to the X-ray treatments, such as mental imbalances and irritability, dizziness, nausea, and loss of appetite. Many were able to maintain a state of well-being. Other research has suggested that even when the radiation is combined with chemotherapy, there are minimal side effects when the Siberian ginseng is used. The recommended dosage during the time of radiation therapy is approximately thirty drops, five times per day.

Siberian ginseng seems to enhance the general resistance to all aspects of the toxic side of anticancer radiation and chemotherapy. My experience in using Siberian ginseng clinically for many years is that it boosts almost every aspect of body function. It is especially good in supporting the endocrine and immune system against physical, emotional, chemical, biological, and radiation stress.

A general dosage to combat stress is 20-40 drops of the liquid extract in room-temperature water three times per day before meals. According to Dr. Schechter, in a personal communication, the extracted, organic form of Siberian ginseng is the most potent form. For children, give one drop for every year of their age, two times a day. When there is no obvious stress, one can take twenty to forty drops one time per day and also take some intervals not taking it at all.

Astragalus and **echinacea** are also very important herbs for supporting the immune system during radiation therapy. These are best taken daily for about one week before and one week afterwards, during the time of radiation. Panax ginseng is also an important antiradiation herb, particularly because of its ability to protect the immune and bone marrow production, as well as its general energizing effect on many organ systems. Chaparral is another excellent herb for helping the body resist the effects of radiation.

Summary of the Radiation Protection Diet

A low-fat, high, natural-carbohydrate, high-fiber, high-sea vegetable, 80% raw, vegetarian diet shifts the body into a slightly alkaline condition that has the effect of optimizing protection from radiation. This type of diet keeps one eating low on the food chain, avoiding all flesh foods and dairy, which are high carriers of iodine-131 and strontium-90.

The radiation protection diet has more emphasis on sea vegetables. For prevention and buildup of a mineral reserve, 3 ounces per week is sufficient. As

402

pollution increases in the ocean, it is important to know whether one's sea vegetables are not contaminated. There is at least one sea vegetable company who checks their sea vegetables for potential pollution at each harvest. It is the Maine Coast Sea Vegetables Company located in Franklin, Maine (207 565-2907). All their sea vegetables come from the still unindustrialized and relatively unpolluted northeastern end of the Gulf of Maine. Their sea vegetables are checked by the Maine Public Health Laboratories for 47 different chemical pollutants. These include PCBs, hydrocarbons, nine different insecticides and 36 different herbicides. No traces of any of these pollutants have ever been detected. The University of Maine's Department of Food Science tests the sea vegetables for lead, arsenic, mercury, and cadmium. As can be expected anywhere in the world, there are some trace heavy metals, but they are very low as compared to the United Nations FAO/WHO codex of tolerable daily intake limits. Tests at the University of Maine show that no harmful organisms, including coliform and e. coli bacteria, or yeast and molds, have shown any unusual microbial activity in the sea vegetables or during the drying, storing, or packaging process.

I regularly eat sea vegetables in their raw state and recommend them on almost a daily basis as part of the general diet. Because each sea vegetable helps remove different radioactive particles, I rotate between kelp, dulse, alaria (wild Atlantic wakame), and laver (Atlantic nori). Some folks report that sea vegetables are something one has to acquire a taste for. Miso is available in an organic and raw form and can be used in soups that are warmed to below 119° F or in tahini sauces or salad dressings. See our recipe section on radiation protection diet for a further discussion of sea vegetables.

The sulfur vegetables come in our sauerkrauts. For those who are sensitive to regular garlic, there are a variety of sun-dried garlics that do not have the irritating and activating effect that the fresh garlic oils may have. Although this diet has plenty of chlorophyll, I do recommend the Algae from Klamath Lake as a general enhancer of the mind-brain and also as a radiation protector. One tablespoon of bee pollen per day is also excellent.

Siberian ginseng is an excellent herb to take. In addition to its power to help one recover and withstand radiation exposure, it helps healing from high stress situations. It is part of my travel and jet lag kit as well.

Yeast is the only food that I do not regularly recommend because it is not a live food, but my impression clinically is that it is useful during times of radiation stress.

Eating the Wild Electron

Light is the basic component from which all life originates, evolves, and is energized. **Light and health are inseparable.** Because we have managed to disconnect ourselves from the sources of light with our fluorescent lights, indoor lifestyles, glasses, contact lenses, sunglasses, tanning lotions, flesh foods, processed foods and even cooked vegetarian diets, many of us suffer from chronic "mal-illumination." Like malnutrition, "mal-illumination" deprives us of a level of nutrients and rhythmic stimulation that is essential for living as fully healthy humans.

Noble Prize Laureate Dr. Szent-Gyorgi describes the essential life process as a little electrical current sent to us by the sunshine. Without light there is no health. This statement is a key in understanding the importance of vegetarian live foods and of other ways of bringing light into our organism. **We are human photocells whose ultimate biological nutrient is sunlight.**

Dr. Szent-Giorgi, when referring to the current of sunshine sent from the sun, is referring to highly charged single electrons that are involved in transferring their energy to our own submolecular patterns without changing our molecular structure. The quantum physics model begins to validate our more intuitive model of vegetarian food as condensed sunlight which then is transferred to our human organism when we eat it. When the energy of the earth's vegetation is transferred to us indirectly through flesh food, much of the bioelectric resonant energy patterns are destroyed. The sunlight energy is also lost if the bio-electric energy patterns of vegetarian foods are disrupted by cooking or processing.

The exciting breakthrough for me is the conceptual synthesis of how our food brings the photon energy of sunlight into our body and how our bodies utilize this energy. I alluded to these concepts when I discussed the research by Dr. Hans Eppinger who found that all cells were essentially batteries which appeared to be charged up when people were healthy. When people were sick, he found their cells to be in a discharged state and poorly functioning.The significant finding is that only uncooked foods were able to increase the cell battery potential.

The next step is understanding cellular metabolism as a battery. The positive pole is energetically fed by oxygen. The negative pole is fed by the high electron photon energy collected from the sun and stored in our vegetarian live food. This high electron food releases its electron energy across the cytochrome oxidase system. The cytochrome oxidase system acts as a step down transformer to turn the electron energy into ATP. ATP is the basic energy storage molecule of biological systems. The biochemical releases of energy from ATP are the fuel for all energy requiring processes at the molecular level in our biological systems.

The electrons are essentially drawn across the cytochrome oxidase system by the oxygen at the positive pole of the intracellular battery. The more oxygen in the system, the stronger the pull. Breathing exercises, eating high-oxygen foods, and living in atmospherically clean, high-oxygen environments increases our overall oxygen content. The key understanding is that the cytochrome oxidase system exists in every cell and requires electron energy to function. This electron energy comes from plant foods as well as what we directly absorb. When the food is cooked the basic harmonic resonance pattern of the living electron energy of the live food is at least partially destroyed. Once understanding this scientific evidence, the logical step is to eat high-electron foods such as fruits, vegetables, raw nuts and seeds, and sprouted or soaked grains.

Dr. Johanna Budwig from Germany holds degrees in physics, pharmacy, biochemistry, and medicine and is one of the first researchers to combine an in-depth knowledge of quantum mechanics and physics with an in-depth knowledge of human biochemistry and physiology. She has concluded that not only do electron-rich live foods act as high-powered electron donors, but **electron-rich foods act as solar resonance fields in the body to attract, store, and conduct the sun's energy in our bodies.** She asserts that the photons of the sunlight are attracted by the sun-like electrons resonating in our biological systems, especially in the double bonded electron clouds found in our lipids. These sun-like electrons are termed pi-electrons. This pi-electron system within our molecular structure has the ability to attract and activate the sun photons. She feels the energy we derive from these solar photons acts as an "anti-entropy factor." Translated into biological terms, entropy means aging. Anti-entropy is associated with the reversal of the aging process. From a quantum physics point of view, photons never become old; they have the same quickness as time. Sun photons transfer a high degree of order (anti-entropy energy) into the pi-electrons of our biological system. The more light we absorb into our system, the more health-restoring and anti-aging energy we bring into our human organism.

Therefore, people who eat refined, cooked, highly processed foods diminish the amount of solar electrons energizing the system and the amount of high solar electrons to create a high electron solar resonance field. According to Dr. Budwig, processed foods may even act as insulators to the healthy flow of electricity. The more we are able to absorb solar electrons, the better we are able to resonate, attract and absorb solar electrons in direct resonance from the sun, other solar systems, and even other galaxies. On a skin-deep level, the more we are able to absorb solar electrons the less sunburn and theoretically, the less skin cancer there will be.

Perhaps the two highest solar electron-rich foods and foods which have the capacity to absorb solar electrons are spirulina and flaxseed in various forms, including flaxseed oil. Dr. Budwig has reported cases of general ill health, and of even cancer, which have been reversed through the use of large amounts of flaxseed oil which has increased the amount of electron energy into the system and therefore created enough energy available to heal the system.

Because spirulina grows at high altitudes in high-temperature environments, it has increased beta-carotene, other carotenoids, enzyme systems, and other biological components to better absorb the intensified solar and cosmic radiations. I discovered that by ingesting spirulina and rubbing the product called Phycotene Cream (developed by Dr. Christopher Hills at Light Force) on myself, other members of our staff, and volunteers, we did not seem to get sunburned working long hours in the sun-filled skies of our mountain mesa at our Tree of Life Rejuvenation Center in Patagonia, Arizona.

Other research has shown that spirulina and Phycotene Creme have been successful in reversing squamous cell skin carcinoma and dissolving pre-cancer squamous cell carcinoma. Other research has found that three-fourths of the people who were hypersensitive to sunlight (suffering from erythropoetic protoporphinaria) were able to increase their exposure time in the sun. Three-fourths of those who improved their tolerance were able to be exposed to sunlight four times longer. For those of us who understand that we are human photocells who often suffer from mal-illumination, this is an extremely exciting finding.

Dr. Budwig also found that when the flaxseed oil is combined with highly charged protein, the three double bonded electron clouds available in the raw flaxseed oil and the protein, make a bi-polar capacitor grid which even better absorbs, stores, and transmits the exchange of solar electrons and enhances the solar resonance. She often uses a type of cottage cheese as a high-protein food to combine with the flaxseed oil. As a nondairy vegetarian, I find that bee pollen and spirulina are perfect high-protein concentrated foods to combine with flaxseed oil.

The discoveries of modern physics and quantum biology, according to Dr. Budwig, suggest there is no other living thing in nature that has a higher accumulation of the sun's electrons than human beings. Humans seem especially aligned with the sun's light. By the same solar electron resonance, our connection to the stars is enhanced by our ability to take in the gift of their light energy and process it biochemically. Light is our umbilical link to the universe.

Our ability to enrich ourselves with solar cosmic energy depends on eating foods with a high solar electron content that resonates with and attracts solar and cosmic rays. Our health and consciousness depends on our ability to attract, store, and conduct electron energy which is essential for the energizing and regulation of all life forces. **The greater our store of light energy, the greater the power of our overall electromagnetic field, and consequently the more energy is available for healing and the maintenance of optimal health.**

A strong solar resonance field promotes the evolution of humanity to reach our full potential as human "sun beings." Light supports evolution and a lack of photons in our bodies hinders it. Light and consciousness are interconnected. As far back as the turn of the century, Rudolph Steiner, the founder of the Waldorf schools, Anthroposophical Medicine, and biodynamic gardening taught that the release of the outer light into our systems stimulates the release of an equal amount of inner light within ourselves. The more we increase our ability to absorb and assimilate light, the more conscious we become. The more we transform **ourselves by enhancing our absorption of light, the more we become that light.** This is the subtle secret of 'conscious eating.'

Part IV

The Art of Food Preparation

The following recipes are based on the principles and conceptual frameworks that have been elaborated in the preceding chapters. I discuss the recipes in what might be considered an untraditional way. I am less concerned whether a recipe is a dessert or a main course, and more with whether a recipe is predominantly acid- or alkaline-producing, possesses omega-3 or omega-6 fatty acids, is heating or cooling, has an effect on the Ayurvedic dosha constitution of the person eating, has a seasonal effect, how it affects different organs, and whether a recipe has antiradiation properties.

In the formulation of these recipes, I have attempted to prepare the foods in such a way so that one can still taste and experience the distinct individual energies of the foods directly. At the same time, however, the food preparations are designed so that they are tasty, artful, interesting, and practical for helping the reader to individualize the diet to his or her own constitution. There is also a brief section on how various herbs affect the Ayurvedic doshas, including whether these herbs are heating or cooling and/or have a digestive-enhancing effect. These recipes also lead us to a slightly new twist on food combining. One does better not to combine two heavy foods together. For example, although avocado is a fruit and theoretically could be combined with other fruits, if it is combined with banana, another heavy food, it will cause an imbalance, especially for kaphas. For a pitta person, one tries not to combine foods that are all pitta unbalancing. Foods with major opposite actions, such as milk and flesh foods, are best not combined. On the other hand, one may chose to combine foods and herbs that modify each other's action. For example, garbonzo beans, which unbalance vata, when combined with tahini, garlic, and lemon, which balances vata, make a good combination which we enjoy as humus. By adding warming herbs (which activate the digestive fire) to vegetables which normally imbalance vata, we are able to broaden the range of foods a vata person can eat without being thrown out of balance. The same principle applies to the kapha and pitta doshas. In this context, food preparation becomes an artful endeavor.

Each recipe section is organized to help readers develop a feeling for developing their own recipes for the particular type of preparation discussed. The recipes are entirely composed of live food preparations without the use of extracted oils, sugar, or dairy. In the recipes there is an occasional use of miso, which although is derived from cooked soybeans, becomes enlivened by a beneficial nonalcoholic fermentation process that creates a lot of enzymes. Miso is very high in many minerals, adds a salty taste, has a strong yang energy, has specific antiradiation effects, and is an excellent nerve and stomach calmer and balancer for vata. Miso balances vata, has a neutral affect on kapha, and if taken in small quantities by pitta, does not cause an imbalance.

Occasionally, honey is suggested in the recipes. Although honey comes from bees and hence does not fit into a strictly vegan concept, honey is highly recommended in the Ayurvedic system as a food that is specifically indicated for balancing the kapha doshas. Paavo Airola, in his book, *Worldwide Secrets For Staying Young,* reports some very interesting longevity research conducted by famed Russian biologist and experimental botanist, Dr. Nicolai Tsitsin. Dr. Tsitsin, who is Russia's chief biologist and botanist in the bee industry, is quoted to have said, after conducting a survey of 150 respondents of 200 Russian people who were all greater than one hundred twenty-five years old,

> "All of the 200 or more people past 125 years old in Russia, without exception, have stated their principle food has always been pollen and honey — mostly pollen."

The honey these Russians ate was not the store-bought, pasteurized, and filtered honey that many of us know of as honey, but an unpasteurized, unfiltered, unprocessed, raw mix of honey and bee pollen found at the bottom of the honey containers. Interestingly enough, many of these Russian centenarians turned out also to be beekeepers. In *Worldwide Secrets for Staying Young,* Airola claims that honey boosts calcium retention, increases red blood cell count for nutritional anemias stemming from iron and copper deficiencies, and has a beneficial effect on arthritis, colds, poor circulation, constipation, liver and kidney disorders, poor complexion, and insomnia.

The knowledge that honey and bee pollen are rejuvenating foods has been known long before the Russians discovered it. Pythagoras, the Greek spiritual teacher and mathematician, used raw foods for healing, and recommended honey for health and long life as far back as 600 B.C. Although honey, strictly speaking, is a bee product and not a plant product, it is possible to find beekeepers who do not engage in an exploitive relationship with their bees by such practices as taking all their honey and feeding them sugar or giving them antibiotics.

Most often, the kind of beekeeper that cares about the welfare of the bees will also sell the kind of honey and bee pollen that is in its unadulterated, totally raw form. For one who adheres to a strict vegan philosophy this may still not feel "correct," but for others who follow the living law of harmony, honey in this context may feel acceptable. As I have discussed earlier, the principle of "harmlessness" is always a relative one in a world where each and every organism takes life in some form in order to survive. My ultimate guide is to eat that which enhances my communion with the Divine and which also does not violate my own spiritual sensitivities in light of the principle of harmlessness. The value and necessity to use honey differs with constitutional types. Honey is drying, warming, and astringent. Those with kapha constitutions are positively balanced and brought into a higher level of harmony and health by the use of honey. Pitta people, on the other hand, can become imbalanced by the use of too much honey. In any case, in the few times where I recommend honey in recipes, apple juice, dates, raisins or figs can usually be easily substituted for honey without affecting the recipes significantly.

An important focus of my concern in the evolution of these recipes was the preservation of both the taste and energetic qualities of the original food. I have also developed the recipes to bring out the energetic interplay of individual foods in conjunction with the properties of herbs. Some of these recipes are those used in the Spiritual Nutrition Workshops that my wife, Nora, and myself developed. Other recipes were developed independently or in collaboration with Eliot Jay Rosen, our first live-food chef for the Spiritual Nutrition Workshops, and Pat Furger, a former food preparation chef, who is presently working on her own live-food recipe book which will include some of these recipes and many more delicious recipes. I also thank Wind D' Golds, who teaches vegan and live-food preparation, for her generous help and contributions to this recipe section. I also extend my gratefulness to Bobbie Sparr, a naturopathic and Ayurvedic practitioner, who double-checked the dosha balancing of these recipes.

I hope to empower the reader with the necessary skills with which to prepare and grow live foods, such as live sauerkraut, sprouts, seed sauces, seed yogurts, and seed cheeses. Also included is a section on dehydrated foods for storage or for traveling and camping trips. These foods are dehydrated at 118° F in order to maximally preserve enzymes. Although dehydration is the most enzyme-conserving and least disruptive of the life energy of the food, according to the Kirlian photography data, the dehydration process reduces the overall energy of the food by about 25%. There is also an inevitable, natural loss of vital energy over time with storage. Because of this energy loss with dehydration and storage, I primarily recommend dehydrated foods for travelling, camping, and situations in which one has to store the food to save it. Dry foods tend to unbalance vata and balance kapha. They may also unbalance pitta if they are dry and heating and not dry and cooling.

My primary goal is to develop an appreciation of the different food and herb energies and to give the reader a basic repertoire of recipes that represent patterns of raw food preparation so that he or she may later begin to create his or her own recipes based on the principles behind these "template" recipes. With a proper understanding of these recipe patterns one can develop a tasty diet which can consistently balance constitutional doshas, maintain a balanced pH, build or cleanse, and heat or cool the body as one chooses. Most of my recipes are designed for one or two servings.

Simple Secrets for Warming, and not Killing, Live Foods

These techniques still preserve the enzymes and other unknown heat-sensitive factors.

1. One easy way to create warmth is to re-warm the plate in the oven or the sun. One can also warm the plate with the food on it for several minutes until warm to the touch.

2. As long as one doesn't go above 118° F for more than 2-3 minutes, one can warm raw soups, grain dishes, and vegetables in a regular sauce pan. An easy rule of the "finger tip" is: if it is warm to the touch of a finger, this is approximately 118° F. Just how much above 118° F, and for how long, is not entirely clear, so I recommend taking away the heat as soon as it becomes warm to the touch.

3. If one is able to find a crock pot which heats at 118° F or below, it is possible to slow-heat certain foods. Small, thinly cut potatoes will actually taste like cooked potatoes after 12 hours in a crock pot. In such a low-heat crock pot it is also possible to make raw stews and vegetable soups. One potential danger to this type of 12-hour, low-heat food preparation is it makes a good medium in which bacteria multiply. With potatoes, this is not particularly a problem, but with soaking vegetables it may be more so. One way to minimize this potential is to scrub the vegetables well before using. Another difficulty to the extended warming approach is that despite the low temperature of the cooking, the food loses its energy over the extended cooking time.

4. Another interesting way to bring external heat to the food is by warming sauces and pouring them over the rest of the food. One can even warm some of the food to 118° F and mix it with the other raw food. This technique is used with the wilted spinach salad.

5. Many foods do not create a marked cooling if they are simply served at room temperature rather than chilling them in the refrigerator before serving.

Balancing Your Doshas While You Eat

There are a number of herbs that specifically enhance digestion, dry or moisten the body, and also heat or cool the body. Many of these herbs are particularly beneficial to the vata and kapha constitutional types whose digestive fire is often low and therefore receive benefit from the heat and digestive stimulating properties of these herbs. There are also some cooling herbs for pitta

410

constitutional types. The interplay of the doshic effect of the foods and the herbs is what gives the balancing effect. Most of this herbal information is taken from my own direct experience as well as the books, *The Yoga of Herbs,* by Dr. Vasant Lad and David Frawley, and *Classical Indian Vegetarian and Grain Cooking,* by Julie Sahni. These healing and culinary herbs are one of the secrets of how one can increase digestive fire and total body heat while eating live foods.

Herbs for Balancing Doshas

In designating the specific effects of a certain herb in the recipes, the word "balances" denotes that the herb brings a particular dosha back into balance. The word "unbalances" means that the herb causes a disharmony in that dosha. For example, a pitta person tends to have their pitta energy more easily imbalanced than a kapha or vata person by heating herbs. Therefore, pittas are more prone to be thrown out of balance by herbs that increase the pitta energy. Likewise, a kapha person who is low in pitta energy will often be brought into balance by the heating energy of the same herb that imbalances the pitta person. For the rest of the recipes, K means kapha, P means pitta, and V means vata. The following are a few commonly used herbs in food preparation:

Allspice is pungent, heating, balances KV, and unbalances the P dosha. It relieves gas, promotes peristalsis, and stimulates metabolism.

Anise is pungent, heating, balances KV, and unbalances the P dosha. It relieves gas and promotes digestion. It comes from the tiny seeds from both Anisum vulgare and Anisum officinalis. In India it is known as foreign fennel.

Asafoetida is pungent, heating, balances VK, and unbalances P. It is a powerful stimulant of the digestive fire and dispeller of intestinal gas, pain, and bloating. It is one of the best herbs for removing V imbalance in the colon. It comes from the dry gum of the living rhizome of several species of Ferula growing in India, Kashmir, and Afghanistan. If available, it is preferable to buy asafoetida in what one might call "lump" form because when it is in powdered form it often has added gum arabic, barley, wheat, or flour. In its lump form it is odorless. When ground, asafoetida gives off an onion-like smell due to the sulfur compounds of its volatile oils.

Basil is pungent, heating, balances KV, and unbalances P if taken in excess. Basil is said to open the heart and mind to the Divine. There are a variety of basil plants. The most famous basil is called Tulsi, or holy basil in India. In India it is said to have an association with Lord Vishnu that dates back to Vedic times. "Holy" basil juice is said to be a longevity drink.

411

Bay leaves are pungent, heating, balances VK, and unbalances P if taken in excess. It stimulates digestion and relieves gas. The Indian bay leaves are the leaf of the cassia tree. The tree grows in India and eastern Asia. American bay leaves, called laurel bay, are more pungent, as well as more expensive.

Black pepper is pungent, heating, balances VK, and is neutral to P, but unbalances P if taken in excess. It is a powerful digestive stimulant that relieves gas, neutralizes toxins, and burns up mucous. It has been used in food and ceremonies since Vedic times in India.

Cardamom is pungent, sweet, heating and balances V. Its sweetness helps to alleviate P if not taken in excess. It is one of the best herbs for enhancing digestion, relieving gas, and strengthening the stomach. Cardamom is the fruit of the plant Elettaria caramomum found in southern India and Sri Lanka. The cardamom pod can be used in its whole form for a mild effect. For a more aromatic effect, the seeds or whole pod can be ground. It comes in three colors: green, white, and black. The white is actually a bleached green. The natural green is preferable. The black cardamom is less spicy.

Cayenne is very pungent and heating, balances VK, and unbalances P. Cayenne can be thought of as containing much sun energy because of its dramatic heating effect. It has the ability to relieve internal and external chilliness. Cayenne also helps to alleviate indigestion, stimulates the digestion, and burns up toxins in the digestive system. It is good for circulation. It is pleasantly warming on a cold winter day. There are many grades of cayenne peppers with different degrees of pungency and heat from the same capsicum plant from which cayenne is taken. Cayenne pepper is a general term for a pepper called "bird chilies" which is also used to make Tabasco sauce. Other red chilies are also given the name cayenne. Dried chili peppers come as pods and also in a powdered form.

Cinnamon is pungent, sweet, astringent, and heating. It balances VK, in excess may unbalance P. Cinnamon's sweet, astringent qualities makes it suitable for Ps who are not in a state of excess. It stimulates digestion and relieves gas. It comes from the bark of the cassia tree, Cinnamomum cassia. This form of cinnamon is stronger than the cinnamon which comes from the bark of the Cinnamomum zylanicum or "sweet" or "true" cinnamon. Cinnamon can be used in whole sticks, crushed or ground.

Clove is pungent, heating, balances VK, and unbalances P. Cloves stimulate digestion and metabolism and eliminate gas. Cloves come from the dried buds of the plant Syzygium aromaticum, a plant native to the Molucca Islands in eastern Indonesia.

412

Coriander is bitter, pungent, and cooling. It balances VPK. A substance that balances VPK is called tridoshic. It helps to cool P aggravations. It is good on a hot summer day. It comes from the plant coriandrum sativum from which the white-colored coriander seeds are taken. The leaves of this plant are highly aromatic. Coriander seeds are a primary spice in curry. The fresh leaves are used in food preparation the way parsley is used. In Chinese and Japanese stores it is also called Chinese parsley. It is also know as cilantro, especially in Spanish and Portuguese-speaking nations.

Cumin is bitter, pungent, and cooling and balances VPK. It stimulates digestion and relieves gas. Cumin comes in white or green seeds from the Cumin cyminum plant. It resembles caraway seeds. Cumin is used in Spanish, Mexican, African, West Indian, and Middle Eastern food preparations. There is also a black or royal cumin which comes from the plant cuminnum nigrum. This variety is more mellow and sweet, grows wild in Iran and in the valleys of Kashmir and is rarer than other types of cumin. Black onion seeds and caraway seeds are often mistakenly referred to as black cumin.

Curry leaf (Neem leaf) is pungent, sweet, and heating. It balances VK and unbalances P. It comes from the aromatic leaf of the plant murraya koeniggi which grows to be six to eight feet tall. Curry leaf is an ancient spice used in Vedic food preparation and comprises the base of the curry powder many are familiar with and commonly use. The fresh leaves keep about two weeks in the refrigerator. They are available as dry leaves, but are about one-third as potent. Curry leaves are frequently used in Indian lentil and vegetable stews. Please note that curry powder, which will be discussed later, is not a single herb but is a "masala" combination. A masala may be made up of a combination of spices, spices and herbs, or spices, herbs, and vegetable seasonings (such as onion or garlic).

Dill is pungent, bitter, and cooling. It balances PK and is neutral for V. Dill helps with digestion and is a good cooling herb for the summer. Indian and European dill are closely related and both can come in either a wild or cultivated form.

Fennel is sweet, pungent, and cooling. It balances VPK. It is good for strengthening the digestive fire without unbalancing P. It helps to cool pitta and relieves gas and digestive slowness. Fennel seeds resemble cumin but are larger. The licorice-like taste of fennel makes it easily distinguishable from other herbs. Fennel is such a good digestive aid that in India it is used as an after dinner "mint."

Fenugreek is bitter, sweet, pungent, and heating. It balances VK and although it slightly unbalances P, it can be taken in small amounts by Ps.

Fenugreek helps digestion. Fenugreek sprouts are good for indigestion. The fenugreek seed is actually a legume or bean.

Garlic is pungent, heating, balances VK, and unbalances P. It is a digestive stimulant, dispels gas, and is a great general healer. It contains all the Ayurvedic tastes but sour. In its sun-dried form, garlic's characteristic aroma and stimulating qualities are significantly diminished so it can be considered more of a sattvic and balancing food than a rajasic, heating, and activating food as when it is in its raw form.

Ginger is pungent, sweet, heating, balances VK, and unbalances P. It stimulates digestion, relieves gas if not taken in excess and helps to detoxify the body, especially the liver. Dry ginger is more balancing for kapha because of its drying qualities and fresh-squeezed ginger is slightly more balancing for vata because of more fluid qualities. It is good for detoxifying during a juice fast. Its sweetness allows Ps to take it in minimal amounts. Botanically, ginger is an aromatic rhizome of the tropical plant Zingiber officinale. A rhizome is a horizontal stem that resembles a root-like structure of a plant which sends out roots from its under surface and stalks from its upper surface. When ginger is organic, freshly picked and young, the skin does not need to be peeled.

Horseradish is pungent, heating, balances VK, and unbalances P. It helps to relieve mucous and stimulates digestion. It is best taken in small amounts. I have used it successfully as an adjunct to helping heal asthma.

Mustard seed is pungent, heating, balances VK, and unbalances P. It stimulates digestion and relieves gas. It comes from the mustard plant, Brassica. Certain mustard seeds are pressed to make mustard oil, which is also heating.

Nutmeg is pungent, heating, and sweet. It balances VK, and unbalances P. It increases food absorption, particularly in the small intestine. It helps to relieve V in the colon. Nutmeg is the nut portion of the Myristica fragrans tree. It is often used along with cardamom. The covering of the nut is a red membrane which is ground and used as a spice called mace. Too much nutmeg has been known to have a disorienting effect on the mind.

Onion is pungent, sweet, and subtly cooling to the digestive tract in its postdigestive effect. In its raw form it balances K, slightly unbalances V, and unbalances P. Its sweetness, watery properties, and postdigestive slowing of digestion may unbalance K if K is already in excess. There are many varieties of onions all possessing varying strengths.

414

Turmeric is bitter, astringent, pungent, and heating. Taken in small amounts it is tridoshic like cumin. It may unbalance VP if taken in excess. It is good for digestion, relieves gas, and increases peristalsis. It improves and balances metabolism in the body. It is the spice that gives curry powder its coloring. It is a rhizome of the plant curuma longa which grows horizontally under the ground. It said to purify the subtle nerve channels of the body.

RAW FOOD RECIPES

• Masala Recipes •

Masala is an Indian word that refers to a seasoning blend that can be any combination of herbs, spices, and vegetables. These already prepared combinations speed up the food preparation process. In India they are often individualized to a particular geographic area or even to a particular food preparer. As one plays with these combinations, I encourage making one's own combinations or varying the proportions of the different combinations according to one's dosha needs.

Purchased masalas often have spices processed in several ways, including cooking in oil. Processing the spices and herbs in this way is said to help preserve the masala because it insulates and dries it. To make your own masala and thereby eliminate the need for excess processing and the use of heated oils, one can mix and dry spices and herbs by putting them in a food dryer at 118° F degrees or lower. The masala recipes below are all raw combinations with the exception of a few already dried spices that one can add to the mix.

Basic Raw, Hot Curry Powder

To make one cup, mix:

1/2 cup coriander seeds
10 dry red chili pods
1 1/2 tsp. cumin seeds
1 tsp. mustard and fenugreek seeds
2 tsp. black peppercorns
20 curry leaves and double if not fresh leaves
3 Tbs. turmeric powder
(typical of South Indian cuisine)

Grind in a blender and store in an airtight jar. Stores well up to three months. For best storage, dry the fresh curry leaves in a dehydrator before using.

Remarks: Imbalances P, balances V and K. A good fall and winter heating masala. Adds taste and heat to sauerkrauts, humus, and seed sauces and salad dressings.

Raw, Mild Curry: same as the basic recipe above, but use only 3 chili pods and 1 tsp. black peppercorns.

Hot and Sweet Raw Curry: same as the basic but add 2 tsp. cinnamon and 1 tsp. cloves.

Basic, Raw Garam Masala

Makes 3/4 cup

1/4 cup cumin
1/4 cup coriander seeds
1 1/2 Tbs. cardamom seeds
2 whole cinnamon sticks
1 1/2 tsp. whole cloves
3 tbs. black peppercorns
4 bay leaves

Blend in a spice mill until a fine powder. Store in an airtight jar.

Remarks: Balances V and K, and unbalances P. Works nicely in all four seasons.

Marathi Hot, Raw Garam Masala

Makes one cup

1/4 cup coriander seeds
4 Tbs. cumin seeds
1 Tbs. fenugreek seeds
1/2 Tbs. cloves
2 Tbs. cardamom seeds
8 broken up bay leaves
8 dry red chili pods, broken up
1/2 cup flaked coconut

Dry at 118° F for 6 hours and blend in a spice mill.

Remarks: Balances K and V and unbalances P. Good for fall and winter.

Nala Masala

1 tsp. cloves
1 tsp. cinnamon
1 tsp. nutmeg
1 tsp. black peppercorns
1 tsp. cardamom

Blend in a spice mill.

Remarks: Balances K and V, and can be used by P in small amounts. Useful in all four seasons. It is nice to add to the soak water for dried fruits to create an overnight spice effect. Good for all seasons.

Curry Masala

2 tsp. curry powder
1 tsp. black peppercorns
1/2 tsp. dried garlic
1/2 tsp. cloves
1 tsp. cardamom

Blend in a spice mill.

Remarks: Heating, balances K and V, unbalances P. Tasty in all seasons. Adds an interesting taste to veggie dips, seed sauces, and seed dressings.

Winter Heat Masala

1 tsp. black peppercorns
1/2 tsp. cayenne
1/2 part dried garlic
1/2 tsp. ginger powder
1/2 tsp. cardamom

Blend in a spice mill.

Remarks: If one has gas difficulties or likes the smell and taste of onions without eating them, add 1/8 tsp of asafoetida (Hing). Hing is balancing to V, especially in terms of lower bowel gas. This is a cold weather masala which can turn almost any salad dressing or vegetable preparation into a warmer and gastric fire stimulator.

Banana Smoothie Masalas

1. Mix 2/3 tsp. cardamom, 1/3 tsp. dried ginger, and 1/3 tsp. cinnamon and blend with 12 oz banana smoothie.
2. Mix 2/3 tsp. powered cardamom, 1/3 tsp. dried ginger, and 1/2 tsp. powdered nutmeg and blend with 12 oz. banana smoothie.
3. Mix 1/2 tsp. each cinnamon and nutmeg, and 1/3 tsp. dried ginger and blend with 12 oz. banana smoothie

Remarks: Taken in small amounts, cardamom and cinnamon do not imbalance P. This masala taken at half the amount of spice per ounce of banana smoothie creates a balanced drink for V, P, and K. This masala is moderately warming, sweet, and stimulating to digestion. It is used comfortably in all seasons.

Pat's Vegetable Cooling Masala

Lemon cucumbers - 50%
Yellow squash - 30%
Green beans - 20%

1. Wash and slice vegetables. Please keep in mind that with dehydration the amount one starts with shrinks drastically. To give you some idea, in the above recipe, start with 5 cups sliced cucumbers, 3 cups sliced squash, and 2 cups sliced green beans.
2. Put entire amount of vegetables into dehydrator and dry for approximately 5-10 hours.

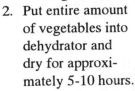

3. After drying put small batches into a mini-food processor or coffee mill and grind to desired grain consistency. Store in jar with tight-fitting lid.

Remarks: This is a cooling masala which balances all three doshas. The dehydrating of the cucumber makes it not unbalancing for K. This is a good masala for late spring and summer and good for P any time.

Heating Vegetable Masala

Prepare the following percentages of vegetables in the same manner as the cooling masala and grind to a powder.

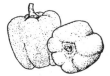

Green bell peppers - 50%
Red peppers   - 40%
Garlic cloves   - 10%

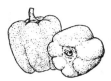

Remarks: This is unbalancing for P, but balancing for V and K. It can be used in all seasons.

Fruit Masala

Apricots -   50%
Kiwis -   30%
Lemon rind - 20%

1. Cut apricots in half, remove pit, then slice each half into 1/2" slices.
2. Peel and slice kiwis.
3. Juice the lemons and store juice in refrigerator for future use.
4. Slice each lemon peel half into 1/2" slices.
5. Put all ingredients into dehydrator and dry for approximately 10-15 hours or more, depending on your dryer.
6. After drying, put ingredients, small amounts at a time, into a coffee mill and grind until small enough for a spice-like consistency.

Remarks: Use with fruit salads or fruit dressings. This also makes a delicious tea; put 1-2 tsp. in a tea strainer and let sit in a large cup of hot water or make a great sun tea by adding 1/4 cup of spice to 1 gallon of water, put in a covered jar and set outside and let the sun shine its love. The fruit masala adds variation to a camping trip. This is a good masala for balancing V, and if used in small amounts, it is tolerated well by P and K. A good one to use in late spring, summer, and early fall.

Pat's Original Harmony Masala

1 bunch celery
2 large bell peppers of each color
4 medium-to-large cucumbers
1 red onion
3 cloves garlic.

1. Slice all vegetables and put into the dehydrator no higher than 118° F.
2. When completely dried put into a coffee mill (a little at a time) and grind until mixture resembles spice.

Remarks: This masala is great for anything from soup to salads. For soups do not grind the vegetable mixture as fine. By leaving it coarser it adds texture as well as taste to soups. This is an all-purpose traveling and camping masala. This is a tridoshic masala and good for all seasons.

Mexican Masala

Tomatoes - 50%
Celery - 20%
Red bell pepper - 20%
Lemon - 10%
Cayenne - 1/4 tsp. or added to taste

1. Slice all vegetables and dehydrate.
2. Put dehydrated veggies into a coffee mill and grind to a spice consistency.

Remarks: Tomatoes unbalance P, and in excess may unbalance V and K. V people do best with tomatoes if the peel and seeds are removed and if it's a sauce, paste, or juice, so this masala form is acceptable for V. This is a warming masala which can be used in any season. This masala, like the other vegetable masalas, can be used in a variety of ways while camping, travelling, or at home. For an instant tomato-celery juice, add 2 Tbs. Mexican masala to one cup of water. Blend or stir for one minute. Let it stand for a minute, add fresh lemon if desired, and drink. For a soup, warm in the sun or heat until hot to fingers. To make a hot tomato dressing, add 2 Tbs. raw apple cider vinegar to 4 Tbs. Mexican masala. Add 1 cup water, 1/4 tsp. cayenne or more to taste, and blend or stir until evenly dispersed. This recipe is extremely heating for camping trips. It is also acidifying.

To make a zingy tomato dip, add 6 Tbs. of the Mexican masala to the juice of one lemon and add water to achieve desired thickness. The lemon creates a more alkalinizing effect and makes it more balancing for V. Let sit in a cool place or refrigerator for a little bit. Serve with dehydrated crackers or slices of cucumber, carrot sticks, or jicama slices.

• Grain Recipes •

It is possible to make raw grains edible by soaking or sprouting them without having to cook them. These grains are turned into biogenic foods when prepared in this way. In their biogenic state, the life force in the seed germ is capable of re-creating a new plant. They are an important food in the live-food approach because they are both high in calories as well as enzymes. Along with the soaked nuts and seeds, they are live foods high in calories which help people gain or maintain their weight. The high enzyme and calorie mixture makes them particularly good for those who, after years of eating cooked foods, have begun to deplete their enzyme systems. They supply a grounding, heating, yang effect. V and P do a little better with grains than Ks. Each grain will affect the doshas differently. Brown rice balances V, but is slightly unbalancing for P and K. Millet, rye, buckwheat, and corn are hot, light, and dry in effect. These, along with barley, are balancing for K, but neutral for V, and slightly unbalancing for P. Wheat is considered cold, heavy, and moist so it unbalances K, but is balancing for V and P. Soaked and sprouted grains support the transition process from cooked foods because they are also more filling for those used to the heavy feeling usually produced by the eating of cooked foods. The high phosphorus content of grains is also good for the nervous system and brain. Although cooked grains have a distinctly acid affect on the system, sprouted or soaked grains run a continuum from slightly acid to neutral, or even slightly alkaline. More research is needed on the acid base properties of soaked and sprouted grains. My own intuition and preliminary research suggests that there is a shift in these grains toward becoming more alkaline-forming, but just how much of a shift the sprouted grains make, and for which grain, cannot be precisely ascertained at this time.

In the soaking or sprouting process, which activates the life-giving enzymatic process, potentially harmful enzyme inhibitors and mineral chelators, such as the phytates, are washed away. The usual method to accomplish this is to soak a grain for one to three days depending on the air temperature. For those grains which sprout, soak for 24 hours and then let them sprout until they are softer and taste edible. The exact length of time depends on the particular grain and the combined effects of the growing/soaking environment. The best grains for sprouting are wheat, rye, and triticale. Rice, sprouting millet, and sprouting oats will sprout, but did poorly on an informal taste test that I conducted. Please note that sprouting oats, which will be described below, are different than whole oat groats, which do not sprout, but do enzymatically change when soaked for 48 hours. The soaked oats are high in enzymes and very tasty.

422

The sprouting grains of wheat, rye, and triticale are similar in the time it takes them to sprout and the length of the sprouting tail, which indicates they are ready to be eaten. The best length of the tail is approximately 1/4", which is the stage which many feel the grain becomes biogenic and reaches its nutritional peak. Sprouted grains can be eaten directly, used in salads, put in the blender to make a cereal or grain drinks, or used to make sprouted breads.

The best grains for soaking are oats, barley, and buckwheat. Hulled raw oats and pearled (hulled) barley become soft and nonstarchy in 36-48 hours at approximately 70° F. Rice may take up to 6 days to turn enzymatically active. Buckwheat can become edible as quickly as 4 to 6 hours. Buckwheat is a good grain for travelling because it takes less than overnight for it to become enzymatically active, soft, nonstarchy, and edible.

The soaking process for all the grains can be accelerated by soaking them in warm water up to 118° F. One can even use a crock pot to do this. I know of at least one crock pot on the market that can be kept at a 118° F or below setting. The warming of the soak water technique is useful when travelling and when one only has one night to activate the grains.

Grandma's Oatmeal Live Porridge

1. Soak one cup of hulled, raw oat groats for 48 hours. Rinse and drain each day.
2. When the oats are soft and nonstarchy, rinse and drain and put in the blender with the juice of three figs which have been soaking overnight. Blend until smooth.
3. Warm to 118° F or when hot to the finger and serve.

Remarks: Oats are sweet warm, heavy, and moist so they are balancing for V and P, but not for K. For an additional heating effect and to make this oatmeal dish balancing for K, soak the grains and or the figs in one of the heating masalas. This presoaking approach allows the masalas to soak into the grain and also permeate the figs and juice. Use approximately 1 tsp. per cup of oats. This adds an unusual taste to the porridge that would even intrigue the three bears. This is a great warm porridge for cold mornings.

Eliot's Tridosha Grain Drink

Makes one serving.

2 oz. hulled, raw oat groats
2 oz. hulled, raw buckwheat groats
1 tsp. flaxseed
1 tsp. sunflower seeds

1. Soak for 48 hours. Changing the water daily is not necessary, but I prefer to.
2. Rinse and blend.
3. This drink can be taken warm or room temperature. To warm, simply heat to finger-hot temperatures in a sauce pan and pour.
4. The grain drink combines well with a banana to make a blended banana drink, especially for V.

Remarks: This mixture is good for V, P, and K. For other variations one may want to add either/or:

a. 1 tsp. miso to the grain drink before one blends. Miso is particularly balancing for V, and acceptable for P. Ks can use miso if 1/2 tsp. is used.
b. 1/4 oz. dulse or other sea vegetables one may like. If the dulse is rinsed, it is balancing for V and neutral in effect on P and K. If it isn't rinsed, the salt unbalances P and K.
c. 1 tsp. of a masala of your choice. The Nala masala is a good one. One's choice of masala can also be added to the soak water for the second day or for both days if one doesn't change the water. This gives it time to permeate the grain. This grain drink can be used in all seasons. It is slightly acidifying to neutral in its effect on pH.

Basic Sprouted Bread Crackers

2 cups winter wheat (or rye) berries

1. Soak wheat berries in a large jar for 12 hours.
2. Drain and rinse and sprout for approximately 2 days or until the sprout tails are approximately 1/4 inch long, draining and rinsing them two times per day.
3. Put the sprouted berries into a food processor or a Champion juicer. It is thick and may strain the juicer. A clicking noise from the Champion means it is overloaded and more than likely it will become quite hot. To eliminate the clicking noise add just a little bit of water into the mouth of the juicer.
4. The Cuisinart food processor is the only piece of equipment that does not require water for the wheat berries. Run the Cuisinart until the berries have a dough-like consistency.

5. Remove dough from processor and knead for a few minutes, if your hands get sticky, wet them with water and start kneading again.

6. Form the sprout dough as one large "bread" and use a rolling pin to spread out the mixture evenly onto the plastic inserts or Saran Wrap that one will be putting on the dehydrator trays. One may place the dough by teaspoonfuls and flatten them lightly onto the dehydrator plastic inserts or Saran Wrap. If using the total dough spread, one can precut them by indenting the crackers with a blunt knife to the size and shape one wants.

7. Place into your dehydrator and set it for 118° F. Dehydrate until crispy. Dryers and room temperature vary so this may take anywhere from 8-12 hours. Usually overnight will do it. The thinner one forms the bread the quicker is the dehydrating time.

8. Two cups of wheat berries will make one pound of dehydrated bread or crackers.

To vary the taste of the crackers or bread you may add one or more of the following to two cups of wheat berries. Add them at the same time you are processing the wheat berries in the blender or Cuisinart.

a. 1 cup dehydrated tomatoes
b. 1/4-1/2 tsp. dehydrated garlic, depending on taste
c. 1/8-1/4 tsp. cayenne, depending on taste
d. 1 1/2 tsp. curry
e. 1 tsp. dehydrated dill with sprouted rye
f. 1 1/2 Tbs. dehydrated onion
g. 1/2 tsp. kelp, depending on taste
h. 1 tsp. basil
i. 1 1/2 tsp. of any of the masalas
j. 1 1/2 tsp. curry and 1 1/2 tsp. dill
k. 1 tsp. caraway seeds
m. 1/2 cup unhulled, soaked sesame seeds
n. 1/2 cup soaked sunflower seeds

Remarks: Drying the wheat into crackers makes the wheat more balancing for K. Normally wheat balances V and P and unbalances K. Rye can also be substituted for wheat in part or completely. Rye is balancing for K but unbalancing for V and P. A 50% rye and wheat cracker comes the closest for balancing all three. These sprouted crackers have a slightly acid to neutral effect on the pH. These crackers can be used all year around. They are particularly good for travelling and camping.

"Thanksgiving Crackers"

2 cups winter wheat (for K use rye)
1 cup raw yams or sweet potatoes
1 cup raisins
1 1/2 Tbs. cinnamon
1 tsp. nutmeg

1. Sprout grains as explained above and mix with yams and raisins.
2. Put through a processor, grinder, or homogenize in the Champion food processor/juicer.
3. Knead for a few minutes.
4. Put into dehydrator by spoonful or rolling pin approach for a whole batch.
5. Leave in the dehydrator at 118° F overnight for 8-12 hours. Checking your crackers half way through the drying period and turning them over will help shorten the drying process.

Remarks: This is a tasty all-seasons cracker which is balancing for V and P and neutral for K if using wheat. It is balancing for K if using rye. This cracker is neutral to slightly alkaline in its affect on pH.

Salsa Cracker

2 cups sprouted winter wheat that has been made into a dough
1/2 onion
2 cloves garlic or 1 tsp. sun-dried garlic
1/4 tsp. cayenne or more, depending on taste
1/2 cup ground, dehydrated tomatoes

Combine all ingredients with the dough base, put into a dehydrator as explained above, and dry for approximately 8-12 hours.

Remarks: This is balancing for V, neutral for K, and slightly unbalancing for P.

Ginger Crisp

2 cups wheat or rye sprouts (for K)
1 Tbs. finely grated, raw ginger

Blend and dehydrate.

Remarks: This is balancing for V, P, and K. The heat of the ginger may unbalance P if eaten in excess. It's nice for cold weather. Slightly acidic or neutral pH.

• Grain Salad Recipes •

Zucchini Barley Salad

1/2 cup soaked barley
1 small zucchini, grated
1 large tomato, diced
1 tsp. cilantro, chopped fine
1 tsp. masala of your choice sprinkled on top

Combine all ingredients and serve.

Remarks: One can serve this cold grain salad on a bed of alfalfa or sunflower sprouts or lettuce. Barley is considered cool, light, and dry. It has a diuretic effect that helps to balance K, but imbalances V. It is also balancing for P. It has a mild laxative effect. This salad can be balancing for V if a warming masala is used. This salad is better for the cooler months, but with a warm masala, it works all year around. The total salad is neutral to alkalinizing on the pH.

Buckwheat-Avo Salad

1/2 cup soaked buckwheat
1/2 avocado
1/2 tsp. crushed garlic or 1/2 tsp. sun-dried garlic

1. Soak and drain buckwheat for 4-6 hours.
2. Cut avocado and mix with buckwheat.
3. Add garlic and mix.

Remarks: Buckwheat is hot, light, and dry. The salad is balancing for K, slightly unbalancing for V and P, and neutral for V. The avocado helps to balance V and P and the garlic helps to further balance the V. This makes a great salad by itself, but is also a great stuffing. To stuff red bell peppers with it, slice off tops of bell peppers, rinse out pepper and stuff with salad, and top with grated carrots. Make a cabbage or nori sea vegetables burrito with it. Lay nori sea vegetable or cabbage flat, add salad and roll it up. Barley can also be substituted for buckwheat.

Spinach-Barley-Seed Salad

1/2 cup sprouted barley
1/4 cup sprouted sunflower seeds
1/4 cup sprouted pumpkin seeds
1 bunch fresh spinach, sliced very thin
1 tomato

1. Soak barley and seeds 36-48 hours and drain.
2. Cut spinach and tomato into bite-sized pieces.
3. Serve with Italian dressing.

Remarks: This salad, if eaten occasionally, is acceptable for all three doshas, although most balancing for K. Better for the summer, and in the winter, a more heating dressing could be used to help K and V. It is slightly acidifying to neutral.

• Sauces, Dressings, Spreads, and Dip Recipes •

Sauces, dressings, spreads, and dips are linked together because they represent a continuum in this system of food preparation. The spreads and dips are essentially the sauces and dressings at different concentrations of liquid. If the seed sauces are left to ferment, they will turn into seed yogurts, and can eventually be turned into live seed cheeses. These seed cheeses represent a high concentration of easily digested, predigested protein. They make a nice addition to salads, tacos, burritos, and soups.

Most of the sauces are seed sauces which are made from soaked seeds or nuts blended with a fruit, juice, or water. Most seeds need to be soaked 6-8 hours and can soak longer if need be. Nuts generally require 12 hours of soaking. To use them on a regular basis, one just has to remember to soak the nuts or seeds the night before. The soaking activates the enzymes and metabolism in the germinal seed or nut as well as washes away inhibitory enzymes. The fats, carbohydrates, and protein in the nuts and seeds become more predigested when soaked. The significance of this is that the seeds and nuts are easier to digest. In the soaked form they become compatible with fruits. The more fat a nut has, the more likely it will unbalance K and P. Some nuts which do this are Brazil, Macadamia, walnuts, and pistachios. Other seeds are warming, such as chia and sesame seed. The soaked seeds and nuts are less concentrated, less heavy, less oily, less sweet, and less dry. Because of this the whole range of soaked nuts and seeds generally becomes neutral to slightly balancing to V, K, and P if not eaten in excess. By blending them and eating them immediately afterwards we further enhance digestion. For some seeds, such as flaxseed, it is difficult to get the full nutrition of the seed without breaking it up by blending. Dehydrating the nuts and seeds tends to make them slightly unbalancing for V if eaten in excess and more balancing for K. Those that are heating for P will become more heating when dehydrated, and thus unbalancing to P if eaten in excess. Soaked nuts and seeds are neutral to slightly acidic in their affect on the pH.

The main seeds and nuts which are commonly used are: sesame, pumpkin, sunflower, chia, flax, and almond (one can soak walnuts, Brazil nuts, etc. but they do not sprout). Chia seeds are particularly heating. After soaking nuts and seeds they become excellent biogenic foods. With unhulled sesame seeds, after soaking overnight, blend the seeds in water for several minutes to break off the hulls. Then strain the mixture through a cheese cloth or special seed bag. What comes through is called a seed milk. One can do this with any seed. Once one has a seed milk, one may creatively combine it in any number of ways using a variety of ingredients. With the exception of unhulled sesame seeds, and perhaps for infants, I do not recommend seed or nut milks because too much nutrient is lost in the straining process. The reason it is particularly important to strain unhulled sesame seeds is that there are high concentrations of oxalates in the hull which may interfere with calcium utilization.

The seed sauce process works quiet well when vegetables as well as fruits are blended with the soaked seeds or nuts. These sauces, as well as the fruit sauces, are basically alkaline in their effect on the body. Whether they are cooling or heating depends on the vegetables, fruits, masala, or spices one adds. For example, a cucumber and dill addition will cause cooling. The addition of ginger and cayenne will cause a heating affect. The usual ratio is between 1/4 to 1/2 cup of seeds or nuts to one cup of liquid. The thinner the sauce, the greater the liquid one must add. Once one makes the sauce, one can drink it directly as a smoothie or it may be poured over a fruit or vegetable salad. Although best consumed immediately, refrigerated seed sauces are an excellent snack for those with hypoglycemia. Seed sauces may last up to 24 hours if kept in the refrigerator.

Sesame Milk

1/2 cup raw, unhulled sesame seeds
4 cups water or more

1. Soak seeds overnight; rinse and drain.
2. Put into blender with water and liquefy.
3. Strain through a large piece of cheesecloth, squeeze gently, and drain the "milk."
4. When finished draining put the milk into a quart jar. If one uses hulled sesame seeds, then one can enjoy a thicker drink because there is no need to strain.

Remarks: Could be unbalancing to P if eaten in excess. Good in all seasons. Warming spices, such as 1/2 tsp. ginger, cardamom, or cinnamon, can make it more warming for the winter. These spices go well with any of these milks. Neutral to slightly alkaline.

Almond Milk

1/2 cup soaked almonds
1 cup water

Instructions are the same as for sesame milk.

Remarks: These traditional milks can be used for a light drink. For a thicker and more nutritious drink just blend without putting through a strainer. With more than a few almonds, it is better to blanch the almonds by letting them sit in boiling water for 30 seconds, quickly drain off the water, and remove the skins by pinching them off. The skins have high concentrations of tannic acid which can have a deleterious effect on the stomach. It has an alkalinizing effect on the body.

Orange Almond Creme Drink

1 cup soaked and blanched almonds
2/3 cup fresh-squeezed orange juice
Optional: 2 dates (for P) or 1/2 tsp. honey (for K)

Blend at least 3 minutes until very smooth and creamy. There should be no grainy taste.

Remarks: This is most balancing for V, but in small amounts because it is soaked and with honey. It is balancing for K, and with dates, for P it is neutral. This can be used as a drink, a sauce over fruit, in a fruit soup or smoothie, or as a topping for the fruit pie (use 1/3 to 1/2 cup). Good for all seasons and is alkalinizing.

Om Sesame Sauce
(Orange-Mango-Sesame)

1/2 cup sprouted sesame seed
2 mangos, peeled, take pit out and use the rest
2 oranges, peeled
Depending on the sweetness, add 2 dates or 1/2 tsp. honey

Put all ingredients into blender and blend on high speed until smooth in consistency. This sauce will take a while to blend because of the sesame seeds, stop the blender often and scrape down the sides with a spatula. Blend for approximately three minutes.

Remarks: Balancing for V and neutral for K and P. Sesame is slightly heating. This is a delightful, all-seasons sauce, slightly alkalinizing.

Classic Banana Sunseed Sauce

1/2 cup soaked sunflower seeds
2 bananas
1/2 cup water (or raw apple juice for a sweeter taste)

Blend and serve over fruit or drink directly.

Remarks: Bananas are sweet, heavy, and cooling. This is most balancing for V. It is unbalancing for K and, if taken in excess, unbalancing for P because of its postdigestive sour effect. This sunseed sauce is one of the main ways I suggest for Vs to put on weight. This sauce supplies a high enzyme content that aids the digestion. This, plus the carbohydrate from the banana and the predigested protein from the seeds, makes it a powerful rebuilder and a good snack for hypoglycemia. It is also helpful for people with poor absorption. It is slightly alkalinizing; good for late spring to early winter.

Spicy Banana Sunseed Sauce

Spice combinations added to the classic banana sunseed:

1. 1/2 tsp. nutmeg and 1 tsp cinnamon
2. 1 tsp. cinnamon and 1 tsp. cardamom
3. 1 tsp. of any of these three spices by themselves

Remarks: These spices make this seed sauce neutral for K and even more balancing for V. It is good for all seasons.

Mango Banana Sesame Seed Sauce

1/2 cup soaked and hulled sesame seeds
1 mango
1 cup water (or 1 cup raw apple juice for a sweeter taste)
2 bananas

Blend and serve.

Remarks: Mango is balancing for V, K, and P. This sauce is neutral to alkaline-forming for the pH. It is an all-season sauce.

• Favorite Flaxseed Recipes •

Flaxseeds are particularly important because they are the best and safest source on the planet of the essential omega-3 fatty acids. One tablespoon of seeds per day is approximately what is needed to supply one's daily need. When combined with sunflower seeds, which supply the essential omega-6 fatty acids, one gets a supply of all fatty acids. The flaxseeds give a creamy texture to whatever they are blended with. Some examples of combinations are below. Do not hesitate to experiment and create one's own unique combinations.

Red Top Salad Dressing

2 Tbs. soaked flaxseed
1 cup carrot juice
1/2 red bell pepper
1/4 tsp. cayenne
Add ingredients and blend
until smooth.

Remarks: This is a heating dressing.
Carrots, cayenne, and flaxseed are all warming. Flaxseed is balancing for V and K, but unbalancing for P. Because of the omega-3 fatty acids the
flax gives relief to all inflammations, and especially joint
and skin inflammations. Just adding flax to several raw food
peoples' diet has rebalanced some V skin conditions. Flax is also
balancing to the bowel by enhancing elimination. This dressing is
alkalinizing and good for all seasons.

Double O-3 Salad Dressing

1 Tbs. soaked flaxseed
1 cup raw apple juice
2 Tbs. raw apple cider vinegar
2 Tbs. raw walnuts

Add ingredients and blend until smooth.

Remarks: This is balancing for V, neutral for K, and unbalancing for P. Because of the walnuts and the apple cider vinegar, this is a particularly acidifying dressing which makes it a choice dressing for those who find themselves too alkaline. It is good for all seasons.

Carrot-Papaya Creme Sauce or Dressing

1 Tbs. soaked flaxseed
1 cup carrot juice
1 papaya
1 tsp. fresh grated ginger to taste

Add ingredients and blend until smooth.

Remarks: This is balancing to V and K, but slightly unbalancing for P. It is alkalinizing. It is slightly warming and good for all seasons.

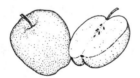

Curry Apple Sunflax Drink

1/2 cup soaked sunflower seeds
1 Tbs. soaked flaxseeds
1/2 tsp. curry
1 cup raw apple juice

Blend.

Remarks: Balancing for V and K, and neutral to slightly unbalancing for P. One clove garlic or 1/2 tsp. sun-dried garlic and 1 tsp. fresh ginger juice heats this drink up for winter months, but makes it more unbalancing for P. It is alkalinizing.

Make Your Own Vegetable Seed Dressing

1/4 to 1/2 cup soaked sunflower seeds (various combinations of pumpkin, sesame, almond, or chia seed can be used). The seeds, including the flaxseed, can be soaked together.
1 Tbs. soaked flaxseed
2 Tbs. raw apple cider vinegar (for alkaline types) or 2 Tbs. lemon juice (for acidic types)
1/4 to 1/2 tsp. cayenne to taste or 1 tsp. masala of choice (optional for Ps)
1/2 cup or more of water or raw apple juice until desired consistency has been reached
1/2 cup cut-up vegetable of your choice

1. Soak flaxseed and sunflower seeds overnight.
2. Drain and put in blender with remaining ingredients.

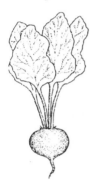

Remarks: This is a basic dressing. One may add one of the following to change the taste and desired effect. During the winter, the more heating masalas are used, such as: Winter Heat, Nala Curry, or Hot Marathi Raw Garam Masalas. In the summer, the cooling masalas or more dill or coriander may be used. The base mixture is balancing to V and K, neutral to unbalancing for P.

Mango-Sesame Seed Sauce

1/4 lb. soaked sesame seed
1 mango
1 Tbs. honey (optional)

1. Put ingredients for mango seed sauce into a blender and blend until very smooth in consistency. Note: sesame seeds take longer to blend, take a test taste every couple of minutes until the sauce is no longer crunchy.
2. Pour mango sesame seed sauce over the fruit.

Remarks: This is balancing for V and K, but slightly heating and slightly unbalancing for P. Ps can enjoy it in small amounts. It is alkalinizing. Good in late spring, summer, and fall.

Sun-Zucchini Dressing

1/2 cup soaked sunflower seeds
1 Tbs. soaked flaxseeds
1 cup raw apple juice
1 cup chopped zucchini
1 clove garlic or 1/2 tsp. sun-dried garlic (optional for P)
1 1/2 tsp. dill
 Blend all the ingredients.

Remarks: This is a mildly cooling, alkalinizing dressing which balances V, P, and K. Good for late spring, summer, and early fall.

Curry Carrot Dressing

a. 1 cup carrots, sliced in chunks and added to blender
b. 1 cup broccoli, cut in chunks
c. 1 clove garlic or 1/2 tsp. sun-dried garlic powder
d. 1 cup beets, cut in chunks
e. 1/2 avocado
f. 1 tsp. grated ginger
g. 1 tsp. or more curry.

Blend.

Remarks: Balancing for V and K, and neutral or unbalancing for P. Ps can have a little, especially if the garlic and ginger is cut in half. It is alkalinizing, and good for winter, spring, and fall.

• Seed Yogurt and Cheeses Recipes •

Seed yogurts and cheeses are variations of the fermentation process of the seed sauce. Once the seed sauce is made, let it stand at a temperature between 70-90 degrees with a screen over the top to protect it from insects flying into it. Friendly airborne lactobacillus will automatically inoculate your blend, but the fermentation process can be aided by using a little of the seed cheese or yogurt from the last batch as a starter. As the fermentation proceeds, health-promoting lactic acid is produced and the predigestion process of the protein, fats and complex carbohydrates occurs. It is thought that the bacteria also produce B_{12}. As the seed yogurt/cheese ripens, the whey (the watery portion) begins to separate. This takes 4-6 hours. At this point what one has created is called a seed yogurt. One may stop the process by putting it in the refrigerator or eating it on the spot.

If one allows the process to continue, after 8-10 hours, the whey completely separates from the seed "curd" and one is ready to make seed cheese from the creation. The whey will be on the bottom and the cheese will be on the top. Seeing bubbles in the cheese and smelling a lemony smell indicates that the seed cheese is ripe for harvesting. To harvest the seed cheese, pour off the whey. A simple way to do this is to take a chop stick and poke a hole in the cheese along the side of the jar. Then gently pour off the whey through this hole. Pour this whey through a sprouting bag or cheese cloth. Following this the rest of the seed cheese will empty into the sprouting bag until all of the whey is eliminated. To further extract the whey from the seed cheese, squeeze the seed cheese, which is now contained in the sprouting bag, to force out the remaining whey. If you squeeze too hard, the bag may burst and the cheese will get "a whey!" If this happens, it is comforting to know you are not the first person in the world to whom this has happened, nor will you be the last. To continue to dry out your seed cheese, wring out by squeezing the seed cheese that is now in the sprouting bag. Then let the sprouting bag or cheesecloth hang on a hook for several hours for any residual whey to drip off.

After drying, the seed cheese can be eaten or stored in the refrigerator for 3-4 days. Seed cheeses make delightful additions to vegetable or fruit salads (it is already predigested so that it combines well with fruits). Since the seed cheese is still soft, it can be molded into interesting shapes and served as a spread with crackers or on vegetables such as celery slices, beet-slice chips, or with carrot sticks.

Seed cheeses can be made even more interesting and intriguing by adding a masala at the original seed sauce stage, such as curry-dill seed cheese below. The choice of herbs makes the seed cheese heating or cooling. Seed cheeses are an acidifying food. They can be eaten in any season.

Curry-Dill Seed Cheese

1 cup water
1 cup sunflower seeds soaked for 6-8 hours or over night
1 1/2 tsp. curry (use 1/2 tsp. for P)
1 tsp. dill

1. Blend all the ingredients.
2. Set out at room temperature with a mesh screen over the top for 8-10 hours.
3. Follow the rest of the steps from the basic seed cheese outline.

Remarks: This is balancing for V and K, and neutral for P if the curry is cut in half. Good for all seasons.

Ginger Seed Cheese

1 1/2 cups soaked sunflower seeds
1 Tbs. finely grated ginger
1/2 cup soaked pinenuts
1 cup water

Blend the ingredients and start the seed cheese process.

Remarks: This is balancing for V and K, but unbalancing for P.

Curried Beet Sun Cheese

1 1/2 cups soaked sunflower seeds
1/4 cup grated beets
1 tsp. curry
1 cup water

Blend ingredients and start the seed cheese process.

Remarks: This is balancing for V and K and unbalancing for P. It is an interesting taste and color for "cheese." It is more of a fall, winter, and spring cheese.

Masala Seed Cheese

1 1/2 cups soaked sunflower seeds
1 tsp. masala of choice

Blend ingredients and start the seed cheese process.

Seed Cheese Wraps

Take any seed cheese and wrap in a nori sheet, cabbage leaf, or put inside 1/2 bell pepper.

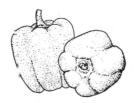

Remarks: The nori is more balancing for P and the cabbage leaf is unbalancing for V, but the overall effect of the dish stays approximately the same. With the cabbage leaves, a V should add more warming and digestively activating herbs.

Almond Miso Sculpture

2 cups soaked, blanched, and peeled almonds
Veggies, fruits or flowers for the chakra 'colors'
2 lemons
1 2/3 ozs. mellow miso

1. Put almonds through Champion Juicer, add the lemon juice and the miso to the almonds, and mix thoroughly and shape.
2. Add veggies, fruit, or flowers for colors and designs and place on the loaf. Surround with bed of sprouts.

Remarks: The miso, almonds, and lemon are balancing for V, neutral to slightly unbalancing for P, and unbalances K. This is alkalinizing and can be eaten in any season. It is a strong builder and nerve tonifier for V. It is good for gaining weight. Better for spring, summer and fall.

• General Commentary on Salad Dressings •

A basic concept behind choosing a particular salad dressing in this live food approach is to use a dressing to balance the salad according to one's dosha and other body needs. For example, adding a masala affects the heating or cooling effects of the food. It directly influences the different doshas. The use of apple cider vinegar makes a salad dressing acid-forming. Using lemon juice in a salad dressing makes it alkalinizing. Soaking seeds and nuts moves these foods in the direction of being neutral to alkaline. If eaten in moderation, soaked seeds and nuts neutralize the potential imbalancing effects on any of the doshas that unsoaked seeds and nuts have. The seed sauces and nuts add considerable building protein and oil to the salad. Walnuts give a specific acidifying effect and add more omega-3 fatty acids. Flaxseed is the main supplier of omega-3 fatty acids, as well as lignands, which boost the immune system.

In this approach to live foods, the addition of a seed dressing transforms a salad into a total balanced meal. When one becomes well-established in live food cuisine, this type of tasty seed sauce/salad becomes a filling meal in itself that simultaneously helps to meet one's minimum protein, fat, and complex carbohydrate needs, as well as biogenic needs. The choice of the masala adjusts the energy of the total meal to one's doshas and the season of the year. If I am not using a seed salad dressing, then I will often add some nuts or seeds, such as walnuts, soaked pumpkin seeds, or sunflower seeds to the salad. Flaxseeds are not well-absorbed unless they are soaked and blended. Powdering the dry seeds in a spice mill and using as a powder also helps assimilation.

The seed and nut sauces and dressings can also be used as soups or even dips by varying the thickness. These sauces and dressings can even be thought of as whole meals in themselves.

Sunny Ginger Tahini Dressing

1/2 cup soaked sunflower seeds
2 Tbs. raw apple cider vinegar (if alkaline)
juice of 1/2 lemon (if acid)
1 tsp. ginger juice
1/2 tsp. mellow miso
2 Tbs. tahini
1/4 tsp. cayenne
1 tsp. curry masala (alternative taste and adds more heat)
1/2 cup raw apple juice or water to right thickness for a soup
1 cup raw apple juice or water for a salad dressing

Remarks: Tahini is heating, oily, and heavy. Although heating, it doesn't necessarily stimulate digestion. Because of all factors in this dressing, it is balancing to V, neutral to K, and unbalancing to P. It is alkaline or acid depending on lemon or apple cider vinegar. This is good for all seasons, particularly winter. This is a good building dressing.

Tahini Ginger Miso Dressing

2 Tbs. raw tahini
1/2 cups water
1 tsp. fresh grated ginger
juice of 1/2 lemon (if acid)
2 Tbs. raw apple cider vinegar (if alkaline)
1 clove garlic or 1/2 tsp. sun-dried garlic (optional for P)
3/4 tsp. mellow miso

Put all liquid ingredients and the ginger into blender first, blend for 30 seconds. Add the rest of the ingredients and blend until smooth.

Remarks: Same as Sunny Ginger, but not as building. For a spicy tahini ginger miso dressing, add 1/2 tsp. black pepper, 1/8 tsp. hing, and 1/4 tsp. cayenne (not for P). Good for winter, fall, and spring.

Three Seed Winter Heat Dressing

Add one heaping Tbs. raw tahini to the Winter Heat Dressing (p. 440). It makes it hotter and adds more oil, which can further imbalance P.

Carrot-Tahini Dressing, Soup, or Veggie Dip

2 heaping Tbs. raw tahini
1/2 tsp. curry
1/4 tsp. black peppercorn
1 cup fresh carrot juice for a dressing
1/8 tsp. hing (good for V)

For a soup add approximately 1/2 cup carrot juice. For a dip, blend in three whole carrots to the soup to increase thickness.

Remarks: Balancing for V and K, and unbalancing for P. This is neutral to slightly alkalinizing, good for any season.

Tahini Ginger Dulse Dressing

1 Tbs. raw tahini
1/2 tsp. fresh, grated ginger
juice of 1/2 lemon (if acid) or 2 Tbs. apple cider vinegar (if alkaline)
small handful dried dulse, which is then soaked and rinsed before using
1/4 tsp. cumin
1/4 tsp. cayenne or to taste
1/3 cup apple juice or water to desired thickness

Blend ingredients in blender or Vitamix until smooth. Serves 1 or 2.

Remarks: It is balancing to V, neutral to K, and unbalancing to P. It is alkaline or acid depending on use of lemon or apple cider vinegar. This is good for all seasons, particularly winter. This is a good building dressing; also a good source of human-active B_{12}.

Winter Heat Dressing

1/2 cup soaked sunflower seeds
1 Tbs. flaxseeds
1/2 cup apple juice or more to desired thickness
2 Tbs. apple cider vinegar (if alkaline)
juice of 1/2 lemon (if acid)
1 tsp. Winter Heat Masala

Blend ingredients and serve.

Remarks: This is a winter dressing that balances V and K and unbalances P. It is acid or alkaline as one chooses.

Acid/Alkaline Sun-Zucchini Dressing

1/2 cup soaked sunflower seeds
2 Tbs. apple cider vinegar (if alkaline)
juice of 1/2 lemon (if acid)
1/2 cup water (or apple juice for a sweeter taste)
1 zucchini
1 tsp. masala of choice

Blend.

Remarks: Zucchini balances V and P, but unbalances K. A hot, dry masala will counterbalance the K. The soaked sunflower seeds neutralize extremes so this is balancing for V and P and neutral for K. This is best in the summer with a cooling masala, but can be used in the winter with a heating masala. It is also a template for making all vegetable dressings by substituting a carrot, beet, broccoli, or other vegetables for the zucchini.

To thicken for a soup, add an additional cup of cut up zucchini to the recipe for sun zucchini dressing. Use 1/2 -1 cup apple juice to the desired thickness for dressing or a soup.

Green Zinger Dressing

1 cup parsley
2 Tbs. raw tahini
3/4 cup water
1/2 tsp. black pepper

Blend and serve.

Remarks: This is balancing for V and K, and neutral for P. Parsley is balancing for all three doshas. The black pepper doesn't unbalance P unless taken in excess.

Sweet & Sour Dressing

1/2 cup sunflower seeds
1 cup water
3 Tbs. raw apple cider vinegar
1 Tbs. honey or 2 dates
1 large tomato
Put all ingredients into blender and liquify.

Remarks: This is balanced for V, neutral for K, and unbalancing for P. It is acidifying and okay for all seasons, but more often used in the summer.

Spanish Salsa Dressing

1/2 cup soaked pumpkin or sunflower seeds
1/2 cup raw apple cider vinegar or lemon juice
3 medium tomatoes
1 clove garlic
1/4 tsp. cayenne pepper or more
1/2 cup fresh chopped coriander

Put first 5 ingredients into blender and liquify.

Remarks: Balancing for V and K and unbalancing for P. More of a fall dressing, but could be used any season. In the summer, increase the coriander and decrease the cayenne.

Curry Apple Dressing

2 Tbs. apple cider vinegar
1/3 cup apple juice
1 Tbs. raw tahini
1/2 tsp. black pepper
1/2 tsp. curry

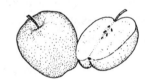

Blend and pour over the salad.

Remarks: Acidifying, balancing for V and K, and unbalancing for P. Good in all four seasons.

Cucumber-Tomato Dressing

1 cucumber, chopped
1/4 cup dried tomatoes
1 cup sesame milk
juice of one lemon (if acid)
2 Tbs. raw apple cider vinegar (if alkaline)
1/2 tsp. mellow miso

Put first four ingredients into blender, blend until smooth. Add miso last and blend for 30 seconds.

Remarks: Cucumber is cooling and sweet, it is balancing to V and P, and unbalances K. Miso is neutral to P, but can imbalance K if in excess. The sourness of apple cider vinegar or lemon imbalances P and K. This dressing is balancing to V, neutral to P, and imbalancing to K. This is a good summer dressing.

Creamy Cuke Dressing

2 heaping Tbs. raw tahini
1 large cucumber
2 tsp. dill
1/3 cup water

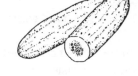

Blend all the ingredients.

Remarks: Balancing to V, P, and neutral to K. Slightly acidifying and cooling. A good summer dressing.

Lemon Tahini Dill Dressing

1 Tbs. raw tahini
1/4 cup lemon juice
1/2 cup water
2 tsp. dill

Blend.

Remarks: This is an alkalizing summer dressing that balances V, K, and P.

Basil-Dill Dressing & Marinade

1/3 cup lemon juice
1/3 cup water
3 Tbs. fresh basil
3 Tbs. fresh dill
1/2 tsp. honey or use 1/2 cup apple juice instead of water

Put all ingredients into a blender and blend until mixed.

Remarks: This is an all-season, alkalinizing summer dressing that balances V, P, and K.

Italian Dressing

2 Tbs. raw apple cider vinegar
1/2 cup water
1 large tomato, quartered
1 tsp. fresh basil
1/2 tsp. fresh oregano
1 clove garlic or 1/2 tsp. sun-dried garlic

Put all ingredients into a blender and blend until smooth. One may need to add more water, depending on the consistency.

Remarks: An acidifying, all-seasons dressing that balances V, K, and slightly unbalances P.

Lemon-Avo Dressing

1 large avocado
2/3 cup water
4 tsp. lemon juice
1 clove garlic or 1/2 tsp. sun-dried garlic

Put all ingredients into blender and blend until smooth in consistency.

Remarks: This is balancing for V, neutral for P, and unbalancing for K. It is alkalinizing and good for all four seasons, but I would add 1/4 tsp. cayenne during the winter.

Lemon Miso Dressing

1/2 cup water
1 Tbs. mellow miso
2-3 Tbs. lemon juice

Put all ingredients into blender. Blend for 30 seconds. This is a simple dressing to sprinkle over veggies or a light salad.

Remarks: Very alkalinizing. Balancing for V, neutral for P, and slightly unbalancing for K. Good for all seasons, but ideal use in the summer.

Sweet Dill Salad Dressing

3 Tbs. raw apple cider vinegar
1 tsp. honey or 2 dates
1 tsp. dill
1 cup water
Put all ingredients into blender and blend for 1 minute.

Remarks: Great on salads and coleslaws. For dill, 1 tsp. coriander or parsley can be substituted. This is a cooling, acidifying, dressing that is good for the summer. It balances V, is neutral for K if honey is used, and neutral for P if dates are used.

Guacamole Dressing

1 avocado, cut into pieces
1 tomato, chopped
1/4 cup lemon juice
1/4 cup water
1 Tbs. fresh coriander
1 clove garlic or 1/2 tsp. sun-dried garlic
1/4 (if P) to 1/2 tsp. cayenne pepper

Put all ingredients into a mini-food processor or mash with a fork and process until coarse in texture.

Remarks: If one needs more acidifying dressing, substitute 2 Tbs. apple cider vinegar for the lemon juice. The lemon juice makes it more alkalinizing. Depending on the amount of cayenne, this dressing can be heating or cooling. It can be balancing for V,P, K depending on the amount of coriander, garlic, and cayenne used. Use during all four seasons.

Sweet-Sour Dressing & Marinade

3/4 cup water
2 Tbs. raw apple cider vinegar
1 tsp. honey or 2 dates depending on sweetness
1 tsp. fresh ginger, grated

Put all ingredients into blender and blend until smooth in consistency. Can also put in a closed jar and shake until ingredients are blended. To use as a marinade, simply put the vegetables in the sauce and let them sit for 4-6 hours.

Remarks: This is an acidifying dressing that is good all year around. It balances V and K, but unbalances P. For a thicker consistency as a dressing, add 2 Tbs. tahini.

445

• Dips •

Like any dip, we can vary its desired effect on the system by the addition of different ingredients.

Sweet Humus

2 cups sprouted garbonzo beans (2-3 days until the sprout is nonstarchy and between 1/2" and 3/4")
juice of 2 lemons
3 Tbs. raw tahini
2 cloves garlic or 1 tsp. sun-dried garlic
1/4 cup raw apple juice
1/4 tsp. cayenne (if P) to 1/2 tsp. (for V or K)
1/8 tsp. hing (if get strong V imbalance from garbanzos)

Blend and serve.

Remarks: Humus is neutral for V. The cayenne, lemon, and garlic help to balance the unbalancing effect of the garbanzos on Vs. Some Vs do get imbalanced with humus. For these folks, 1/8 tsp. hing keeps the humus from having an unbalancing effect. P and K are also balanced by humus. The apple juice is sweet and balancing to P and K. Humus is good in all seasons. During the winter, more cayenne and garlic might be needed. Adding 4 raw olives to the recipe can bring the olive oil taste to the raw humus. Humus is one of the few raw beans I recommend for sprouting. Many of the raw sprouted beans tend to unbalance V and cause gas. One reason is that the trypsin and other enzyme inhibitors are still partially active in a raw sprouted bean. The more it is sprouted, the more the enzyme inhibitors are inactivated and washed away so the easier it is to digest. Garbanzo beans from which humus is made are cool and dry. Their dryness helps to balance K. The sesame in humus brings more heat and oil which is balancing to V. To these base recipes one can also add 1 tsp. of a masala of choice for variation. Humus is nice to eat with crackers, on top of sliced tomatoes or vegetable cuttings, on top of salads, or in sea vegetables and cabbage tacos. Raw humus, along with avocado and sprouts, makes a nice filler to be stuffed in bell peppers.

Sour Lemon Humus

2 cups sprouted garbanzo beans (sprout 2-3 days until nonstarchy and sprout is between 1/2" and 3/4")
juice of 2 lemons
3 Tbs. raw tahini
2 cloves garlic or one tsp. sun-dried garlic
1/4 -1/2 tsp. cayenne to taste
water to desired thickness, up to 1/4 cup

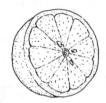

Blend and serve. I try to use no
water to keep it as thick as
possible.

Remarks: This is more
alkalinizing and the
lemon helps to
balance V.
Otherwise
it is the same
as sweet humus.

Acidifying Humus

2 cups sprouted garbanzo beans (sprout 2-3 days until nonstarchy and sprout is between 1/2" and 3/4")
3 Tbs. tahini
1/3 cup raw apple cider vinegar
2 cloves garlic or 1 tsp. sun-dried garlic
1/4 tsp. cayenne

Blend and serve.

Remarks: Same as sweet humus, but acidifying.

Curry Humus

Add 2 tsp. curry to 2 cups of any raw humus mix.

Beet Spread

1 1/2 cups grated beets
1 1/2 cups sprouted sunflower seeds
juice of 1/2 lemon plus the pulp
1 Tbs. raw tahini
1/2 tsp. dill
1/2 tsp. coriander
No water to 1/4 cup water or less depending on the thickness desired
1/4 tsp. cayenne

Blend and serve.

Remarks: Beets sweeten, warm, and moisten. They balance VK and unbalance P, although still help with liver conditions in P people. The coriander and dill help to balance P in this recipe which is balancing for V and K and neutral for P. This is good in all seasons.

Humus Spread

1 cup sprouted garbanzo beans (sprout 2-3 days until nonstarchy and sprout is between 1/2" and 3/4")
1/2 cup grated beets
4 Tbs. raw tahini
3 Tbs. raw apple juice
2 Tbs. raw apple cider vinegar (if alkaline) or lemon juice (if acidic)

Blend and serve.

Remarks: Essentially the same as sweet humus except the beet helps to balance the V and thus makes this combination easier for Vs.

Spanish Spread

1 cup sprouted garbanzo beans (sprout 2-3 days until nonstarchy and sprout is between 1/2" and 3/4")
1 avocado
2 medium tomatoes
3 Tbs. fresh cilantro (coriander)
2 cloves garlic or 3/4 tsp. sun-dried garlic
1/4 tsp. cayenne or more to taste

Blend and serve.

Remarks: The avocado is more balancing for V and P and unbalancing for K; the tomato is mildly unbalancing for V, P, and K, but some of its effects are neutralized by coriander. The result of this combination is balancing for V, P, and K.

Tahini Mango Fruit Dip

1 mango
3 Tbs. tahini
2 tsp. finely grated ginger

Blend.

Remarks: Mango is balancing for V, P, and K; tahini and ginger together unbalance P and balance V and K. This dip is balancing for V and K and slightly unbalancing for P. Depending on how much ginger, it can be a cold or warm weather dip, although with 2 tsp. ginger it is particularly good for fall. It has a neutral pH effect.

Almond Guacamole Dip

1/2 cup soaked and blanched almonds
1 avocado
1 tomato, cut in pieces
juice of 1 lemon
2 Tbs. basil
small amount of cilantro for decoration on top
1/4 (for P)-1/2 tsp. cayenne

1. Soak almonds for 12 hours and then heat in boiling water for 30 seconds, strain off the water quickly and then pop the skins off the almonds using thumb and index fingers. Aside from a creamier taste and purer white color, the main reason we blanch almonds is that almond skins have a lot of tannic acid. Tannic acid is found in black teas and is a stimulant and irritant to the system. Four cups of almonds recommended in this recipe would contain a substantial amount of tannic acid if skins were not removed.
2. Put the blanched almonds, avocado, tomatoes, cut up basil, and lemon juice through the Champion Juicer processor.
3. Sprinkle with chopped cilantro. If you do not have a Champion Juicer you can use a mini-food processor. Serve with salad; this also can be used as a spread on crackers or bread.

Remarks: This is unbalancing for K and P, and balancing for V. It has a neutral pH effect. Almond guacamole dip can be used year around and its strong balancing of V makes it especially good for fall.

449

Spinach Avocado Dip

1 avocado
3 cups chopped spinach
1/2 tomato
2 Tbs. lemon juice
1/2 tsp. dill
1/4 tsp. nutmeg
1/8 tsp. hing

Blend and serve.

Remarks: Spinach is cooling, light, dry, with a warming aftereffect on the body. In small amounts it is tolerated by V and P, but will unbalance if too much is eaten. Spinach is balancing to K. This combination is balancing to V, P, and K. It is alkalinizing. Good in all seasons.

• Vegetable Dish Recipes •

Burrito a la Nori

One sheet uncooked nori
1/2 cup guacamole
1 handful alfalfa sprouts
1/2 tomato, diced
1/4 cup sprouted peas

First put on the guacamole which moistens the nori sheet; then add on the rest of the contents and roll up.

Remarks: This is neutral to P, K, and V if not eaten in excess. Peas are cool, heavy, sweet, and astringent and are balancing for K and P. This is an alkalinizing combination that is best in the summer. Humus can be used instead of guacamole if desired. It will make it more balancing for K, but less balancing for V unless hing or some heating herbs are added.

Beet Nori Burrito

1/4 cup beet slaw (see below for recipe) on nori. This can also be tastefully done with carrot slaw or cabbage slaw.

Avo-Cabbage Taco

1 tomato
1 large carrot
1 large cabbage leaf
1 avocado sliced into 1/2" pieces or 1/2 cup guacamole
1/2 cup Mexican masala

1. Grate carrots.
2. Chop tomato into bite sizes.
3. Put 1/2 cup guacamole on several cabbage leaves which are used as a taco shell.
4. Then add the tomatoes and grated carrots.
5. Pour Mexican masala over the top.

Remarks: Cabbage is not the best choice for V. It is balancing for P and K. Vs can enjoy the cabbage taco if it is heated with spices to increase digestive fire and hing is added to neutralize the gas-producing aggravation of cabbage and the rest of the cabbage family such as broccoli, cauliflower, Brussel sprouts, and kale. The avocado and carrot make this combination more neutral for V. The combination is balancing for K and P and neutral for V. It is alkalinizing and good in all seasons but better in the summer and not for the fall for Vs.

Humus Taco

1. 2 tomatoes chopped into bite-sized pieces
2. 2 large carrots grated
3. Handful alfalfa, clover, or sunflower sprouts
4. 1/2 avocado cut into bite-sized pieces.
5. 1/2 cup humus
6. Several large cabbage leaves

Spread out cabbage leaves, coat with humus and add on avocado, tomato bits, then sprinkle grated carrots and sprouts on top.

Remarks: Balancing for P and K, but neutral to unbalancing if eaten in excess by V. It is alkalinizing or acidifying depending on the type of humus. It's good in all seasons.

Veggie Boats

Use the same combinations as in the humus or cabbage tacos, but put into the half shell of one half bell pepper or a butter lettuce leaf.

Cabbage Coleslaw

1 1/2 cups each of shredded purple & green cabbage
1 cup shredded Chinese cabbage
1/2 cup shredded celery
oriental dressing

Combine all ingredients and store in refrigerator for 1 hour for the blending of flavors. Serve on individual cabbage leaves.

Remarks: This is balancing for P and K and unbalancing for V. It is good for summer and is alkalinizing.

Carrot Slaw

1 cup green cabbage, slice thin
1 cup purple cabbage, slice thin
1 cup grated carrots
Dressing: 3 Tbs. raw apple cider vinegar and 1 tsp. honey (or 2 dates) and blend.

Combine all ingredients and toss with dressing.

Remarks: This is balancing for P and K, and unbalancing for V. The carrots and apple cider vinegar help to balance V but is best taken by V in small amounts. It is a good summer salad which is acidifying.

Beet Slaw

1 cup grated beets
1 cup green cabbage, slice thin
1/2 cup grated jicama

Combine all ingredients and toss with apple cider vinegar and sweet dressing.

Remarks: Same as carrot slaw.

Chopped Broccoli with Ginger and Garlic

1 cup chopped, fresh broccoli
2 cloves garlic, chopped fine or 1/2 tsp. sun-dried garlic
1 Tbs. fresh ginger juice

Toss together with your favorite dressing. The broccoli ginger/garlic also makes a nice sauce if blended with water or apple juice to desired thickness.

Remarks: This is balancing to V, P, and K but V may unbalance in excess. Alkalinizing and good for all seasons, especially the winter.

452

Pat's Pesto

1/2 lb. sweet basil
2/3 lb. shelled walnuts
1/3 lb. pine nuts
3 large cloves garlic or 1 1/2 tsp. sun-dried garlic

Put all ingredients through "Champion" homogenizer. This homogenizer is also used to make seed and nut butters. It produces a much finer blend than a blender or an osterizer.

Remarks: This is balancing for V and slightly unbalancing for P and K. It is acidifying and good in all seasons, especially the fall. This raw pesto is great to use on raw vegetable slices such as cucumbers, carrots sticks, or beet slices. Another delightful approach is to fill a bell pepper or large red pepper with pesto and add sprouts on top The pestos are slightly heating and acidifying.

Tomato Pesto

To Pat's pesto mix add 1/2 cup dehydrated tomatoes and put them through the Champion homogenizer with the rest of the ingredients.

Remarks: Same as Pat's Pesto.

Three Nut Carrot Loaf

3/4 cup walnuts
1/2 cup sunflower seeds
1/4 cup pine nuts
1/2 large avocado
1 1/2 cups grated carrots
1 cup parsley
1 tsp. black pepper
1 clove garlic or 1/2 tsp. sun-dried garlic (onion may be used instead of garlic)
1 cup sprouts
1/2 red and yellow pepper
Nori sheets (optional)

1. Soak nuts and seeds for 12 hours and rinse.
2. Blend all ingredients until slightly chunky.
3. Mold into a shape.
4. Garnish with red and yellow pepper slices.
5. Optional choice to wrap in dry nori sheets to make a roll.

Remarks: This is balancing for V, neutral for K, and unbalancing for P. It is acid to neutral for pH. Good for all seasons. Recipe is for 2-4 people.

Avo-Sun Seed Pate

2 large avocados
1 1/2 cup sunflower seeds
1/4 cup lemon juice
1/2 cup parsley
1/4 tsp. cayenne
1 handful sunflower sprouts

1. Soak the sunflower seeds for 6 hours.
2. Blend all ingredients and mold into a shape.
3. Sprinkle the sunflower sprouts over the pate.

Remarks: This is balancing for V and neutral for P and K. It is neutral to slightly alkalinizing and good for all seasons. Recipe is for 2-4 people.

Veggie Pate

1 cup soaked sunflower seeds
1/2 cup chopped broccoli
1/2 cup chopped carrots
1/4 bunch cilantro
1 Tbs. lemon juice
1 clove garlic or 1/2 tsp. sun-dried garlic
1 Tbs. mellow miso

1. Add all ingredients except the miso to a blender and blend until semi-smooth.
2. Add miso and mix.
3. Mold into a form that makes one happy.

Remarks: This is balancing to V, P, and K. A K might do better by cutting the amount of miso in half. This is alkalinizing and good for all seasons. Recipe is for 2-4 people.

Veggiekraut

The sauerkrauts are acidifying, fermented foods which help repopulate the colon with health-promoting, lactic acid-producing bacteria. Raw sauerkraut has these healthy bacteria but store-bought, pasteurized sauerkraut does not. Raw sauerkraut has no salt or vinegar in it. It is allowed to ferment in its own juices. The only thing that is added is certain herb seasonings. Depending on the spices and vegetab.es used, the sauerkrauts can be heating or cooling, but are a primarily cooling summer food. The fermentation process makes it easier to digest for V so if some warming spices and V balancing vegetables are used the krauts are balancing for K, neutral for V if not eaten in excess, and neutral to slightly unbalancing for P because of the acidity. They are good in all seasons, but best for the summer.

Materials needed:
1. a large crock or stainless steel container
2. a plate which will just fit inside the crock
3. a jar filled with water to use as a weight to fit inside the crock to press down on the dish
4. a towel or cloth to fit over the crock
5. a Champion Juicer, food processor, or appropriate equipment which will break down the veggie fibers

Directions:
1. For sauerkraut, use 3 large heads of red or green cabbage or a combination of both. You can also make a smaller amount, but it should be enough to fill a small jar or crock so the fermenting process can happen.
2. For veggiekraut use hard, fibrous vegetables—carrots, beets, broccoli, cauliflower, turnips, and, of course, cabbage.
3. All herbs and spices are optional; ginger, cayenne or red pepper, dill, curry, garlic, hing, and horseradish have all been used with a positive taste success; let your imagination be your guide. Grated dulse or kelp, can also be used to create a "salty" taste, add minerals, and for radioactive protection.
4. Remove the outer cabbage leaves and save them for use later to put on top of the sauerkraut mix. Wash and clean other veggies.
5. Cut cabbage and veggies in small pieces to fit into a champion juicer or whatever appliance or technique used to crush and cut up the vegetables. Whether using a Champion Juicer, or another grater or food processor, the main idea is to produce as much juice as possible. The juice is the medium which activates the fermentation. With a Champion use the "blank" instead of the grater, this produces more juice.
6. Put all ingredients into a crock and repeatedly push down to remove all air from the veggies. Pack down the veggies until the surface is smooth and has a least 1/8 inch of juice on top of it.
7. Cover the surface with the outer cabbage leaves that had been saved.
8. Put a plate on top of the leaves inside the crock.
9. Put the weighted jar on top of the plate.
10. Cover with the towel and set in a location which is approximately room temperature. The fermentation process takes 4-7 days. On warm-to-hot

days, the process may take only 4 days, however on cold, winter days it would be wise to leave it sit for 7 days. Occasional tastes will be the main way one knows if the batch is ready. If the fermentation goes too long it will have a more spoiled taste. A good sauerkraut taste will be a little on the zingy side.

11. Uncover after approximately 7 days and skim off the cabbage leaves and small layer underneath the cabbage leaves.

12. Transfer the veggiekraut to a glass container, cover and refrigerate. The sauerkraut is always fermenting and if left outside of the refrigerator, this fermentation process will accelerate. The refrigerator greatly slows or stops the fermentation process. Fermented sauerkraut can be stored for several months in a cold enough refrigerator. If they get fizzy then they are spoiled and should not be eaten. I've purchased several raw veggie krauts from the store which fizzed and expanded when they were opened. This means the fermentation process has gone too far and they need to be added to the compost.

Sauerkraut

This is the basic recipe. Explore the different tastes by adding ginger, garlic, curry, or dill to different batches. It seems best to not use more than two spices. Usually one spice in good measure gives the best results. Curry and dill used in equal amounts give a special taste. My favorite seasoned sauerkrauts using only one spice are **cabbage curry kraut and ginger kraut.** These both have heating qualities that help to balance V. One can also play with the different purple and red cabbage colors. If one is eating in a Rainbow Diet pattern, the purple cabbages make a nice addition to dinners in the evening when purple foods are best eaten.

Curry Carrot Veggiekraut

1 small head cauliflower
1 small head red cabbage
3 cups carrots
2-3 cloves garlic or one tsp. sun-dried garlic
2 Tbs. curry

Remarks: Balancing for K, neutral for V if not in excess, and slightly unbalancing for P. This is a good winter kraut.

Carrot-Beet Kraut

2 heads green cabbage
2 cups carrots
2 cups beets

Remarks: This is balancing for K and V if not in excess and neutral for P. For an unusual taste that will clear the sinuses, add 1 tsp. raw horseradish either before or after the main fermentation The horseradish is good for balancing V and K, but will unbalance P.

Ginger Zucchini Kraut

2 heads green cabbage
4 cups zucchini
To each 2 cups of this mixture add 1 Tbs. ginger juice

Remarks: This is balancing for K, neutral for V if not in excess, and slightly unbalancing for P. It's a nice one for all seasons.

Pesto Kraut

4 cups purple cabbage
1 bunch fresh basil
3 cloves garlic or 1 Tbs. sun-dried garlic

Remarks: This is balancing for K, neutral if not in excess for V, and slightly unbalancing for P. Good for all seasons.

Daikon Ginger Kraut

4 cups purple cabbage
2 cups diakon
2 tsp. fresh ginger juice.

Remarks: This is balancing for K and V, if not in excess, and unbalancing for P. It is a good fall and winter kraut.

• Salad Recipes •

There is an infinite number of vegetable or fruit salads that can be made. My approach is to find a balance between a few components which one can clearly taste, yet with enough variety to continue to be quite tasty and interesting each day. There are three approaches that enable one to continue to taste each vegetable or fruit in a salad. One is to put each one of them on the salad plate separately and put the salad dressing over each separately. Another approach is to cut the vegetables in big enough pieces that it is readily identifiable and tasty. A third approach is to grate one major foreground component such as a beet or a carrot and put it over a background component. The main two background components I use are a nest of sprouts in the bottom of the salad or several different lettuces to hold the foreground component such as the grated beet or carrot. This approach allows one to experience a predominant taste above others in a salad. I then add in one or two secondary components such as: avocado squares, hot peppers, bell peppers, almonds, walnuts, sunflower seeds, and tomatoes. I may then add one pungent herb or vegetable such as arugala or kale. These salads can be in a bowl or spread out on a plate.

My choice of the secondary tastes and energies are influenced by the chosen dressing of the day. If the dressing is a seed sauce, I usually do not use nuts and seeds on the salad. If the dressing is a thin or light dressing, or even a thin tahini dressing, then I might use nuts or seeds in the salad. If there is a need for a more acidifying salad I will use walnuts and an apple cider vinegar dressing and the seeds and nuts will not be soaked. If I want it to be more alkalinizing, then I will use soaked nuts and seeds, lemon-based dressings and no walnuts.

Salads are mostly light and cool which make them especially balancing for P and K and a pleasant summer meal. However, with the masalas like winter heat used in dressings there is no salad alive that will not warm one to the core and also be balancing for V. During the cold seasons, the salads are balancing for P and V; and for K with the addition of heating dressings. Cooling dressings will be okay for pittas in the winter, but may imbalance V and K. In the summer, I mostly use cooling dressings and the salads are balancing for P, V, and K. A heating dressing in the summer may unbalance a P. Salads are easiest for P and K to assimilate, but V will also do fine with salads if they use more oily, warming dressings, avocados, and soaked nuts and seeds (the additional water and oil component of the soaked nuts and seeds keeps Vs from getting too dry and flatulent). Warming vegetables, like beet and carrot, also help to balance V and K. Cooling vegetables, such as zucchini, squash, and cucumber, help to balance P. Dressings with a little hing added will also help prevent a wind imbalance for V.

Most of these salads take about ten minutes to prepare. For myself, I don't really use "set" recipes. I begin by intuiting my "color needs" in a *Rainbow Diet* way. I then ask myself "Do I want to pick a beet or carrot from the garden? Is the arugula ready to harvest?" Whether I choose a cooling or heating dressing will depend on how I feel at the time. Since the salad is the only food I eat at lunch and is usually my last meal for the rest of the day, I give it considerable attention as far as completeness and appropriateness to my needs at the time. **Salads can be a complete balanced meal.**

BAK Salad

1 medium-sized beet
1 avocado
1/2 handful kale
alfalfa, clover, and sunflower sprouts to cover the bottom of the salad bowel 1/2" to 1" deep

1. Cover the bottom of the bowel with sprouts.
2. Grate up beet and leave in a mound in the center of the sprouts.
3. Cut up the avocado into 1/2" pieces and place on the mound.
4. Pour on Winter Heat Masala Dressing (see dressing section).

Remarks: Balancing to V, P, and K. Kale has 14 times more iron in it per weight than beef plus many other nutrients. It is light and pungent with a heating aftereffect. Like many of the other dark leafy greens, such as collards, arugula, dandelion, and mustard greens, it is good for the liver and immune system, and skin, eyes, and mucous membranes because of its high nutrient and vitamin A content. This salad is alkalinizing and good for all seasons, especially the summer.

Carrot Tomato Salad

3 carrots
1 tomato
1/2 handful arugula
Sprouts or lettuce to cover the bottom of the dish or salad bowl by 1/2 to 1"
1/2 cup curry masala sun dressing

Cover bottom of the bowel or dish with sprouts or lettuce greens.
Grate three carrots and place in a mound in the center.
Add arugula in 1-2" long parts of the plants.

Remarks: This is balancing to V and K and neutral for P because of the heating effect of the carrots, tomato, and arugula. The arugula adds a bitter, pungent, heating effect that makes it good for all seasons, especially the fall, winter, and spring cleaning. This is an alkalinizing salad. Like the rest of the bitter and pungent greens, arugula is most balancing for K.

Spinach Salad

1 handful spinach
1/2 cup coarsely ground cauliflower
1 carrot
10 walnuts
Add your favorite dressing

1. Put spinach into individual salad plates or bowls.
2. Put cauliflower into mini-food processor and grind until coarsely ground, sprinkle over salads.
3. Add grated carrots and walnuts on top.

Remarks: This is balancing for V, P, and K. Spinach is cool, light, and dry with a slight heating aftereffect. It can be unbalancing to P and V if eaten in large amounts. The walnuts help to keep this salad from being too alkalinizing as they are so acidic. This is a good summer salad.

Spinach Avocado Salad

1 avocado
1 bunch spinach
3/4 handful dulse
1 tomato
1/3 cup apple curry dressing
1 handful alfalfa sprouts

1. Put spinach in bottom of the salad bowel.
2. Add the sprouts.
3. Cut the avocado into 1/2" pieces and spread out on salad.
4. Soak the dulse in water to get off the salt, rinse and drain and add to the salad.
5. Cut the tomato into 1/2" pieces and sprinkle on salad (one carrot can be used instead).
6. Add 1/3 cup apple curry dressing (see section on salad dressing).

Remarks: This is balancing for V, K, and P. The avocado adds to the balancing effect on V. Sprouts are most balancing for P and K as they are light and cool. By themselves sprouts can be taken by V in moderate amounts, but may unbalance in excess. Alfalfa, clover, and seed sprouts can be eaten in normal amounts by V when they are combined with balancing foods such as heating vegetables, herbs, salad dressings, soaked nuts and seeds, and avocado. When alfalfa, clover, and seed sprouts are well-balanced the combination is able to be eaten in normal, meal-size amounts by Vs. Some sprouts, such as radish, are more heating and balancing for V. This is a summer, alkalinizing salad that is good all year around.

Wilted Spinach Salad

Same recipe as above, but warm some apple cider vinegar honey dressing in a sauce pan until hot to touch. Turn off heat and drop in 6 spinach leaves for 30 seconds. Then put them on the spinach salad and pour the hot dressing over the whole salad. The spinach leaves wilt easily. This is a warm salad which still remains essentially raw, give or take a few enzymes.

Carrot and Fresh Dill Salad

1 cup grated carrots
1/2 cup grated jicama
1 Tbs. fresh dill

Enjoy with your favorite dressing.

Remarks: This is a cooling summer salad that helps to balance pitta in the summer. Although jicama is balancing for P and K and unbalancing for V, the overall effect of the salad is balancing for V, K, and P. A warm dressing will help to balance V. It is alkalinizing. This is good for all seasons, especially summer.

Daikon Ginger Salad

1/4 cup finely grated fresh ginger
1/3 cup fresh lemon juice
1/4 tsp. cayenne
1 daikon, grated

1. Let the grated ginger sit in the lemon cayenne juice for several hours.
2. Pour the grated ginger and marinade over the grated daikon and serve.

Remarks: Daikon is unbalancing for P in large amounts so this salad is balancing for V and K, and unbalancing for P. It is a good winter and spring salad. It is alkalinizing.

Lemon Jicama Appetizer

1 jicama, grated
1/4 cup lemon juice
1/4 tsp. cayenne (less for P)

Pour cayenne lemon juice over the grated jicama and serve.

Remarks: Jicama is unbalancing to V and balancing for P and K. The lemon juice and cayenne help to calm and warm V so that this is neutral for V, and balancing for P and K. This is alkalinizing and a good summer appetizer.

Sprouted Pea Salad

1 handful arugula
1 cup sliced carrots (dice if they are large)
1/2 cup sprouted peas (sprouting section)
1 handful alfalfa or clover sprouts
1/4 cup sprouted pumpkin seeds (sprout section)
1/2 cup guacamole

Remarks: Peas are cooling, heavy, sweet, and astringent. They are neutral to V and balancing to P and K. A hot guacamole helps to make this combination balancing for V, P, and K. This is an alkalinizing summer salad.

Daikon Cucumber Salad

1 cucumber cut into 1/8" rounds
1 daikon finely grated
1/4 cup tahini lemon dressing

Spread the daikon over the cucumber slices and pour the dressing over the combination.

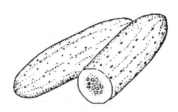

Remarks: Balancing for V and K and neutral for P. An alkaliniz-ing summer salad.

Mixed Greens and Sprout Salad

4 leaves each Romaine, butter, and red leaf lettuces, and arugula
1 tomato cut into bite sizes
1/2 handful chopped parsley served on top
1 handful of a mixture of alfalfa, sunflower, buckwheat, and clover sprouts
1/3 cup seed dressing of choice
1 avocado

1. Cut the lettuce and arugula into 3" sizes.
2. Slice up the avocado into 1/4 to 1/2" bite-sized pieces.
3. Cut up a quarter handful of parsley.
4. Add the seed dressing and mix.

Remarks: This is balancing for V, P, and K. Parsley is a slightly warming diuretic which balances K, unbalances P, and can be tolerated by V in small amounts. The avocado and seed dressing helps to balance V and P. A good all-season alkalinizing salad. For the fall and winter, choose a heating seed dressing to further help calm V.

California Hot Corn Salad

1 cup mixed greens as in mixed green salad
1 cup fresh, raw white corn, removed from the cob
1 avocado cut into 1/2" cubes
1/3 cup diced, red, hot peppers
1/2 cup avocado or Mexican masala dressing

1. Line a small glass salad bowl with the corn by pressing the corn to the sides firmly with your hand.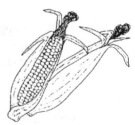
2. Toss mixed greens, red cabbage and yellow bell pepper together and put into the center of the bowl.
3. Add the dressing.

Remarks: Corn is warm, light, dry, sweet, and astringent. Its dry, astringent warmth makes it good for K. If it is fresh corn that still is moist, it is neutral for V and slightly unbalancing for P. Corn in a dry form, as in chips, popcorn, or tortillas, is unbalancing for V. The peppers make this a heating salad that balances K and V, but unbalances P. It is an alkalinizing salad.

463

Seven Spears Salad

7 raw asparagus spears
1/2 avocado cut in 1/2" pieces
1/4 cup sweet dill dressing
handful of sprouts

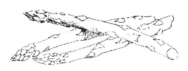

Place spears and avocado on
a bed of sprouts and pour
the dressing on top.

Remarks: Asparagus is balancing to V, P, and K. It is sweet, bitter, astringent, cool, light, and moist. A slightly acidic salad because of the dressing. Some books suggest asparagus is acidifying as well. This is a summer salad.

Marinated Cucumber and Tomato Salad

1 large cucumber
1 tsp. fresh dill
4 cherry tomatoes
1-2 cups apple cider
    vinegar dressing

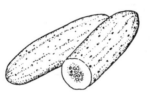

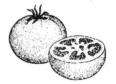

1. Slice cucumber and toss with
   the dill and tomatoes. Add enough apple
   cider vinegar dressing to thoroughly cover the
   vegetables.
2. Let sit several hours or overnight.

Remarks: This is balancing for V and P, and neutral for K. It is an acidifying summer salad.

Kale-Avocado-Sunsprout Salad

1 handful kale
1 avocado
1 handful sunflower sprouts
1/3 cup soaked sunflower seeds
1/2 cup tahini ginger dressing or favorite dressing

1. Wash and cut fresh kale.
2. Toss with sunflower sprouts and put in a large salad bowl.
3. Decorate with sliced avocado in a pinwheel design and sprinkle sprouted sunflower seeds on top.

Remarks: This is balancing to V, P, and K. It is an alkalinizing four-season salad.

Underground Salad

1 daikon
1 beet
1 carrot
1/4 cup tahini ginger dressing

Grate the beet, daikon, and carrot; mix and pour the dressing over the mix.

Remarks: This is balancing for V and K, and unbalancing for P. It is an alkalinizing fall and winter salad.

Walnut Salad

1/4 cup walnuts
1 cup thinly sliced Chinese cabbage
1 cup finely grated carrots
1/2 cup apple cider vinegar honey dill dressing

Combine ingredients, toss with dressing or dressing of choice.

Remarks: This is balancing for V and K, and neutral for P. It is an acidifying summer salad.

• Fruit Salads •

Many fruits can be eaten by all three doshas. Their ability to be eaten by all three depends on being ripe and sweet. If an apricot, for example, is not ripe and sweet, it will unbalance P, but if it is sweet, it will balance. It is difficult to include all these nuances in the Ayurvedic charts. Some fruits, such as banana, may need a little spice, such as dry ginger, to balance for K and tumeric to balance for P. Mangos, soaked raisins, sweet purple grapes, sweet cherries, sweet apricots, fresh sweet berries, and pineapple (in small amounts for K) do not unbalance any of the doshas. Apple, which is good for P and K, with the addition of cinnamon, will balance V. Fresh figs balance V and P, but need some dried ginger to balance K.

Melon Ball

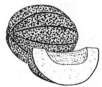

1 canteloupe
1 honeydew melon

Make small, ball-shaped pieces of the melons. Scoop out most of watermelon and cut edges into design of your choice. Fill watermelon with balled melons.

Remarks: This is balancing for P and V and unbalancing for K. This is an alkalinizing summer salad.

Mango Sesame Fruit Salad

1 large banana
1 red apple
1/2 cup oranges, kiwis, and
    other seasonal fruit
1/3 cup Mango Sesame Seed Sauce
1/4 cup soaked raisins

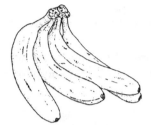

1. Cut all fruit into
   1/2" bite sizes and mix.
2. Pour mango sesame seed
   sauce over the fruit.

Remarks: This is balancing for V and P and neutral to slightly unbalancing for K. This an alkalinizing combination that can be used in all seasons, but is best in spring, summer, and fall.

Cambodian Papaya Salad

1 green papaya
1 carrot
1/8 cup fennel
1/4 cup basil-dill dressing as desired

1. Grate the papaya and carrot into long, thin strips.
2. Mix the papaya and carrot strips together with the fennel and add the dressing.

Remarks: This is balancing for V and K and neutral for P. It is an alkalinizing salad for all seasons. A little cayenne will warm it up for the winter.

Ganeshpuri Breakfast

1 large papaya sliced in half
2 bananas
1 lemon or lime

Slice the bananas and put in the center of the papaya half and squeeze lemon over the combination.

Remarks: Balancing for V and slightly unbalancing for P and K. An alkalizing summer or fall treat.

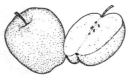

Apple-Strawberry Delight

1 apple, cored and cut in cubes
1 cup ripe strawberries
1/4 cup sprouted almonds
1 Tbs. grated coconut

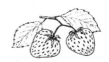

1. Put strawberries and almonds through champion juicer or mini-food processor.
2. Mix cubed apples and strawberry mixture in a bowl and serve in individual small bowls. Sprinkle with grated coconut.

Remarks: This is balancing for V and neutral for P and K. It is an alkalinizing summer treat.

Banana-Apple-Seed

2 apples
2 bananas
1/3 cup soaked sunflower seeds
1 Tbs. cardamom
1/2 tsp. cinnamon
1/4 cup soaked raisins

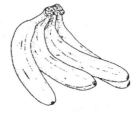

1. Juice the apples.
2. Put juice in the blender with the bananas, cardamom, and cinnamon.
3. Pour the sauce over the apple sauce that came from the two apples that were juiced. This system conserves food.
4. Sprinkle on the raisins.

Remarks: This is balancing for V, P, and K. It is alkalinizing and good for all seasons. Although some books suggest apples are unbalancing to V because of their dryness, tartness, and astringent skin, this may be more true of the Indian apples, which taste like wood. The organic apples, such as the red McIntosh, are juicy and sweet and so are balancing for V. Some American apples are more bitter and dry and they would be more unbalancing for V.

• Smoothie Recipes •

There is a great number of smoothies that can be created with or without soaked seeds. A smoothie can be a whole meal in itself if sprouted seeds are added.

Tropical Delight

1 small canteloupe
1 fresh pineapple
1 cup raw apple juice

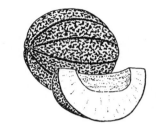
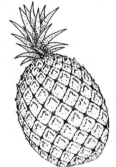

1. Juice canteloupe and
   pineapple.
2. Add raw apple juice (add
   cinnamon for V).
3. For a more frothy drink, blend
   2 cups in a blender.

Remarks: Raw apple juice without any
herbs is balancing to K and P, but slightly unbalancing to V. A sweet canteloupe is balancing for V and P,
but unbalancing for K. This smoothie is balancing for P, and
neutral for V and K. It is an alkalinizing summer drink.

Citrus Smoothie

8 oz. freshly squeezed, sweet orange juice
4 oz. pineapple juice
1 banana

Put all ingredients into blender and blend until smooth.

Remarks: This is balancing for V, neutral for P, and unbalancing for K. It is an
alkalinizing, all-season fruit drink that is best in summer and fall.

Papaya Delight

1 fresh papaya
8 oz. raw apple juice
2 dates or 1/2 tsp. honey (if sweeter drink desired)

Put all ingredients into blender and blend until smooth. Add honey or a date only
if you like it sweeter.

Remarks: This is balancing for V and neutral for P and K. It is an alkalinizing,
all-season fruit drink.

Papaya Zinger

1 fresh papaya
2 bananas
1 tsp. ginger powder

Blend ingredients.

Remarks: This is for the Ks, who like bananas and papaya. It is balancing for V and K and unbalancing for P.

Apple-Banana-Strawberry Smoothie

8 oz. raw apple juice
1 banana
1 cup fresh strawberries
1/2 tsp. ginger powder (for K)

Put all ingredients into blender and blend until smooth.

Remarks: Balancing for all three doshas. An alkalinizing summer drink.

Omega 36 Banana Flax Smoothie

2 bananas
1 Tbs. flaxseed
1/2 cup sprouted sunflower seeds
1 heaping tsp. cardamom
1 tsp. cinnamon
1/2 cup raw apple juice or more to desired thickness

Put all ingredients into blender adding apple juice slowly until desired thickness has been reached.

Remarks: Balancing to V, P, and K. An alkalinizing, all-season drink.

Carrot-Avocado Drink

2 cups fresh carrot juice
1 avocado

Put all ingredients into blender and blend until smooth. This can also be a soup if you only use 1 cup carrot juice.

Remarks: Balancing for V, P, and K. An alkalinizing all-seasons drink.

Banana "Nut" Shake

1 cup sesame or almond seed drink
1 banana
3 dates (for P and V) or 2 tsp. honey (for K)
1/2 tsp. cinnamon (for P and K)

Put all ingredients into a blender and blend till smooth.

Remarks: Balancing for V, neutral for K, and neutral to slightly unbalancing for P in excess.

• Soup Recipes •

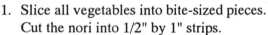

5-Minute, Warm, Enzyme-full, Raw Vegetable Soup

1 carrot, chopped
1 grated beet
1/4 head purple cabbage
1/4 handful sunflower or alfalfa sprouts
1/4 tsp. ginger
3 cups water
1-2 sheets nori
1/8-1/4 tsp. cayenne to taste (less for P)

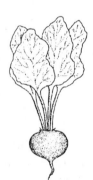

1. Slice all vegetables into bite-sized pieces. Cut the nori into 1/2" by 1" strips.
2. Add to 3 cups water that has been heated to 118° F (to estimate 118° F without a thermometer, stick finger in until it begins to be warm).

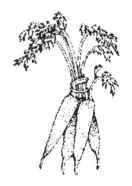

3. Turn off the heat and let it sit until it is cool, then heat it back to 118° F again and eat.
4. Top off with a small handful of alfalfa or sunflower sprouts.

Remarks: Balancing for V and K and unbalancing for P. It is an alkalinizing, all-season soup that is best in fall and winter.

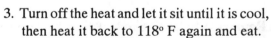

Warm, Raw Veggie Soup

8 cups water
2 potatoes
3 carrots
2 celery stalks
2 zucchini
1 tsp. winter heat masala (use just a touch for P)

1. Slice all the vegetables into 1/4" sizes.
2. Let sit in sun all day or put in a slow cooker (not above 118° F).

Remarks: Balancing for V, P, and K. A good alkalinizing soup for any season. This is great stock for soup or broth to drink plain. For a broth, pour soup through a strainer to remove the vegetables.

AMZ Soup

1 avocado
1/2 tsp. mellow miso
1 medium-large zucchini
2/3 cup water
1 tsp. heating or cooling masalas

1. To a blender add zucchini, avocado, and water.
2. Heat to 118° F.
3. Take a small amount of soup mixture and add the miso; put miso mixture back into the soup and blend.

Remarks: This is balancing for V and P and unbalancing for K. It is an alkalinizing summer soup.

Hot Spice Corn Soup

corn kernels from three fresh corn cobs
1 hot red pepper
1/2 tsp. fresh ginger juice
2 Tbs. dulse cut into strips that have been soaked and rinsed
2 cups water heated to 118° F

Blend and eat. Serves 2-4.

Remarks: This is balancing to V and K and imbalancing to P. Without the ginger or red pepper, it is neutral for P.

Spinach Soup

1 bunch fresh spinach
1/2 cup parsley
1 avocado
1/2 to 1 cup water, depending on desired thickness
1 Tbs. lemon juice

Add ingredients and blend. For a warm soup, add water heated to 118° F.

Remarks: This is balancing for K, and neutral for V and P. It is an alkalinizing summer soup.

Sprout Soup

1 cup buckwheat sprouts
1 cup sunflower sprouts
1 large avocado
1 cup water
1 tsp. masala of choice
1/4 handful parsley

1. Blend ingredients together.
2. Garnish with parsley.
3. Serves 2-4.

Remarks: The avocado oil balances this soup for V and the sprouts balance it for K. It is balancing for V, P, and K. Unless a hot masala is added, this is a cooling summer soup with alkalinizing qualities.

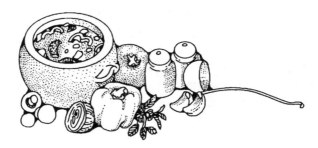

Vegetable Stew

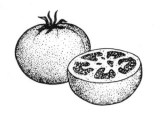

4 cups water
2 cups potato, chopped semi-fine
3/4 cup dehydrated cherry tomatoes
1/2 tsp. curry
1/8 tsp. cayenne
1 handful raw dulse, kelp, or alaria
(it is helpful to experiment with the different taste effects)

1. Soak the dulse or alaria in room temperature water for 10 minutes to remove the sea salt and possible seashells.
2. Put all ingredients into a slow cooker (not above 120° F) for 6-8 hours. If it goes longer than 8 hours, there is the possibility that bacteria can grow in it at these low temperatures.
3. When finished, take approximately 1 1/2 cups of the vegetables and put into blender; blend for 30 seconds; put back into the stew. This blend thickens the soup. Serves 4-8.

Remarks: This is balancing for V, P, and K. It is an alkalinizing, all-seasons soup.

Upbeet Soup

2 cups carrot juice
1 avocado
1/2 cup grated beets
1/2 cup grated carrots

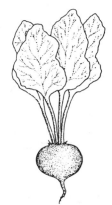

1. Juice carrots.
2. Put all ingredients into blender and blend until smooth.
3. If you prefer a more chunky soup, reserve 1/4 cup grated beets and carrots; add to soup last; mix well and serve.
4. Put all ingredients into blender. Put into bowl and stir. Garnish with buckwheat sprouts. Serves 3-4 people.

Remarks: This is balancing for V and K and neutral to slightly unbalancing to P if taken in excess. This is an alkalinizing, all-seasons soup. On a cool winter day, one might want to add 1-2 tsp. of a heating masala.

Creamy Borscht

2 cups beet juice
1 avocado
1 cup grated beets to thicken (optional)
1 sheet of nori cut into 1" by 1/4" strips

Blend, add the nori strips on top, and serve.

Remarks: This is balancing for V and K and neutral for P. It is an alkalinizing, all-season soup that is particularly nice in the summer and fall.

Sunflower-Squash Soup

1 cup sunflower sprouts
1/4 cup soaked sunflower seeds
1 Tbs. soaked flaxseeds
1 medium yellow squash
2 Tbs. raw apple cider vinegar
1 cup or more of water until desired consistency has been reached
1 clove garlic, crushed, or 1/2 tsp. sun-dried garlic to taste
1 tsp. basil

1. Put all ingredients, including the drained, soaked seeds into a blender.
2. Add water slowly until desired soup-like consistency has been reached. The apple cider vinegar gives this soup a more acidifying effect. If water is used instead of apple cider vinegar, then it will be more alkaline. Serves 2-4.

Remarks: This is a cooling soup that is balancing for V and P and neutral for K. It is a summer alkalinizing soup.

Tomato Soup

1 qt. fresh tomato juice
1 avocado
2 med. tomatoes, chopped
2-3 Tbs. chopped coriander
1/4 tsp. cayenne(for P) to 1/2 tsp.
1 tsp. basil

1. Blend tomato juice and avocado together.
2. Add the rest of the ingredients to this blend and mix thoroughly with a spoon. Serves 2-4.

Remarks: Neutral for V, K, and P. It is an alkalinizing summer soup that can be "souped" up for the winter with a hot masala such as winter heat. It would be unbalancing for P, but balancing for V and K.

Tomato Sea Vegetable Soup

Tomato soup from previous recipe
1/2 handful raw dulse or 1/2 handful raw kelp

1. Cut the kelp and dulse into 1/4" by approximately 1" strips.
2. Soak in water for 10 minutes and pour off the water.
3. Marinate in lemon juice for 1 hour.
4. Add the marinade and the four sea vegetables to the tomato soup.

Remarks: This is an alkalinizing and mineralizing soup that is neutral for P, V, and K. It is alkalinizing Like the tomato soup, it can be modified for all seasons. The amount of cayenne will determine if its heating or cooling.

Three-carrot Soup

3 carrots, sliced
1 cup carrot juice
1 avocado
1 tsp. cumin

Blend and serve.

Remarks: Balancing for V and K and slightly unbalancing for P. An alkalinizing summer and fall soup.

Carrot Sprout Soup

1 cup carrot juice
1 avocado
1 handful sunflower, alfalfa and clover sprouts.
1 tsp. masala of choice (optional)

1. Put avocado and carrot juice into blender and blend until smooth.
2. Although this soup is delicious as it is, one can add 1 tsp. of a masala of choice or various sea vegetables to create an additional variety of soup. Try it on its own first, before adding to it.

Remarks: This soup is balancing for V and K and slightly unbalancing for P. This soup is an alkalinizing, slightly cooling summer and fall soup.

Heavenly Garden Soup for 25

1/4 lb. sweet potato
1/4 lb. yam
3/4 lbs. purple potato
1 1/2 Tbs. dill
1 yellow finn potato
3/4 lb. carrot
1 qt. water
1/4 bunch celery
1/2 large head green cabbage
1/4 head cauliflower
1/4 bunch spinach
3 oz. light miso
2 cloves garlic or Panax
1/4 bunch cilantro
1/4 tsp. ginger
1/4 lb. Shitake mushrooms
1 tsp. basil
2 gallons water

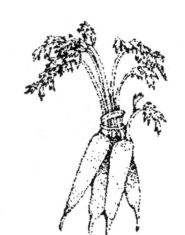

1. Slice all vegetables into bite-size pieces.
2. Chop garlic.
3. Heat water to 118° F; do not boil.
4. Add all ingredients except miso and cilantro.
5. Keep the water on warm and let vegetables marinate in water for 3-4 hours. Add cilantro during the last 1/2 hour.
6. When soup has finished, take 1 cup of the broth and put in a bowl; add the miso, stirring it into the broth; put this back into the pot.
7. Take 2 cups of the soup from the pot put into a blender, blend for 30 seconds and add this mixture back to the soup pot.

Remarks: This is balancing for V, P, and K. It is an alkalinizing, all-seasons party soup.

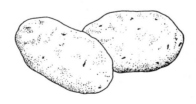

Kale and Barley Soup

1 qt. water
3 cups finely chopped kale
2 celery stalks, finely chopped
2 Tbs. finely chopped coriander
3/4 cup sprouted, organic barley
2 tsp. oregano

1. Add all ingredients to a slow cooker (not above 118° F).
   Slow heat for 8-10 hours.
2. Put 1/3 amount of soup into a blender and blend for 30 seconds; add back to remaining soup.
3. Mix miso with small amount of soup; add back to remaining soup and serve.

Remarks: Barley is cool, light, and drying. Barley is good for K and P, and slightly unbalances V. Combined with kale, this soup is balancing for K and P and unbalancing for V This soup is neutral to slightly alkalinizing. It is for all seasons. Serves 4.

Apple Spinach Cosmic Soup

1 cup cut spinach
1/2 apple
1 cup carrot juice
1/2 carrot
1/2 avocado
1 cup sprouts
1/2 tsp. nutmeg

Blend and serve with some sprout garnish on top.

Remarks: This is balancing for V, P, and K. It is an alkalinizing, all-seasons soup.

• Dehydrated Foods •

Dehydration is the best way to store food in terms of minimizing energy loss and preserving enzymes. It maintains the food in its essentially live state. However, as previously pointed out, there still is an estimated energy loss of approximately 25%.

The dehydration process is a basic one that has been used for thousands of years in the form of sun drying of foods. In addition to sun dehydrators that one can build or buy, there are also electrically heated, warm-air-blown dryers that work quite well. The most primitive, and by far the least expensive, drying system besides the sun, is a 250 watt sun lamp used as a food drier. It is a thrifty idea created by Joanna Brick, and jointly modified by the two of us. Place the sun lamp about 18" above the food to be dried. Although the food can be left on a flat cookie pan, one can also elevate the food to be dried on a screen so there is air circulation underneath.

Dehydrated food is the best way to go for storage, camping, and travel. Dehydration can also make some foods quite tasty and make some tasty non-sugar cookies as well. I do not, however, recommend it as a substitute for fresh live foods. Dehydrated foods, because of their dryness, are more balancing to K and may unbalance V if taken in excess. Dried foods are generally more warming, particularly if a heating masala is used with them.

Besides dehydrating fruits and vegetables for storage, leftover seed sauces and grain blends can make tasty crackers when they are dried. The general process is to put some Saran Wrap or stable plastic sheets over a screen and pour on the sauces. Dehydrate until sauce is dry enough to turn over on the screen and pull off the Saran Wrap or plastic sheet. This allows air circulation to speed up the drying process. When the seed sauce becomes hard like a cracker, then it is ready to eat. These can then be broken into smaller crackers for travelling. These will keep for several weeks. Contrary to fruits and vegetables, which are better to eat after they have been rehydrated by soaking in water, the crackers are best eaten in their cracker form.

Spicy Sprouted Seeds

1. Put sprouted seeds (can be sunflower, pumpkin or almonds) in a covered container and sprinkle on a masala, cayenne, or whatever particular individual spice one wants.
2. Shake the mixture and spread out on a screen to be dehydrated in the sun, or a dehydrator.
3. Dehydrate until seeds are dry and crunchy.

Remarks: These dried seeds and nuts with herbs make an excellent substitute for the salted chip habit. The dryness and heat unbalances V and P and is better for K. Depending on how the seed or the nut affects the doshas, it will be shifted by the dryness. For example, dried sesame will become imbalancing for V and balancing for K. Dried foods are good for the rainy seasons and less useful in the hot, dry season.

Dehydrated Seed, Nut, and Fruit Cookies

General Instructions:

1. Soak the seeds or nuts overnight. At least 6 hours for seeds and 12 hours for nuts.
2. Mix with a fruit such as raisins(soaked or unsoaked) or dates.
3. Put through the homogenizer of the Champion juicer, or a food processor, or blender. The Champion homogenizer makes the smoothest blend.
4. Drop onto a plastic sheet or a fine mesh screen in teaspoon sizes.
5. Put into the dehydrator at 118° F.
6. When the cookies are just dry enough to turn over, scrape them from the cookie screen or plastic sheet and turn over to increase the drying rate. This also keeps them from getting stuck on the plastic. The drying usually takes overnight, approximately 10-14 hours.

Another method of making these cookies is to make them in a total connected sheet. For this process:

1. Spread the whole batter on a fine mesh screen, and fold one half of the screen over the cookies
2. Take a rolling pin to flatten the batter to a smooth surface 1/8" to 1/4" thick
3. Gently try to unfold the top of the folded screen
4. Put into the dehydrator
5. When the batter is dry enough, turn over and free the batter from the screen with a spatula or just pull off
6. This seed fruit "cookie" can be cut into squares at one time or just pulled off in strips as desired

Sunrays

2 cups sprouted sunflower seeds
1/3 cup soaked raisins without the water

Prepare as per the general instructions for dehydrating above.

Remarks: This is balancing to P and K, and neutral to V in moderation. It is neutral to alkalinizing in pH effect. A great standard cracker for all seasons, dips, snacks, camping, and travelling.

Omega 36s

2 cups sprouted sunflower seeds
1/3 cup raisins
2 Tbs. soaked flaxseeds

Prepare as per the general instructions.

Remarks: Supplies both the omega-3 and omega-6 fatty acids. It is balancing for P and K, and neutral to V in moderation. It is neutral to alkaline in pH effect. Good for all seasons.

Almond Date

1 cup soaked almonds
1/4 cup dates

Prepare as per the general instructions.

Remarks: Almond in moderation is okay for V, but unbalancing for P and K. Dates make it more unbalancing for K and more balancing for P and V. This cookie is balancing for V and neutral for P and K. It is alkalinizing and good for all seasons. Other fruit and nut or seed combinations which work well are almond-raisin and sunflower-date. Different spices, such as cardamom or cinnamon, can make for an interesting and warming taste.

Sunny Sea Crackers

1 cup sunflower seeds, soaked to slightly sprouted
1 tsp. dulse cut into fine strips after they have been soaked and drained

Prepare as per general instructions.

Remarks: Same as Sunrays.

Wind's Almond Fig Spice Cookie

2 cups soaked almonds
1 cup soaked figs
1 tsp. cardamom
1/2 tsp. cinnamon
1/2 tsp. nutmeg

Prepare as per the general instruction. Brazil nuts make an interesting substitution for almonds.

Remarks: This is balancing for V, neutral to K and P. It is for all seasons and is alkalinizing.

Banana Nut Cinnamon Treat

1 cup sprouted almonds
1 ripe banana
1 tsp. cinnamon

Prepare as per general instructions.

Remarks: This is balancing for V and unbalancing for P and K. It is alkaline and for all seasons.

Pinenut Apple Cookie

1 grated apple
1 cup pine nuts, soaked
1 tsp. cinnamon

Prepare as per general instructions.

Remarks: This is balancing for V, P, and K. It is neutral to alkalinizing in pH effect. It is good for all seasons.

Zucchini Chips

1 zucchini
1/4 tsp. cayenne

Slice zucchini, sprinkle cayenne over the batch, then dehydrate.

Remarks: It is neutral to balancing for V, P, and K. It is an all-seasons, alkalinizing chip.

Sun and Sea Crisp

2/3 cup soaked sunflower seeds
1/3 cup soaked sesame seeds
1/2 cup shredded carrot
2 Tbs. shredded dulse that has been soaked and rinsed
Choose a masala of choice if you can tolerate, and like, more heat

Prepare as per general instructions, except use a tablespoon to make the patties about the size of a half dollar and 1/4" thick.

Remarks: This is a more heating crisp. It is balancing to V and K and slightly unbalancing for P. It has a neutral to slightly alkaline effect on pH.

Wind's Sweet Grain Crisps

2 cups rolled oats
1 cup barley flakes
1 cup raisins
1 apple
1 1/2 tsp. cinnamon

1. Soak grain for 48 hours and change the water two times per day.
2. Soak the fruit for 4 hours.
3. Blend grains and fruit.
4. Spread evenly on tray and dehydrate.

Remarks: This is balancing for P and K, and neutral for V. It is acidifying and a good winter cookie.

Rye Wheat Onion Cracker

1 cup rye sprouts
2 cups wheat sprouts
1/2 onion
2 pinches thyme and savory
2 cups water

Blend ingredients and spread on trays to dehydrate. Takes 12-24 hours.

Remarks: This is balancing for V, P, and K. It is an alkalinizing cracker and good-for-all-seasons.

Eliot's Spiritual Nutrition Fruit Seed Pie

Crust for a 9" pie dish:
3 cups soaked sunflower seeds
1 cup seeded dates or soaked raisins. Any date is good except bread dates.

1. Put through a champion juicer or food processor (Cuisinart). For the Champion no water is needed unless the juicer starts to get hot and clicks. The food processor does need about 2 oz. water
2. Flatten the seed crust on a pie form, making thicker around the edges and 1/4 inch on the bottom

Fruit Filler

Whatever tasty fruit is in season (bananas, persimmons, peaches, apricots, cherries). Banana is a good thickener to any of these. Four medium-sized bananas will fill a 9" pie dish. Adding a little apple juice to the bananas makes it move easily enough in the blender to make a blend.

1. Blend well and pour over the crust just before ready to serve about 1/2" deep.
2. Decorate the pie, if you wish, with artistically cut pieces of fruit. Another tasty form of decoration is to pour another blended compote on top of the filler.

Remarks: This is balancing for V, and neutral for P and K. It is alkalinizing and for all seasons and festive occasions.

Persimmon Fruit Pie

6-8 ripe persimmons without seeds

1. Prepare crust as per the general instructions for Eliot's Fruit Seed Pie above.
2. Blend the persimmons until smooth and pour over the crust.
3. Add the orange almond creme drink recipe, but use 1/3 to 1/2 cup of fresh orange juice instead of 2/3 cup. Swirl this in a vortex in the center of the pie on top of the filler.

Remarks: Persimmon is balancing for K and unbalancing for V and P. However, because of the sunflower seeds and date crust this delight is neutral for V and P and is balancing for K. This is alkalinizing and for the persimmon season.

• Sea Vegetables •

Many people are unfamiliar with sea vegetables. People all over the world have been eating sea vegetables for thousands of years. Four varieties of sea vegetables have been found in Japanese burial grounds that were 10,000 years old. The Australian Aborigines use three different types of sea vegetables. The Native American Indians have included alaria (wakame-like), nori (laver), and kelp in their traditional diets. The Atlantic coastal people of Scandinavia, France, and the British Isles have been eating sea vegetables for hundreds of years. The vegetarian movement in America, particularly macrobiotics, has brought attention to the tremendous health benefits of sea vegetables. Gram for gram, they are higher in minerals and vitamins than any other class of food. They are rich in A, B, C, and E, and human-active vitamin B_{12}. One half ounce of alaria contains 2.15 ug of human-active B_{12} which is 10 times more B_{12} than the daily minimum requirement. Dulse has the least amount of human-active B_{12}, but the amount of B_{12} in one half ounce of dulse is .29 ug. which is still a little more than the minimum daily need. One half ounce of kelp has .48 ug, approximately 1-2 times the daily minimum, and laver (nori) has .74 ug., or 2-3 times the daily minimum.

The minerals in the sea vegetables are found in similar ratios to those in the blood. They produce substantial amounts of proteins, complex carbohydrates, carotenes, and chlorophylls. For example, dulse and nori respectively, have 21.5 and 28.4 grams of protein per hundred grams of sea vegetable. They have approximately 2-4.5% fat, and 40 to 45 gms. of carbohydrate per hundred grams of sea vegetable. Alaria (essentially identical to the Japanese wakame) and kelp are extremely high in calcium. All of them seem to be high in potassium with kelp being the highest, followed by dulse and alaria. Alaria and kelp are high in magnesium, each having three times th RDA estimated daily dose of magnesium per 100 grams. Kelp and alaria have very high amounts of iodine. One hundred grams of kelp has approximately ten times the estimated RDA amount. One hundred grams of alaria and nori have approximately 8487 and 4266 iu. of vitamin A per hundred grams. One hundred grams of most of the sea vegetables has about one third the RDA of the B vitamins, one tenth the RDA of vitamin C, and about one third the RDA of vitamin E. As pointed out earlier, these sea vegetables also contain chelating agents which are effective for protection against the absorption of radioactive particles.

Sea vegetables are something for which one often has to acquire a taste. I find that they taste excellent in their raw leaf form. Although I have never enjoyed raw granular kelp or kelp in tablet form, eating the actual kelp frond is a tasty addition to salads and soups. It is best to eat the sea vegetables in their raw form after the sea salt and occasional sea shells and animals has been rinsed off. It takes about ten minutes of soaking and rinsing to do this. After the raw sea vegetables are soaked, one can eat them right away or can marinate them in vinegar or lemon juice. I enjoy adding a variety of masalas to the marinade.

Basic Land and Sea Vegetable Salad

Cut, soak, and drain 1/2 handful of dry sea vegetables, such as alaria, kelp, dulse, or nori, to any salad and mix. Nori sheets are best added dry and cut up into bite-sized strips.

Remarks: Soaked sea vegetables are balancing to V and neutral to P and K. They are alkalinizing and good for any season. I like to rotate my sea vegetables each day to give a nutritional and taste variety

Basic Sea Vegetable Miso Soup

1 handful dulse, alaria, kelp, or nori or a mixture of the four
1/2 tsp. mellow miso
1 1/2 cups water heated to 118° F
1 tsp. fresh ginger root

1. Soak and drain the sea vegetables
2. Add to the warm water
3. Dissolve the miso in a quarter cup warm water and add to the soup

Remarks: This is balancing to V, neutral to K, and unbalancing for P. It is a highly alkalinizing, cool- or wet-weather drink that is excellent for building digestive fire.

Cucumber-Kelp Pickles

1 handful kelp
1 cucumber
1 Tbs. masala of choice
1/2 glass apple cider vinegar
1 cup water to cover the cucumber slices
1 red chili pepper (not for P)

1. Cut the kelp into small strips and the cucumber into bite-sized rounds.
2. Cut the chili pepper into 1/4 inch pieces.
3. Add ingredients to a masala that has been mixed into the apple cider vinegar and water and let it sit overnight or 4-6 hours.
4. Drain and serve.
5. Use drain for a light salad dressing.

Remarks: This is balancing for V, neutral for P, and unbalancing for K. It is acidifying and best in the summer.

Carrot Dulse Salad

1 handful dulse
1/4 cup raisins, soaked
1/2 cup walnuts
2 carrots
tahini ginger dressing

1. Cut up the dulse and soak.
2. Grate the carrots.
3. Mix all ingredients and add the tahini ginger dressing.

Remarks: The overall effect of this combination is balancing for V and K, and neutral for P if not taken in excess. It is slightly acidifying and a warming, all-seasons salad.

Tomato Nori Appetizer

1 sheet nori
1 tomato

1. Cut the nori into 1" squares and put a slice of tomato on each square.
2. Dehydrate.

Remarks: This is balancing for K and unbalancing for V and P.

Zucchini-Dulse Dance

2 small zucchinis
1/4 cup cut up dulse
1 tsp. each of basil and parsley
3 Tbs. apple cider vinegar
1/2 tsp. honey (optional)

1. Cut up the zucchini into bite-sized pieces and put in a bowl.
2. Mix the other ingredients in a cup and pour over the zucchini.

Remarks: This is balancing for V, P, and K. It is an acidifying summer salad.

Nori-Ginger Tahini Dip

1/2 cup powdered dulse
1/2 cup raw tahini
3 Tbs. raw ginger juice

Mix ingredients and blend.

Remarks: This is balancing for V, neutral for K, and unbalancing for P. It is alkalinizing, heating, and an all-seasons dip. Add water to make it thinner for a sauce.

Sweet and Spicy Alaria

3 cups apple cider vinegar
1/2 tsp. celery seeds
1/2 tsp. black pepper
1 Tbs. whole cloves
1 tsp. honey or 2 dates
2 cups dried alaria cut into 1" strips

1. Soak the dried alaria and rinse.
2. Add to the other ingredients and let marinate for 24 hours in the refrigerator.

Remarks: This is balancing for V and K and neutral for P. It is slightly acidifying and an all-seasons condiment.

Avocado Sea Wrap

1 avocado
Nori sheets or dulse strips

1. Cut the avocado lengthwise.
2. Lay avocado strips inside the nori or dulse strips and wrap.

Remarks: This is balancing to V and P and slightly unbalancing to K. This is neutral to alkaline and good for all seasons.

Hijiki Carrot Salad

3 medium-sized carrots
1/4 cup dried hijiki
1/2 cup soaked pine nuts
1 red bell pepper
1 handful alfalfa sprouts
1/2 avocado
juice of one lemon and water to make 1/2 cup total liquid
1/4 tsp. cayenne

1. Soak hijiki overnight and drain.
2. Cut the carrots into 1/4" rounds or grate.
3. Slice the bell pepper into 1/8" strips.
4. Blend the 1/2 avocado and cayenne with the diluted lemon juice.
5. Put the alfalfa sprouts in the bottom of the bowl and add the rest of the ingredients on top.
6. Pour the lemon avocado dressing over the top.

Remarks: This is balancing to V and K, and neutral for P. It is alkalinizing and an all-seasons combination.

Sesame Sea Seasoning

1 cup black sesame seeds
2 sheets of nori or 1/2 handful of dulse in dry form
1 Tbs. ginger powder

1. Grind the sea vegetables into a powder.
2. Add the sesame seeds and blend.

Remarks: This is neutral to V and K and unbalancing for P. It is slightly alkalinizing and good for all seasons.

Avocado Sea Dressing

1 avocado
1/2 cup lemon juice
1 clove garlic or 1/2 tsp. sun-dried garlic
1 Tbs. caraway seeds
1 Tbs. Sesame Sea Seasoning (see recipe above)

Blend all the indredients.

Remarks: This is balancing for V, neutral for K, and unbalancing for P. It has a neutral to alkaline effect on pH. It is tasty for all four seasons.

Dulse and Dine Dressing

1/2 handful dried dulse
1/4 tsp. ginger
3/4 cup apple juice
1/4 cup water
1 Tbs. organic apple cider vinegar

1. Soak 5-10 minutes and rinse the dulse.
2. Blend all the ingredients.

Remarks: Balancing for V, neutral for K, imbalancing for P. This is an acidifying dressing. To make it alkalinizing, delete the apple cider vinegar and add juice of 1/2 lemon. If you want a thicker dressing, add 1 or 2 Tbsp. organic, raw, sesame tahini according to your taste. This same recipe can be tastefully repeated using 2 sheets of powdered dry nori instead of the dulse.

Dulse Chips

2 handfuls dried dulse
1/4–1/2 tsp. cayenne

1. Soak and rinse the dulse.
2. Mix with cayenne.
2. Put in a dehydrator until dry, approximately 4 hours.

Remarks: Balancing for K, neutral for V, and unbalancing for P.

Dumus

2 cups humus
1 handful dulse

Soak and drain the dulse and blend into the humus.

Remarks: Balancing for P and K, and neutral for V. Hing, 1/8 tsp., helps to balance V. This is acidifying or alkalinizing depending on lemon or apple cider vinegar used to make the humus. It is good for all seasons. Can be eaten with dulse chips, vegetable sticks, etc.

Dumus Nori Roll

1 sheet raw nori
3 Tbs. dumus
1/2 avocado
1 handful sunflower seed sprouts
1/2 tomato

1. Spread the dumus on the nori.
2. Add strips of avocado cut lengthwise.
3. Cut the tomato into 1/4" pieces.
4. Put sprouts on top and roll up the nori.

Remarks: This is balancing to V, P, and K . Good for all seasons and acid or alkaline depending on recipe.

• Sprouting •

Sprouting is a wonderful way to optimize life force and nutrient content of a seed. As the seed or nut sprouts it becomes more alkaline and transforms itself into a new life form. A wheat seed trasmutates into a wheat sprout from which one can make sprouted wheat bread. If left to sprout for a week it turns into wheatgrass, a highly nutritious food in itself. This can be juiced to produce the powerful healing, alkalinizing, and cleansing wheatgrass juice. Most seeds can sprout. Some of the grains, such as oats, millet, and buckwheat groats, become enzymatically active but do not actually grow a sprout. It is possible to get certain types of oats, rice, and millet that actually sprout, but they are not very tasty.

The Basic Sprouting Technique

1. Soak the seeds or nuts overnight in water. Fill a quart-sized, wide mouth jar 4 inches above the seed level. The seeds expand and absorb the water. Depending on the temperature, seeds usually take 6 hours; almonds need about 12 hours; oats and rice need 48 hours; buckwheat groats need 4-6 hours; garbanzo beans need 48-72 hours. Besides garbonzo and mung beans, I do not recommend eating a lot of other beans because they do not digest well and bring on gas, especially for those with a vata imbalance. In small amounts, however, some of the bean sprouts can be tasty.
2. Put a wire screen mesh on top of the jar. Some lids are designed to screw on. Other mesh material can be secured with a rubber band. For beans, a flaxseed bag can be used. There are a variety of other seed soaking devices, at various levels of cost, that can be used.

3. After the initial overnight soaking, pour off the soak water and rinse three times or more until clear. The soak water can be used to water plants. Soak the seeds in a dark area for 24 hours and then expose to sunlight. Rinse several times during the day. A tilted rack, such as a dish rack, provides a good drainage system for the sprouting jars.
4. When the sprouts reach their specific length, then store in the refrigerator to slow their growth and preserve their freshness.
5. People often enjoy growing a variety of sprouts in the same jar or basket. Alfalfa and clover is one combination; mung, fenugreek, and radish is another.

Growing Wheatgrass

The same technique for growing wheatgrass also can be applied to growing buckwheat and sunflower sprouts.

1. Soak organic wheat berries for 12 hours and sprout for 12 hours in the dark Rinse several times during the day.
2. Prepare one inch of compost rich soil and dampen.
3. Sprinkle wheat berries over this soil in a thin layer, and cover them with a thin layer of soil. One cup of wheat berries will fill a 10" by 14" inch tray.
4. Gently water each day.
5. Grow at room temperature in indirect sunlight. Keep the soil moist. A mist sprayer can be used.
6. When the sprouts reach seven inches, which usually takes one week, they are ready for harvest.
7. To harvest, cut as close to the soil as possible because the nutrients are most concentrated in the stem near the soil.
8. Sprinkle the cut greens on a salad or juice them. You need a specific wheat-grass juicer for this. The juice should be drunk immediately, but the cut greens can store for up to one week.
9. *Survival Into the 21st Century,* by Viktoras Kulvinskas, or Ann Wigmore's book, *The Hippocrates Diet,* has elaborate instructions on sprouting. The best teacher, however, is one's own direct experience.

Sprouting Tip: Sometimes in humid, hot weather, mold may grow on the sprouts. The best prevention is to rinse frequently and to spray regularly with a 3% hydrogen peroxide mist.

Food Preperation Index

Bibliography For:
Conscious Eating, by Gabriel Cousens, M.D.

Aihara, Herman. *Acid and Alkaline.* George Ohsawa Macrobiotic Foundation: Oroville, California, 1986.

Airola, Paavo. *Are You Confused.* Health Plus Publishers: Phoenix, Arizona, 1971.

_____. *How to Get Well.* Health Plus Publishers: Phoenix, Arizona, 1974.

_____. *Hypoglycemia- A Better Approach.* Health Plus Publishers: Phoenix, Arizona, 1977.

_____. *How to Keep Slim, Healthy and Young with Juice Fasting.* Health Plus Publishers: Phoenix, Arizona, 1971

_____. *Worldwide Secrets for Staying Young.* Health Plus Publishers: Phoenix, Arizona, 1982

Albert, Mathan & S.J. Baker. "Vitamin B12 Synthesis by Human Small Intestinal Bacteria." *Nature.* Vol 283, 781-782, February 1980.

Altchuler, S. "Dietary Protein and Calcium Loss: A Review," *Nutritional Research,* 2:193, 1982.

Baker, Herman, PhD, Frank, Oscar, PhD, Khalil, Fikry, PhD, DeAngelis, Barbara, BA and Hutner, Seymour, PhD. "Determination of Metabolically Active B_{12} and Inactive B_{12} Analog Titers in Human Blood Using Several Microbial Reagents and a Radiodilution Assay." *Journal of the American College of Nutrition.* Vol 5:467-475, 1986.

Baker, Herman, PhD. "Analysis of Vitamin Status," *The Journal of the Medical Society of New Jersey.* Vol. 80, 633-636, August 1983.

Baker, Herman, PhD and Oscar Frank, PhD. "Why Blood Vitamin Analyses are Better Indicators of Viamin Status than Functional Analyses." *Townsend Letter for Doctors.* Issue No. 36, April 1986.

Baker, Herman, PhD and Oscar Frank, PhD. "Vitamin Assays Using Micro-Animals Compared with Functional Analyses." *American Clinical Lab.* Issue 8, 32-37, Feb. 1989.

Baker, Herman, PhD and Oscar Frank, PhD. "Our Experiences with Vitamin Malabsorption: An Overview." *Survey of Digestive Diseases.* Vol 1, 203-216, 1983.

Baker, S.J., M.D. and D.L. Mol in, M.D."The Relationship Between Intrinsic Factor and the Intestinal Absorption of Viatmin B12."*British Journal of Haematology,* 46-51, n.d.

Baker, S.J. and E.M. DeMaeyer. "Nutritional Anemia: It's Understanding and Control with Special Reference to the Work of the World Health Organization." *The American Journal of Clinical Nutrition.* Vol: 32, 368-417, Feb. 1979.

Baker, S.J., M.D. and V.I. Mathan, M.D. "Evidence Regarding the Minimal Daily Requirement of Dietary Vitamin B12." *The American Journal of Clinical Nutrition.* Vol. 34, 2423-2433, November 1981.

Ballentine, Rudolph, M.D. *Transition to Vegetarianism.* The Himalayan International Institute of Yoga Science and Philosophy of the U.S.A. Honesdale, Pennsylvania, 1987.

Banerjee, D.K. and J.B. Chatterjea, "Vitamin B12 Content of Some Articles of Indian Diets and Effect of Cooking On It." *British Journal of Nutrition.* Vol. 17, 385-389, 1953.

Bennett, John G. *Long Pilgrimage.* The Rainbow Bridge: San Francisco, 1965.

Beral, V., S. Evans, H. Shore, and G. Milton. "Malignant melanoma and exposure to fluorescent light at work." *Lancet,* ii: 290-292, 1982.

BIBLIOGRAPHY

Berger, Stuart M. *Forever Young.* Avon Books: New York, 1989.

Bieler, Henry G., M.D. *Food is Your Best Medicine.* Ballantine Books: New York, 1966.

Bitar K., Reinhold J.G. "Phytose and Alkaline Phosphatase Activities in Intestinal Mucosae of Rats, Chicken, Calf and Man." *Biochimica et Biophysica Acta,* 268:442-52, 1972.

Black, Dean, Ph.D. *Regeneration: China's Ancient Gift to the Modern Quest for Health.* The BioResearch Foundation: Springville, Utah,1988.

Blauer, Stephen. *The Juicing Book.* Avery Publishing Group, Inc: Garden City Park, New York, 1989.

Bragg, Paul, N.D. Ph.D. and Patricia Bragg, Ph.D. *Bragg Apple Cider Vinegar System.* Health Science: Santa Barbara, California, 1977.

_____. *Apple Cider Vinegar Health System (Revised).* Health Science: Santa Barbara, California, 1989.

_____. *The Miracle of Fasting.* Health Science: Santa Barbara, California, 1989.

_____. *Toxicless Diet* Health Science: Santa Barbara, California, 1987.

Britt, R.P., Christine Harper and G.H. Spray. "Megaloblastic Anaemia Among Indians in Britian." *Quarterly Journal of Medicine, New Series.* XL, No. 160, 499-520, October 1971.

Brody, Jane. "How to Make Sure Your Water is Fit to Drink," *The New York Times,* November 14, 1979.

Buchinger, Otto, M.D. *About Fasting.* Steinhage, Bad Pyrmont, Germany, 1988.

Burkus, J. *Terese Neumanaite.* Suduvox Press: Chicago, 1953.

Burrows, Millar. *The Dead Sea Scrolls.* Viking Press: New York, n.d.

Cahill, Greg. "Foul Play in the Chicken Industry." *Pacific Sun, Project Censorship.* June 8, 1990.

Carter, Vernon Gill and Tom Dale. *Topsoil and Civilization.* University of Oklahoma Press: Norman, 1981.

Chancellor, Philip, M. *The Handbook of the Bach Flower Remedies.* The C. W. Daniel Company LTD: London, 1971.

Chopra, Deepak, M.D. *Perfect Health.* Harmony Books: New York, 1990.

Clement of Alexandria, *The Instructor.* n.d.

Collin, Jonathan, M.D. "The New England Journal of Medicine Examines Vitamin B12 (Fairly!)" *Townsend Letter for Doctors.* #61/62 371-372, Aug/Sept. 1988.

Cook, J.D., Noble N.L. and Morck, T.A., et al. "Effect of Fiber on Nonheme Iron Absorption," *Gastroenterol* 85:1354-58, 1983.

Cott, Allan, M.D. *Fasting as a Way of Life.* Bantam Books: New York, 1977.

_____. *Fasting: The Ultimate Diet.* Bantam Books: New York, 1975.

Cousens, Gabriel, M.D. *Sevenfold Peace.* H.J. Krammer: Tiburon, California, 1990.

_____. *Spiritual Nutrition and The Rainbow Diet.* Cassandra Press: Boulder, Colorado, 1986.

Crawford, M.A., "A Re-evaluation of the Nutrient Role of Animal Products," Proceedings of the Third World Conference on Animal Production, ed. R.L. Reid, Sydney University Press, 24,1975.

Culhane, J. "PCB's: The Poisons That Won't Go Away," *Reader's Digest,* 113-115, Dec. 1980.

Davidson et al, *Human Nutrition and Dietetics,* 94-95, n.p., n.d.

Diamond, Harvey and Marilyn Diamond. *Fit for Life.* Warner Books: New York, 1985.

_____. *Living Health.* Warner Books: New York, 1987.

"Diet and Stress in Vascular Disease" *Journal of the American Medical Association.* Vol. 176, No. 9, 806, June 3, 1961.

Dinshah, H. Jay. *Out of the Jungle.* The American Vegan Society, New Jersey, 1975.

Duggan, R., "Dietary Intake of Pesticide Chemicals in the United States (11), June 1966-April 1968," *Pesticides Monitoring Journal,* 2:140-52, 1969.

Eckart, Dennis E. "How EPA Fails to Guard Our Water Supply," Member of Congress, 11th District, Ohio. Letter to *The New York Times,* November 8, 1984.

Eisman, George. "B_{12} or not B_{12}?" *Vegetarian Voice.* Vol. 15, No. 3, 1, 3 and 11, February 1989.

Ellis, F., et al. "Incidence of Osteoporosis in Vegetarians and Omnivores," *Amercian Journal of Clinical Nutrition,* 25:555, 1972.

"Environmental Quality - 1975, "The Sixth Annual Report of the Council on Environmental Quality, Washington, D.C., 369, Dec 1975.

"Environmental Quality - 1979, "The Tenth Annual Report of the Council on Environmental Quality, Washington, D.C., Dec 1979, "A Plague on Our Children," NOVA, WGBH Educational Foundation, Boston, 1979. Severo, R., "Two Studies for National Institute Link Herbicide to Cancer in Animals," *New York Times,* June 27, 1980.

Ewing, Upton Clary. *The Prophet of the Dead Scrolls.* Philosophical Library, Inc: New York, 1963.

Fisher, Irving, "The Influence of Flesh Eating on Endurance," *Yale Medical Journal,* 13(5):205-221, 1907.

Gerson, Max, M.D. *A Cancer Therapy- Results of Fifty Cases.* Totality Books Publishers: Del Mar, California, 1958.

Gofman, John W., M.D., Ph.D. and Egan O'Connor. *X-Rays Health Effects of Common Exams.* Sierra Club Books: San Francisco, 1985.

The Gospel of the Holy Twelve. Edited by "A Disciple of the Master." HealthResearch: Mokelumne Hill, California, 1974.

Gurudas. *Gem Elixirs and Vibrational Healing, Vol. 1.* Cassandra Press: Boulder, Colorado, 1985.

_____. *Gem Elixirs and Vibrational Healing, Vol. 2.* Cassandra Press: Boulder, Colorado, 1986.

_____. *The Spiritual Properties of Herbs.* Cassandra Press: Boulder, Colorado, 1988.

Haas, Elson, M.D. *Staying Healty with the Seasons.* Celestial Arts: Millbrae, California, 1981.

Hallberg L., and L. Rossander. "Improvement of Iron Nutrition in Developing Countries," *American Journal of Clinical Nutrition* 39: 577-583, 1984.

Hamaker, John D. *The Survival of Civilization.* Hamaker-Weaver Publishers, Seymour, Missouri, 1982.

Hastings Encyclopedia on Religion and Ethics. Charles Scribner Sons: New York, n.d.

BIBLIOGRAPHY

Hardinge, M., et al. "Nutritional Studies of Vegetarian: Part V, Proteins..." *Journal of the American Dietic Association,* Vol. 48, no 1, 27, Jan 1966.

_____. "Nutritional Studies of Vegetarian: Part I...."*Journal of Clinical Nutrition,* Vol 2, no 2, 81, March-April, 1984.

Harris, S., "Organochlorine Contamination of Breast Milk."*Environmental Defense Fund,* Washington, D.C., Nov 7, 1979.

Hausman, P. "Protein: Enough is Enough." *Nutrition Action,* 4, Oct. 1, 1977.

Hazelwood, Carlton, "A View of the Significance and Understanding of the Physical Properties of Cell Associated Water," *Cell Assoicated Water,* Editors: Drost-Hansen, W. and James Clegg, Academic Press: New York, 1979.

Hegsted, D., cited in Register, U.D., et al. "The Vegetarian Diet," *Journal of the American Dietetic Association,* 62(3):255, 1973.

Herbert, Victor, M.D. "Vitamin B_{12}: Plant Sources, Requirements and Assay." and "Recommended Dietary Intakes of Vitamin B_{12} in Humans." *American Journal of Clinical Nutrition.* 1988: Vol 48, 852-8 and Vol 45, 671-8, 1987.

Herbert, Victor, M.D., G. Drivas, C. Manusselis, B. Mackler, J. Eng, and E. Schwartz "Are Colon Bacteria a Major Source of Cobalamin Analogues in Human Tissues?"*Transactions of the Association of American Physicians.* Volume XCVII, 161-171, 1984.

Heyssel, R.M., M.D., R.C. Bozian, M.D., W.J. Darby, M.D. and M.C. Bell, PhD. "Vitamin B12 Turnover in Man." *American Journal of Clinical Nutrition.* Vol. 18, 176-184, March 1966.

"Hold the Eggs and Butter," *Time,* 56-63, March 26, 1984.

Howell, Dr. Edward. *Enzyme Nutrition, The Food Enzyme Concept.* Avery Publishing Group, New Jersey, 1985.

_____. *Food Enzymes for Health and Longevity.* Omangod Press: Woodstock Valley, CT, 1946.

Hur, Robin. *Food Reform: Our Desperate Need.* Heidelberg Publishers: 95,1975.

Immerman, Alan. "Vitamin B12 Status on a Vegetarian Diet."*World Review Nutrition and Diet.* Vol 37, 38-54, 1981.

_____. "Evidence for Intestinal Toxemia - An Inescapable Clinical Phenomenon." *The ACA Journal of Chiropractic,* April 1979.

"Infant Abnormalities Linked to PCB Contaminated Fish," *Vegetarian Times,* 8, Nov 1984.

Ioteyko, J., et al, *Enquete scientifique sur les vegetariens de Bruxelles,* 50, Henri Lamertin, Brussels, n.d.

Jacobson, S., "The Effect of Intrauterine PCB Exposure on Visual Recognition Memory, *Child Development,* Vol 56, 1985.

Jensen, Dr. Bernard. *Foods that Heal.* Avery Publishing Group: Garden City park, New York, 1988.

Jones, Susan Smith, Ph.D. *Choose to Live Peacefully.* Celestial Arts: Berkeley, California,1990.

_____. *Choose to Be Healthy.* Celestial Arts: Berkeley: California, 1987.

Kamen, Betty, Ph.D. *Startling New Facts About Osteoporosis.* Nutrition Encounter: Inc., Novato, CA, 1989.

Kenton, Leslie & Susannah. *Raw Energy.* Century Arrow: London, 1984.

Kenton, Leslie. *Ageless Ageing.* Grove Press, Inc: New York, 1985.

Kervran, Louis C. *Briological Transmutations.* Swan House Publishing Co: Brooklyn, New York, 1972

Klapper, Michael, M.D. *Vegan Nutrition: Pure and Simple.* Gentle World, Inc.: Umitilla, Florida, 1987

Kirschner, H.E., M.D. *Live Food Juices.* H.E. Kirschner Publications: Monrovia, California, 1975.

Koch, Glenn Alan. *A Critical Investigation of Epiphanius' Knowledge of the Ebionite; A Translation and Critical Discussion of "Panarion30."* University of Pennsylvania, (Unpublished), 1976.

Kondo, Haruki, Binder, M. J., Kolhouse, J.F., Smythe, W.R., Podell, E.R. and Allen, R.H. "Presence and Formation of Cobalamin Analogues in Multiviamin-Mineral Pills." *Journal of Clinical nvestigations.* Vol 70, 889-898, October 1982.

Kouchakoff, Paul. "The Influence of Cooking Food on the Blood Formula of Man," Proceedings: First International Congress of Micro Biology, Paris, 1930.

Kulvinskas, Victoras. *Survival Into the 21st Century.* 21st Century Publishing: PO Box 702, Fairfield, Iowa, September 1975.

Kushi, Michio. *Natural Healing Through Macrobiotics.* Japan Publications, Inc: Tokyo, 1978.

Lad, Dr. Vasant. *Ayurveda, The Science of Self-Healing.* Lotus Press: Santa Fe, New Mexico, 1984.

Lad, Dr. Vasant and David Frawley. *The Yoga of Herbs.* Lotus Press: Santa Fe, New Mexico, 1986.

Langley, Gill, Ph.D. *Vegan Nutition, A Survey of Research.* The Vegan Society: Oxford, 1988.

Langley, Gill, PhD and Victor Herbert, M.D. "The B$_{12}$ Controversy Continues... Letters to the Editor."*Vegetarian Dietetics.* Volume III, Number 2, 1-6, Winter 1989.

Lee, Lita Ph.D. *Radiation Protection Manual.* Grassroots Network, Redwood City, California, 1990.

Leaf, A. *National Geographic, 143:93, 1973.

Levine, Stephen, Ph.D. and Parris Kidd, Ph.D. *Antioxidant Adaptation.* Biocurrents Division, Allergy Research Group: San Leandro, California, 1985.

Liberman, Jacob, O.D., Ph.D. *Light, Medicine of the Future.* Bear & Co: Santa Fe, N.M., 1991.

The Lost Books of The Bible and The Forgotten Books of Eden. The World Publishing Company: New York, 1972.

Marsh, A.G., et al. "Vegetarian Lifestyle and Bone Mineral Density," *American Journal of Clinical Nutrition.* 48, 1988:837.

Mazess, R. "Bone Mineral Content of North Alaskan Eskimos, *"Journal of Clinical Nutrition,"* 27:916, 1974.

Mead, Nathaniel. "The Champion Diet."*East West Journal,* 44-50, 98-104, September 1990.

BIBLIOGRAPHY

Meyerowitz, Steve. *Water - Pollution - Purification.* The Sprout House,Inc.,Great Barrington, Massachusetts, 1990.

"Milk: Why is the Quality So Low?"*Consumer Reports* 70-76, January 1974.

McCabe, Ed. *Oxygen Therapies.* Energy Publications: Morrisville, New York, 1988.

McDougall, J.A. "Should You Take B$_{12}$ Supplements?"*Vegetarian Times,* 53, June Issue, n.d..

Molholt, Bruce, Ph.D. "Water Fact Sheet," *Cancer Forum:* Box HH, Old Chelsea Station, New York, New York, 10011, n.d.

Morningstar, Amadea with Urmila Desai. *The Ayurvedic Cookbook.* Lotus Press: Santa Fe, New Mexico, 1986.

Morter, Dr. M. Ted, Jr. *Your Health Your Choice.* Fell Publishers, Inc: Hollywood, Florida, 1990.

_____. *Correlative Urinalysis: The Body Knows Best.* B.E.S.T. Research, Inc: Rogers, Arkansas, 1987.

Mott, Laurie and Karen Snyder. "Pesticide Alert," *The Amicus Journal,* Spring 1988.

Muhaiyaddeen, M.R. Bawa. *The Tasty Economical Cookbook, Vol. II.* Fellowship Press: Philadelphia, PA, 1981.

"National Institutes of Health, Consensus Conference: Osteoporosis," *Journal of the American Medical Association* 252, 799, 1984.

"New Danger in Mother's Milk," *Time,* 31, April 7, 1986.

New England Journal of Medicine. A Study on Contamination in Mother's Breast Milk, March 26, 1981.

Ni, Hua-Ching, *Heavenly Way, The Union of Tao and Universe.* The Shrine of Eternal Breath of Tao: Los Angeles, California, 1989.

Nilas, L. "Calcium Supplementation and Postmenopausal Bone Loss," *British Medical Journal,* 289:1103, 1984.

Oldfield, Harry and Coghill, Roger. *The Dark Side of the Brain.* Element Books: Great Britian, 1988.

Ott, John N. *Light Radiation and You.* Devin-Adair Publisher: Greenwich, Conneticut, 1982.

_____. *Health and Light.* Simon and Schuster Pocket Books, New York, 1973.

_____. "Color and Light: Their Effects on Plants, Animals and People Part 1," *International Journal of Biosocial Research 7,* Special Subject Issue - 1985 and "Color and Light: Their Effects on Plants, Animals and People Part 4," *International Journal of Biosocial Research 10,* Special Subject Issue - 1988.

Pasternak, B. S., N. Dubin and M. Moseson, Maalignant melanoma and exposure to fluorescent light at work. *Lancet,* i:704, 1983.

Phillips, R. "Coronary Heart Disease Mortality Among Seventh Day Adventists with Differing Dietary Habits," *Abstract American Public Health Association Meeting,* Chicago, Nov 16-20, 1975.

"Poor Toxic Monitoring Seen as a Threat to Water," *The New York Times,* B13, October 25, 1984.

Pottenger, F.M. "The Effect of Processed Foods and Methabolized Vit. D Milk on the Dento-facial Structure of Exposed Animals," *American Journal Orthodontics and Oral Surgery,* August, 1946.

Ray, Sondra. *The Only Diet There Is.* Celestial Arts: Berkeley, California,1981.

Regenstein, L., *How to Survive in America the Poisoned,* Acropolis Books, n.p., 103, 1982.

Richards, Evan. *The Complete Guide to Raw Cultured Vegetables.* Rejuvenative Publishing: Santa Cruz, California, 1987.

Richards, B., "Drop in Sperm Count is Attributed to Toxic Environment," *Washington Post,* September 12, 1979.

Rigel, D.S., Friedman, R.J., Levenstein, M., and Greenwalk, D.I. Malignant melanoma and exposure to fluorescent lighting at work. *Lancet,* i:704, 1983.

Riss, B., Thomsen, K. and Christiannsen, C. "Does Calcium Supplementation Prevent Postmeno-pausal Bone Loss?" *New England Journal of Medicine* 316, 173, 1987.

Robbins, John. *Diet for a New America.* Stillpoint: Walpole, New Hampshire, 1987.

Roberts, Rev. Alexander, D.D. and James Donaldson, LL.D. *The Ante-Nicene Fathers: The Clementine Homilies.* Wm. B. Eerdmans Publishing Compnay, Grand Rapids, Michigan, n.d.

Robin, Rhona. "Protecting You from Toxic Substances," *NRDC Newsline,* 122 E. 42nd St., New York, New York, 10168, n.d.

Rosen, Steve. *Food for the Spirit.* Bala Books: N.Y., N.Y., 1987.

Rudd, Geoffrey. *Why Kill For Food?* The Vegetarian Society: Wilmslow, Cheshire, England, 1956.

Rudin, Donald O., M.D. and Clara Felix. *The Omega 3 Phenomenon.* Rawson Associates: New York, 1987.

Rumi, *Open Secret.* Translated selections by Coleman Barks and John Moyne. Threshold Books, Putney, Vermont, n.d.

Sai Baba, "An Article on Food and Health." *Discourse on Health.* n.p., October 8, 1983.
Saenz de Rodriguez, Dr. C.A., *Journal of the Puerto Rican Medical Association,* O., as per note 3, 186-187. Feb 1982.

Sanders, T.A.B. and F.R. Ellis. "Haematological Studies on Vegans." *British Journal of Nutrition.* Vol 40, 9-15, 1978.

Santillo, Humbart, B.S., M.H. *Food Enzymes, The Missing Link.* Hohm Press: Prescott Valley, Arizona, 1987.

Santora, A.C. "The Role of Nutrition and Exercise in Osteoporosis," *American Journal of Medicine* 82, 73, 1987.

Shannon, Sara. *Diet for the Atomic Age.* Avery Publishing Group, Inc: Wayne, New Jersey, 1987.

Shaw, Spencer, M.D., E. Jayatilleke, M.D., S. Meyers, M.D., N. Colman, M.D., B. Herzlich, M.D. and V. Herbert, M.D. "The Ileum is the Major Site of Absorption of Vitamin B_{12} Analogues." *The American Journal of Gastroenterology.* Vol. 84, 22-26, No. 1, 1989.

Scharffenberg, John A., M.D. *Problems With Meat.* Woodbridge Press Publishing Company: Santa Barbara, California, 1979.

Schechter, Steven, N.D. *Fight Radiation with Foods, Herbs and Vitamins.* East West Health Books, Brookline, Massachusetts, 1988.

_____. "The Radiation Threat." *East West Journal,* 36-42, November 1987,

Schell, O., *Modern Meat,* Vintage Books, Random House, 283-284, 1985.

Schmidt, Gerhard. *The Dynamics of Nutrition.* Bio-Dynamic Literature: Wyoming, Rhode Island,

BIBLIOGRAPHY

1980.

Schwartz, Richard H., Ph.D. *Judaism and Vegetarianism*. Micah, Marblehead, Massachuetts, 1988.

Sheldrake, Rupert. *A New Science of Life*. J.P. Tarcher: Los Angeles, 1981.

Smith, R. "Epidemiologic Studies of Osteoporsis in Women of Puerto Rico and Southeastern Michigan..." *Clin Ortho*, n.p. 45:32, 1966.

Specker, Bonny L., PhD., Miller, D., MS., Norman, E.J., PhD, Greene, H., M.D. and Hayes, K.C., DVM, PhD. "Increased Urinary Methylmalonic Acid Excretion in Breast-Fed Infants of Vegetarian Mothers and Identification of an Acceptable Dietary Source of Vitamin B12." *American Journal of Clinical Nutrition*. Vol 47, 89-92, 1988.

Steinberg, K.K. "A Meta-Anaylsis of the Effect of Estrogen Replacement Therapy in the Risk of Breast Cancer," *JAMA*, 265 (15): April 17, 1991.

Steinman, David. *Diet for a Poisoned Planet*. Harmony Books: New York, 1990.

Stevenson, J.C. "Dietary Calcium and Hip Fracture," *Lancet* 2, 1988:1318.

Stewart, Alice M. "Delayed Effects of A-bomb Radiation: A Review of Recent Mortality Rates and Risk Estimates for Five-Year Survivors." *Journal of Epidemiology and Commnity Health*, 36, 80-86, 1982.

Stewart, J.S., Roberts, P.D. and Hoffbrand, A.V. "Response of Dietary Vitamin B12 Deficiency to Physiological Oral Doses of Cyanocobalamin." *The Lancet*. 542-545, Sept. 12, 1970.

The Surgeon General's Report on Nutrition and Health. Washington, D.C., U.S. Department of Health and Human Services, Public Health Service, 1988.

Svoboda, Dr. Robert E. *Prakruti, Your Ayurvedic Constitution*. Geocom: Albuquerque, New Mexico, 1989.

Swank, Roy, M.D., Ph.D. *The Multiple Sclerosis Diet Book*. Doubleday & Company, Inc: Garden City, New York, 1977.

Szekely, Edmond Bordeaux. *The Discovery of The Essene Gospel of Peace*. International Biogenic Society, U.S.A., 1989.

_____. *The Essenes by Josephus and His Contemporaries*. International Biogenic Society, U.S.A., 1971.

_____. *The Essene Gospel of Peace, Book One*. International Biogenic Society, U.S.A., 1981.

_____. *The Essene Gospel of Peace, Book Two*. International Biogenic Society, U.S.A., 1981.

_____. *The Essene Gospel of Peace, Book Three*. International Biogenic Society, U.S.A., 1981.

_____. *The Essene Gospel of Peace, Book Four*. International Biogenic Society, U.S.A., 1981.

_____. *The Essene Science of Fasting and The Art of Sobriety* International Biogenic Society, U.S.A., 1971.

_____. *The Essene Teachings of Zarathustra*. International Biogenic Society, U.S.A., 1971.

_____. *The Essene Way - Biogenic Living*. International Biogenic Society, U.S.A., 1989.

_____. *From Enoch to the Dead Sea Scrolls*. International Biogenic Society, U.S.A., 1981.

_____. *Search for the Ageless - Volumne Three: The Chemistry of Youth*. International Biogenic Society, U.S.A., 1977.

_____. *Scientific Vegetarianism.* International Biogenic Society, U.S.A., 1971.

Thakkur, Dr. Chandrashekhar. *Introduction to Ayurveda.* Shri Gulabkunverba Ayurvedic Society, Jamnagar, India, 1975.

Tierra, Michael, C.A., N.D. *Planetary Herbology.* Lotus Press: Santa Fe, New Mexico, 1986.

Tilden, J.H., M.D. *Toxemia Explained.* Keats Publishing, Inc: New Canaan, Connecticut, 1981.

Toben, Robert. *Space, Time and Beyond.* New York: E.P. Dutton and Co., Inc: n.p., 1975.

Tompkins, Peter & Christopher Bird. *The Secret Life of Plants.* Harper & Row: London, 1973.

Treadway, Scott and Linda, Ph.D.'s. *Ayurveda & Immortality.* Celestial Arts: Berkeley, California, 1986.

Vaclavik, Charles. *The Vegetarianism of Jesus Christ.* Kaweah Publishing Company, Three Rivers, California, 1986.

Vermes, G. *The Dead Sea Scrolls.* Penguin Books, London, 1987.

Walford, Roy, M.D. "Beyond the Longevity Taboo." *East West.* 55-58, 95-98. December, 1989.

_____. *The 120-Year Diet.* Simon & Schuster Pocket Books: New York, 1986.

Walker, A. "The Influence of Numerous Pregnancies and Lactations on Bone Dimensions in South African Bantu and Caucasian Mothers," *Clinical Science,* n.p., 42:189, 1972.

Walker, N.W., D.S. *Raw Vegetable Juices.* Pyramid Books: New York, 1972.

Wasserman, Harvey. *Killing Our Own: the Disaster of America's First Experience with Atomic Radiation*

Recommended Reading List

General Diet:

Airola, Paavo,Ph.D. *Are You Confused.* Health Plus Publishers, Phoenix, Arizona, 1971.

_____. *How to Get Well.* Health Plus Publishers, Phoenix, Arizona, 1974.

_____. *Hypoglycemia: A Better Approach.* Health Plus Publishers: Phoenix, Arizona, 1977.

Bragg, Paul, N.D. Ph.D. and Bragg, Patricia, Ph.D.*Apple Cider Vinegar Health System (Revised).* Health Science: Santa Barbara, California, 1989.

Cousens, Gabriel, M.D. *Spiritual Nutrition and the Rainbow Diet.* Cassandra Press: Boulder, Colorado, 1986

Diamond, Harvey and Marilyn. *Fit for Life.* Warner Books: New York, 1985.

Klapper, Michael, M.D. *Vegan Nutrition: Pure and Simple.* Gentle World, Inc.: Umitilla, Florida, 1987

Kulvinskas, Viktoras, M.S. *Survival Into the 21st Century.* 21st Century Publishing: PO Box 702, Fairfield, Iowa, September 1975.

Kushi, Michio. *Natural Healing Through Macrobiotics.* Japan Publications, Inc: Tokyo, 1978.

McDougal, John, M.D. *The McDougal Plan.* New Wind: Clinton, New Jersey,1983

Robbins, John. *Diet for a New America.* Stillpoint: Walpole, New Hampshire, 1987.

Steinman, David. *Diet for a Poisoned Planet.* Harmony Books: New York, 1990.

Wigmore, Ann. *The Hippocrates Diet.* Avery Publishing Group: Wayne, New Jersey, 1984.

Fasting:

Airola, Paavo,Ph.D. *How to Keep Slim, Healthy and Young with Juice Fasting.* Health Plus Publishers: Phoenix, Arizona, 1971.

Bragg, Paul, N.D. Ph.D. and Bragg, Patricia, Ph.D. *The Miracle of Fasting.* Health Science: Santa Barbara, California, 1989.

Cott, Allan, M.D. *Fasting: The Ultimate Diet.* Bantam Books: New York, 1975.

_____. *Fasting as a Way of Life.* Bantam Books: New York, 1981.

Kirschner, H.E., M.D. *Live Food Juices.* H.E. Kirschner Publications: Monrovia, California, 1975.

Szekely, Edmond Bordeaux. *The Essene Science of Fasting and The Art of Sobriety.* International Biogenic Society, U.S.A., 1971.

Walker, N.W., D.S. *Raw Vegetable Juices.* Pyramid Books: New York, 1972.

Ayurvedic:

Chopra, Deepak, M.D. *Perfect Health.* Harmony Books, New York, 1990.

Lad, Dr. Vasant. *Ayurveda, The Science of Self-Healing.* Lotus Press, Santa Fe, New Mexico, 1984.

Svoboda, Dr. Robert E. *Prakruti, Your Ayurvedic Constitution.* Geocom, Albuquerque, New Mexico, 1989.

General Health:

Cousens, Gabriel, M.D. *Sevenfold Peace.* H.J. Krammer: Tiburon, California, 1990.

_____. *Spiritual Nutrition and The Rainbow Diet.* Cassandra Press: Boulder, Colorado, 1986.

Diamond, Harvey and Marilyn Diamond. *Living Health.* Warner Books: New York, 1987.

Jones, Susan Smith, Ph.D. *Choose to Live Peacefully.* Celestial Arts, Berekely, California, 1987

_____. *Choose to Be Healthy.* Celestial Arts: Berkeley, California, 1987.

Essene:

Szekely, Edmond Bordeaux. *The Discovery of The Essene Gospel of Peace.* International Biogenic Society, U.S.A., 1989.

_____. *The Essenes by Josephus and His Contemporaries.* International Biogenic Society, U.S.A., 1971.

_____. *The Essene Gospel of Peace, Book One.* International Biogenic Society, U.S.A., 1981.

_____. *The Essene Gospel of Peace, Book Two.* International Biogenic Society, U.S.A., 1981.

_____. *The Essene Gospel of Peace, Book Three.* International Biogenic Society, U.S.A., 1981.

_____. *The Essene Gospel of Peace, Book Four.* International Biogenic Society, U.S.A., 1981.

_____. *The Essene Science of Fasting and The Art of Sobriety.* International Biogenic Society, U.S.A., 1971.

_____. *The Essene Teachings of Zarathustra.* International Biogenic Society, U.S.A., 1971.

_____. *The Essene Way - Biogenic Living.* International Biogenic Society, U.S.A., 1989.

_____. *From Enoch to the Dead Sea Scrolls.* International Biogenic Society, U.S.A., 1981.

_____. *Search for the Ageless - Volumne Three: The Chemistry of Youth.* International Biogenic Society, U.S.A., 1977.

_____. *Scientific Vegetarianism.* International Biogenic Society, U.S.A., 1971.

RECOMMENDED READING LIST

Vegetarianism/Religion:

Schwartz, Richard, Ph.D. *Judaism and Vegetarianism*. Micah Publications: Marblehead, Massachusetts, 1988,

Vaclavik, Charles. *The Vegetarianism of Jesus Christ*. Kaweah Publishing Company: Three Rivers, California, 1986.

White, Ellen. *Counsels on Diet and Foods*. Review and Herald Publishing Association, Takoma Park, Washington, D.C., 1938.

Enzymes:

Howell, Dr. Edward. *Enzyme Nutrition, The Food Enzyme Concept*. Avery Publishing Group, New Jersey, 1985.

_____. *Food Enzymes for Health and Longevity*. Omangod Press, Woodstock Valley, CT, 1946.

Santillo, Humbart, B.S., M.H. *Food Enzymes, The Missing Link*. Hohm Press, Prescott Valley, Arizona, 1987.

Living Foods:

Cousens, Gabriel, M.D. *Spiritual Nutrition and The Rainbow Diet*. Cassandra Press: Boulder, Colorado, 1986.

Kenton, Leslie & Susannah. *Raw Energy*. Century Arrow, London, 1984.

Kulvinskas, Viktoras, M.S. *Survival Into the 21st Century*. 21st Century Publishing: PO Box 702, Fairfield, Iowa, September 1975.

Wigmore, Ann. *The Hippocrates Diet*. Avery Publishing Group, Wayne, NJ, 1984.

Acid/Base:

Cousens, Gabriel, M.D. *Spiritual Nutrition and The Rainbow Diet*. Cassandra Press: Boulder, Colorado, 1986.

Morter, Dr. M. Ted, Jr. *Your Health Your Choice*. Fell Publishers, Inc Hollywood, Florida, 1990.

Radiation:

Schechter, Steven, N.D. *Fighting Radiation and Chemical Pollutants with Foods, Herbs, and Vitamins—Documented Natural Remedies that Boost Your Immunity and Detoxify*. Vitality, Ink., Encinitas, California, 1990.

Recipe Books:

Acciardo, Marcia. *Light Eating for Survival*. 21st Century Publications: Fairfield, Iowa, 1978.

Kulvinskas, Viktoras. *Love Your Body*. 21st Century Publications: Fairfield, Iowa, 1972.

Wigmore, Ann. *Recipes for Longer Life*. Avery Publishing Group: Wayne, New Jersey, 1978.

Glossary

Abstinence-restraint of appetite or desires, especially of food and drink thought to be harmful

Acidosis-a physical and mental state when the body pH becomes too acidic

Acidotic coma-a comatose state which happens when the body becomes too acidic

Adaptogen-a substance which increases resistence to a broad range of biological, environmental, psychological, and chemical stresses

Adulterate-to make impure or make inferior by adding extraneous or improper ingredients

AEC-Atomic Energy Commission

Aerobic Exercises-exercises which tonify the cardiovascular and respiratory system

Affirmations-positive statements that are repeated regularly to create a positive effect

Alchemical-the transformation of substances into new substances by subtle means

Alkalosis-a physical and mental state which the body pH has become excessively alkaline

Alzheimer's Disease-pre-senile dementia

Amino acids-the building blocks which make up proteins

Amoebas-protozoan of the genus Amoeba which occur in water, soil, and as internal animal parasites; characteristically having an undefined and changing shape

Amylase- enzyme used for the digestion of complex and simple carbohydrates

Amyloid-a hard protein deposit resulting from the degeneration of tissue; usually associated with aging

Analogues-a compound that appears structurally similarly, but is not the same and has a different affect on the body

Anemia- a deficiency of normal red blood cells due to a variety of factors including an iron deficiency of a B12 deficiency

Anion- a negatively charged ion that migrates in solution to a positively charged pole; Chloride ion(Cl-) and (iodine(I-) are examples

Anorexia-loss of appetite; a mental imbalance in which the person eats less than they need because of trying to achieve a distorted body image which they perceive as healthy, but which is usually considerably underweight.

Anti-oxidant-a substance that neutralizes the action of free radicals in the body

Anti-oxidant enzyme-an enzyme which protects the body from free radical damage by neutralizing free radicals

Aspirants- one who aspires for achievement; a spiritual student

Astringent an herb or medicine that constricts, drys, or draws the body tissues together

Atrophic gastritits-chronic inflammation of the stomach with atrophy of the mucous membranes of the stomach

Aura-the energy field around a person which some people can see with the naked eye and which now can be photographed with special cameras

Autolysis-the process of self-digestion of body wastes and dead cells

Autonomic nervous system-the part of the nervous system which works independently of conscious control of the mind

Autotoxemia-making one's own body full of toxins by diet and life style; a state in which the body cells begin to die because of so many toxins in the system

Auxones-plant hormones

Ayurvedic-the 5000 year old science of medicine from India

ben Nachman, Moses- Spanish Talmudist, kabbalist, and Bible commentator(1194-1270)

Betaine hydrochloride-a supplement that increases the amount of hydrochloric acid in the stomach

Basri, Hazrat Rabia -a sufi mystic who was vegetarian

Bile-a bitter, alkaline, greenish-yellow fluid made in the liver and secreted by the liver gallbladder system into the small intestine which contains bile salts, cholesterol, lecithin, fat, bile pigments, and mucin. ·

Bio-electric- electric phenomena occurring in living tissue

Bio-spiritual-the transforming effect of spiritual energy on the human body and mind

Bioactive- live, organic foods that are fully matured and which add energy to the human organism and have a positive affect on the human mind and body

Biocidic-a category of cooked foods that are stale, processed, adulterated,commercially grown with herbicides, insecticides, pesticides; foods which have a deleterious affect on the body and mind when eaten

Biogenic-live, organic foods which are not fully grown and are filled with much regenerative energy which add more energy and have a more postive affect on the human body and mind than any other food category

Blood sugar imbalances-see hypoglycemia

Bodhi tree- the tree under which Buddha was said to be sitting when he became enlightened

Bodhisattva-one whose essence is enlightenment

and who out of compassion works to uplift humanity

Brahmin priests-priests of the Hindu tradition

Brassicae family-the brocoli and cabbage family of vegetables

Campylobacter-a pathogenic bacteria found in 80% of chickens and 90% of turkeys in typical slaughter house situations; it is associated with acute gastrointestinal infections with symptoms similar to that of Salmonella infections

Candida albicans- a fungal or yeast infection usually of the colon or vaginal areas, but also found throughout the whole system

Carbohydrate-an organic food substance belonging to a class of compounds represented by sugars, starches and celluloses. Complex carbohydrates are starches and the simple sugars are the breakdown products of the digested starches such as glucose or fructose.

Carbonic acid-an acid produced by normal body metabolism

Carcinogenic- cancer causing

Carnivorous-one who eats flesh food

Catabolic-the destructive phase of metabolism involved with the breaking down of the body tissues

Catalase-an anti-oxidant enzyme that breaks down peroxidases

Catalyst-a substance which increases the rate of enzymatic reactions

Cathartic-a medicine used as a purative to clean out the bowel

Cation- a positively charged ion which is attracted to the negative pole; calcium(Ca^{++}) and magnesium(Mg^{++}) are examples

Cellular metabolism-normal metabolic processes of the cell

Cerebrospinal fluid- the fluid which surrounds the spinal cord and the brain

Certified organic- although different in various states, means food that has been ground in soils in which no chemical fertilizers have been used for three years and have not received spraying of any herbicides, pesticides or any synthetic chemical

Chelating-the use of substances to draw radioactive materials and other toxins out of the intestinal tract, blood stream, or tissues.

Chlorella-a blue-green algae

Cholinesterases- an enzyme found in the blood and nervous system which plays an important role in the transmission of nerve impulses.

Cis-the curved biochemical structure of a fatty acid which is biologically active; it is fatty acids as they are found in their natural state

Clostridum perfringen enterotoxin-a bacteria that grows in wounds and gives off a toxin that causes gas gangrene

Co-enzyme- factors that aid the functioning of enzymes

Coagulate-to clot

Cognizant-fully informed

Colchicine-a medicine for the treatment of gout

Colloid-a fluid solution in which the particles are evenly distributed

Commercial foods-foods which have been grown in soils in which chemical fertilizers have been used and foos which have received pesticide, herbicide, pesticide treatment or have gone through other forms of procession g so that the food is not in its natural state.

Compulsions-repetitive actions that one feels psychotically compelled to take

Constitution- the basic genetic psycholological and physiological make up with which one is inherently endowed

Convulsions-an involuntary paroxyysm of muscle contractions which may be related to as brain seizure, metabolic imbalance, or other causes

Cornaro, Luigi-a person who lived to 102 years by undereating; developed the concept of sobriety in eating

Coronal-the energy around the body that looks like a halo; usually referred to as around the crown of the head

Cosmic-relating to the universe as a whole

Cosmic energy-energy that permeates the whole universe

Cross-linking-when free radicals react with the protein molecules in a cell or in the tissues, the protein chains became linked together and tangles in a way that disrupts their function

that a family of plants, usually referred to the mustard family which has a strong pungent or bitter taste

Cytoplasm-the protoplasm of a cell which is outside of the nucleus

Dark field microscope-a high powered microscope that is able to see much details about cells and organisms in the blood

Dead Sea Scrolls-scrolls discovered near the Dead Sea found near the remains of the ancient Qumran community; these scrolls are thought to be written by the Essenes and tell much about their life and offers insights into the Torah and the New Testament

Degenerative diseases-the result of a chronic disease process in which the body is slowly breaking down or malfunctioning; arthritis is an example

Deionization-a process usually referred to treating water in which all the ions are removed so that the water is essentially distilled

Denatured-usually refers to protein which has been heated and lost the required shape needed to function properly; in essence, having lost its nature

Detoxifiers-substances or healing processes that

help the body let go of its toxins

Deranged-insanity; not working properly

Developmental abnormalities-abnormalities which happen while in the uterus

Diabetic acidosis-the acidosis that occurs when diabetes is out of control

Disciples-students of a teacher; often refers to the 12 disciples of Jesus

Divine Cosmic Energy-the universal energy of God

Disaccharides-two simple monosaccarides that are linked together

Diverticulosis-an infection in the pockets of the colon

Dosha-one of the three forces called vata, pitta, and kapha which go out of balance.

Dosha personality/constitution- the constitutional characteristics of a person that tend to go out of balance the easiest; also the personality characteristcs of a person which tend to go out of balance the easiest

Dysfunctional- that part of the organism or personality which is not working properly

Dyslexia- impairment of the ability to read

Electrocardiogram- a test of the electrical patterns of the heart

Electroluminescence- the light given off by a living organism; the electromagnetic energy given off by the cells which can be measured by Kirilian photography

Electrolyte- soluble minerals in the body that are capable of carrying a current; soluble minerals in the body which are essential for the functioning of the cells

Elixir- a special preparation that brings good health

Endocrine glands-glands such as the adrenal, pituitary, and thyroid whose secretions pass directly into the blood stream

Endotoxin- toxins produced within the microorganism which does not leave the the cell until it disintegrates

Enteric- pertaining to the intestine; usually referring to a coating on a pill that protects it from being digested before it gets to the small intestine

Entropy- part of the second law of thermodynamics which says that structures become progressively chaotic' in reference to biologica systems it is the progressive disordering of the human organism we call aging

Enzyme- a biologically, chemically, and energetically active protein complex that is made by a living organism which accelerates metabolic processes, digests food, helps to detoxify the body, and protects it against free radicals.

Epidemiology- the study of the occurrence and distribution of disease

Equilibrium- the balanced state of all the biological, emotional, and psychological processes of the human system

Esoteric- secret knowledge

Essenes- a Jewish sect that goes back to the time of Enoch and which formed communities several hundred years B.C.; spiritual community in which Jesus was raised and became the leading teacher of vegetarians and against animal sacrifice; experts in how to live a healthy life

Essene Tree of Life-the symbolic Tree of Life found in the garden of Eden with its roots grounded in the seven earthly natural angelic forces : mother nature, angel of the earth(topsoil and regeneration),universal life force, joy, sun, water, and air; and the branches reaching to the seven heavenly and angelic forces: God, angel of eternal life, creative work, peace, power, love, and wisdom; humanity is put in the trunk or the very center of these forces.

Essential amino acids-those amino acids that the body can not produce on its own and must take in by diet

Essential fatty acids-those fatty acids that the body can not produce on its own and must take in by diet

Essential minerals-those minerals that the body must have for health

Etheric-refers to the subtle energy body that can be measured and occasionally seen that directly surrounds the physical organism

Extracellular fluid-the fluid in the body which is outside of the cells ; the inner ocean of the body that bathes and nourishes the cells

Extracellular-that which is outside of the cells

Fermented foods-that which is the predigestion of foods by the enzymatic action of bacteria; these ferments not only are easier to digest but contain lactic acid produced by the bacteria that is healthy for the body

Flavonals-raw food components that enhance health

Fletcherizing-chewing your food until it becomes liquid

Flight or fright gland-the adrenals

Food enzyme stomach-that part of the stomach where the food digests itself from the live intracellular enzymes within the food. No gastric secretions take place there; the uppermost part of the stomach

Four Transition Stages-four stages of becoming a vegetarian

Free radicals-a type of atom that is highly reactive because it is electrochemically unbalanced due to an odd electron; this electron reacts with the electrons of the atoms in the cell structures and other biological elements in a way that disrupts their process

Free radical scavengers-biochemical components

that nullify free radicals

Frutarian-a person who only eats fruits

Gandhi-the father of modern India; a proponent of ahimsa or dynamic non-violence

Gastroenterology-the study of the stomach, the intestine,and their diseases

Gastrointestinal toxin- toxins in the intestines produced by bacteria growing on incompletely digested food

Genetic mutation-the disruption of the normal genetic material or DNA in a way that it communicates a new biological message; often this new message results in biological defects

Gibberellins-a class of plant hormones which have an enhancing affect on the human immune system

Glutathione peroxidase-an anti-oxidant, anti-free radical enzyme

Gnosticism-the doctrine of early some early Christian sects that valued inquiry into spiritual truths above faith

Goitrogenic-anti-thyroid factors

Gonadotropin-a gonad stimulating hormone

Greenhouse effect-the excessive release of carbon dioxide into the atmosphere which is resulting in the warming of the global temperatures

Guru Nanak-the founder of the Sikh religion

Hatha yoga-the part of yoga that focuses on limbering, strengthening, and breathing exercises

Hemagluttins-a special immunological biological protein that causes the clumping of red blood cells

Hemoglobin-the iron carrying part of the red blood cell

Hesperin-a active part of the vitamin C complex as it is found in nature

High redox potential-a molecule that has a high amount of energy to transfer to other molecules

Hijiki- a sea vegetable

Hinduism-the main religion of India

Histamine-a protein complex associated with allergy reactions

Holistic-the approach that a healthy person needs to be healthy in body, mind, and spirit

Homeopathic-the medical science that uses the theory that like heals like when miniscule doses of medicine are used

Homeostasis-the maintenance of a steady balanced state in the individual by coordinated physiological processes in the body

Hunzakuts-a predominantly vegetarian people living in the Himalayas mountains who are famous for their good health and longevity

Hydration-the amount of water in the body

Hydrocarbons-the atomic building blocks of organic materials

Hypertrophy-enlarged from overuse

Hypochondria-excessive worry about ones health

Hypoglycemia-a physiologic imbalance in which the body is not able to balance the blood sugar; it

results in physical, emotional, and mental symptoms

Immune system- the part of the organism which resists invasion and infection from elements foreign to the natural elements of the body

Indican-a substance occuring in the urine that comes from intestinal putrefaction and is a measure of bowel toxicity

Indole-a substance produced by putrefying bacteria in the colon; it breaks down to indican

Inhibitory enzymes- those enzymes that inhibit the activity of other enzymes

Inorganic mineral salts-minerals found in nature which do not have any life force or are not in an organic complex.

Interstitial-the area inbetween parts' the finest connective tissue of an organ or inbetween cells

Intracellular-that which is found in the cell

Intrinsic factor- a substance excreted by the stomach wall that is needed for the absorption of B_{12}

Ionizing-that which produces ions; often used in the term ionizing radiation in which ionic particles are produced by high intensity radiation

Irradiated- that which had been subjected to radiation

Irradiated foods-an example of humanity being out of touch with nature

Isotopes-radioactive elements

Jainism- a religion in India that is intensely focused on ahimsa or dynamic non-violence

Jaundice-a diseased condition of the liver in which bile pigments are released into the system and the person looks yellow

Judaic Christians-the early followers of Jesus; they were vegetarians and often Essenes

Kapha-a dosha energy that is related to the energy of water and mucous

Kelp-a sea vegetable

Ketones-breakdown products from the metabolism of fats and alcohol

Kirlian photography- a special photographic process that can photograph the electromagnetic field of bio-luminescence around an animal or plant

Klamath Lake- the location in Oregon where the blue green algae called Aphanizomenon flos-aqua is harvested

Kosher-the rules for what foods one can eat and how to prepare them in the Jewish religion

Koran-the Islamic holy scriptures

Krebs cycle- the final metabolic path through which foods are processed to produce energy, water, and carbon dioxide

Krisha- a Hindu deity

Lacto-vegetarian- a vegetarian diet that includes dairy products

Lankavatar- a Buddhist holy scripture

Nori(laver nori)- a sea vegetable

Law of Adaptive Secretion-only the digestive enzyme concentration that is needed is secreted

Law of Moses-Ten Commandments and other laws from the Five Books Moses

Leukocytosis-an increase in the white blood cell count in the blood

Lignands- a special plant fiber that boosts the immune system

Linoleic acid-an unsaturated essential fatty acid; an omega-6 fatty acid

Linolinic acid=an unsaturated essential fatty acid; an omega-3 fatty acid

Lipase-a class of enzymes that digests fats and oils

Muhaiyadeen, Bawa-a vegetarian, considered an Islamic saint

Macrobiotic-a way of eating the balancing of the yin and yang in the foods at 50/50; roots from Japan, but developed in this country since the early 60's

Mahaparinirvana sutra-a Buddhist scripture

Maimonides, Moses -a great Jewish sage, physician, rabbi, and Torah scholar who lived first in Spain and then Egypt(1135-1204); also known as Rambam

Materialistic-mechanistic theory of nutrition-a theory of nutrition developed in the early 1800's which is the predominant theory of nutriton today; it sees food in mechanical terms rather than energetic terms

Melancholia-a state of being depressed

Melantonin-a substance produce by the pineal gland that helps us adjust to the cycle of the day;it had functions we do not fully understand yet

Meridien-energy circuits in the human body according to acupuncture

Meso-health-the state of appearing in good health on the surface, but not actually being in optimal health; it leads to early onset of degenerative diseases

Messianic Epoch-the time during which the Messiah comes to earth and guides the whole planet into the golden age of peace and God

Metabolic-the biochemical process within the cells which produces energy for the body

Metabolic heat-the actually heat given off by the process of metabolism

Methionine reductase-anti-oxidant enzymes which neutralize free radicals

Methoxylated bioflavonoids-live food factors; a class of flavonals which are thought to have a strong anti-inflamatory effect than cortisone,ar good for removing heavy metals, car exhaust, and decrease red blood cell clumping; part of the vitamin C complex

Methylmalonic acid-if blood levels are elevated, it suggests a deficiency of B_{12}.

Microbe-a small organism that lives in the body naturally or by invasion; bacteria, virus, fungus, amoeba

Milk intolerance-a bad reaction from drinking milk usually from allergies or absence of the enzyme lactase needed for milk sugar digestion

Midrash-the discovery of meaning other than literal in the Bible

Miso-a fermented soybean paste

Molecular bonding-bonding between molecules

Monoamine oxidase-an enzyme found in high concentrations in the neurological system

Monosaccharides-a simple carbohydrate that is made of only one building block; glucose is an example

Monosodiumglutamate(MSG)-a taste enhancer that has been associated with allergic and neurological reactions

Montanists-a follower of Montanus, a Bishop of the second century who claimed that the Holy Spirit dwelt in him and used him as an instrument for guiding people in Christian life

Morphogenic field-an archtypical species thoughtform field that shapes all of a species from the present into the future; it has shape but not energy

Multiple sclerosis-a degenerative disease of the nervous system

Mutagenic-substances or processes which cause genetic mutation

Myelinization-the process of building myelin during the development and repair of the nerves

Myristicin-the liquid constituent of nutmeg oil

Nadis-the subtle nerve channels in the Yogic system

Nazarenes-thought to be a subgroup of the Essenes

Neuralgias-pain in the nerves

Neurotoxcity-poisonous to the nerves

Neurotransmittors-the neurochemicals that are involved in the transmission of nerve impulses

Nobelitin-a methoxylated flavonal

Orthomolecular-the use of vitamins and minerals to improve mental and emotional states

Osteoporosis-calcium loss from the bone structure

Ostego vision-vision by Helen White in 1863 which forms the core of the Seventh Day Adventist diet and health practices

Ovo-lacto-vegetarian-one who eats eggs, dairy, vegetarian foods, but no fish, chicken, or red meat

Oxalic acid-a substance found in certain foods like spinach and beet tops that temporarily combines with calcium

Oxidation-the process of combining with oxygen

Paciferans-live plant factors which are an antibiotic like substance

Para-amino salicylic acid-an anti-microbial drug, especially for tuberculosis

Paracelsus-a famous Swiss physician of the

sixteenth century

Parasite-an organism that grows on another organism

Parseeism-the name given to the religion of followers of Zoroaster who live in India

Progenitor Cryptocides-a mutable organism that is thought by some to be the cause of cancer

Polycholorinated biphenyls-an environmental toxin

Pepsin-a digestive enzyme

Peptide bonds-links between small chains of amino acids

pH-the measure of acidity or alkalinity

Peristalsis-the muscle contractions of the gastrointestinal tract

Phenol-a toxic chemical that is sometimes produced with bowel toxicity

Phlegm-mucous

Phobias-specific fears

Photosynthesis-the process of plants using sunlight to make simple carbohydrates from carbon dioxide and water

Phytase=the enzyme made by the body that dissolves phytate complexes

Phytates(phytic acid)-a substance found in different vegetables, beans, and grains which bind certain mineral, especially zinc

Philo of Alexandria- a historian who studied the Essenes

Picocurie-100 of a microgram

Pitta-the dosha energy associated with fire; metabolism

Pliny the Elder-naturalist and historian who studied the Essenes

PMS-premenstral syndrome; the occurrence of symptoms such as bloating, swelling, irritability, sadness, and breast tenderness before the onset of menses

Prakruti-an individual's inherited constitution; inborn tendencies which influence personality

Prana-another name for energy; often associated with breath, but can refer to cosmic energy

Precondition-conditions that are necessary for something to happen

Precursors-that which comes before in a chain of steps

Prostaglandins-biochemical agents that are thought to mediate most of the body processes; particularly associated with the immune system, inflammations, and allergies

Protease-an enzyme group that digests protein

Psycho-spiritual danger-a factor or energy that is a threat to the mind and the spirit

Psychophysiology-that which pertains to the functioning of the body and the mind

PUFA-polyunsaturated fatty acids

Ptylin-enzyme in the stomach that digests starches

Psychosomatic complex-that which pertains to connection between mind and body

Pylorus-the bottom part of the stomach and specifically the value that opens from the stomach into the small intestine

Pyorrhea-infection of the gums

Pyridoxine-vitamine B_6

Pyroracemic acid-a normal organic acid in carbohydrate metabolism

Pythagoras-a Greek sage, philosopher, scientist, mathematician and inventor of the Pythagorean theorem who advocated a live food vegetarian diet;his disciples had to fast forty days on water before he would initiate them into the higher teachings

Qurban-dietary laws in Islam

Rabbi Abraham Isaac Kook-Chief Rabbi of Palestine from 1921 until 1935; taught vegetarianism

Rajasic-a diet and life style that leads to out going and/or aggressive activity

Rama-a Hindu deity

Rambam-another name for Moses Maimonides

Rutin-part of the vitamin C complex; strengthens vein walls

Saccharomyces cerevisiae-yeast that can be eaten

Sadduce-a Jewish sect

SAT-scholastic aptitude test

Sattvic-a diet and life style that supports the spiritual life

Saturated fat-fat which has all its carbon chains filled with hydrogens; usually is opaque

Satya Sai Baba-one of the few Indian teachers today who has transcended cultural limitations to support a live food diet

Sentient-living organism

Shivapuri Baba-an Indian mystic who ate vegetarian raw foods for almost his whole life and life to be 137 years

Sikhism-an offshoot of Hinduism founded in the 1500s that abolished the caste system

Skatole-a bowel toxin

S.O.D. (superoxide dismutase)-an anti-oxidant enzyme that destroys free radicals

Solanin-a toxin found particularly in potatoes which have turned green after exposure to sunlight

Somato-nervous system-that which applies to the body mind system

Spiritualization process-the movement of the Divine energy in the human organism in a way that accelerates the healthy flow of energy in the body, mind, and spirit; the energy that enhances the transformation of the person into a spiritual being on every level

Stages 1-4-ar the basic evolutionary changes one makes when one becomes a vegetarian

Stasis-stuck movement

Structured water-water which has the highest energy;usually found in fruits and vegetables

Subtle Organizing Energy Fields(SOEFs)-the energy matrix that connects the organism to the cosmos and is the template for the physicalization of the human body

Sulfonolipids-lipids with sulfur in them; often found in blue-green algae

Superconductor-a medium that conducts energy with no resistence to slow it down or make it lose energy through friction

Surangama Sutra-Buddhist scriptures

Symbiotic-two living organisms that live in conjunction with each other

Szent-Gyorgyi-a Nobel laureate; Hungarian biochemist who first isolated vitamin C

Traditional Chinese Medicine(T.C.M.)-the traditional system of Chinese medicine based on acupuncture and herbs

Tagamet-a drug for ulcers

Tahini-seasame nut butter

Talmud-commentaries on the Five Books of Moses

Tamasic-a life style and diet that creates a negative, lethargic, anti-social attitude and mind

Tangeretin-a life food element found in tangerines that prevents blood sludging

Tannic acid-an astringent substance used to tan leather which is also found in certain foods

Taoists-a spiritual path originating in China which is based on continually moving toward harmony with the universal and natural forces; it used the principles of yin and yang as a guide

Tarahumara Indians-a vegetarian culture noted for its longevity

THM's(Trihalomethanes)-a cancer causing group of chemicals formed by the interacting of the chlorine in chlorinated water with tiny decaying organic elements in water

Thymus gland-an important gland for the immune system; located in the upper chest above the heart

Tikkum-the teaching that humanity must work with God to uplift the world

Torah-the Five Books of Moses; the most sacred scriptures in the Jewish tradition

Toxemia-excess of toxins in the system

Toxoplasmosis-a disease caused by the protozoan Toxoplasma; in children it often takes the form of an infection in the brain

Trans fatty acids-fatty acids that have been processed and changed from their biologically active curved shape to a biologically inactive straight shape

Trappist- an order of monks associated with the Catholic Church; they have a tradition of vegetarianism

Trichinosis-a disease caused by the ingestion of pork containing Trichinella spiralis; characterized by painful swelling and stiffness of the muscles, exhaustion, fever, and diarrhea

Tridosha-includes all three doshas; a food that balances all three doshas

Triglyceride-a combination of glyceride and three fatty acids

Tryamine- a protein complex that causes constriction of the blood vessels and uterus

Trypsin-a digestive enzyme for the digestion of protein that is released in the small intestine

Tryptophan-an amino acid widely distributed mostly in animal protein but a little in plant protein; it has been used to aid sleep

Undulant fever-Brucellosis; often caught from livestock

Unstructured water-water that holds the least amount of energy; distilled water in highly unstructured

U.S.D.A.-United States Department of Agriculture

Ultraviolet light(UV)-light that is beyond the violet part of the spectrum; has an extremely short wave length; specifically needed to stimulate certain physiological processes in the body

Vata-the dosha associated with the air element in the body; movement of muscles and nervous system and activity of large intestine

Vedas-the most ancient of the Hindu scriptures

Vegan-a person who eats no flesh food dairy, or eggs or used any product from an animal

Vilabamban Indians-a vegetarian group of people living in Ecuador who are noted for their good health and longevity

Virulent-a strong infective agent

Viscosity-how easily a liquid flows

Wakame-a sea vegetable

Yang-associated with heat, moist, activity of mind and body, aggressiveness, male energy

Yin-associated with cold, dry, quiet mind and body, passive, female energy

Yogananda, Paramahansa- a teacher from India who settled in the Los Angeles area and who included many of the teachings of Jesus and devotion to Jesus in his work

Zeta energy-the energy associated with the degree of structure in a colloidal system

Zend Avesta-the main scripture of Zoroastrinism

Zero Point Process-a seminar which teaches a person how to dissolve all limiting thoughts and identities; the wisdom part of the Tree of Life seminars.

Zoroastrianism-the religion of the Persians before their conversion to Islam

Zoroaster(Zarathustra)-the one who started Zoroastrianism

Index

INDEX

Join the Support Network for Conscious Eating

The **Conscious Eaters Newsletter** is available by subscription; the cost is $5.00 for your biannual newsletter for a year (Canada and outside US, $8.00). To receive it, please send the enclosed cut-out slip with your name, address, and telephone number. The newsletter will have articles, a question and answer column, new recipes, and a listing of the Tree of Life Seminars and schedule.

You are welcome to write to find out how to get products mentioned in the book. Please share your experience with the **Conscious Eaters Approach**. *I will only answer letters that are short and less than one page. Please send a stamped, self-addressed envelope.* I will try to answer general questions raised in your letters in the **Conscious Eaters Newsletter**. I will not be answering personal medical questions or attempting to give specific medical advise in my responses to you. Please address your letters to Tree of Life Rejuvenation Center, PO Box 1080, Patagonia, AZ 85624.

> Peace Be With You,
> Gabriel Cousens, M.D.

Other Books by Gabriel Cousens, M.D.

Spiritual Nutrition and The Rainbow Diet. Cassandra Press: Boulder, Colorado,1986.

It is considered by *Meditation Magazine,* as "The best book on diet from both a health and spiritual point of view ever to see print." This book describes in detail how proper diet can be an excellent aid to spiritual life. It presents a new scientific model and way of thinking about nutrition that includes the subtleties of human life, the energies of the food we take in, and of spiritual life. *Spiritual Nutrition and The Rainbow Diet* addresses the spiritual, scientific, intuitive, and subtle aspects of nutrition. The book is available at your local bookstore on request or it can be directly ordered from Essene Vision Books, PO Box 1080, Patagonia, AZ 85624 or by calling 800-754-2440 or 602-394-2060. Cost is $11.95 plus $2.50 for shipping and 90 cents tax if you live in California.

Sevenfold Peace, H.J. Kramer, Inc. Tiburon, California, 1990.

According to Robert Muller, former Assistant Secretary General of the United Nations and Chancellor of the University of Peace, *Sevenfold Peace* , "...gives us golden keys to human fulfillment: body, mind, and soul in harmony with humanity, the earth, and the heavens. It is an excellent manual for our evolutionary transcendence into the third millennium. I love *Sevenfold Peace!"* *Sevenfold Peace* integrates the ancient wisdom of the Essenes with the urgent need of humanity today to understand how to live in a peaceful way. Sevenfold Peace is a holistic approach to peace that includes peace with: God, the earth, culture, community, family, mind, and body. It helps you become a peacemaker by learning how to create peace in every aspect of your life. Ask for this book at your local bookstore or you can order it from Essene Vision Books, PO Box 1080, Patagonia, AZ 85624 or by calling 800-754-2440 or 602-394-2060. Cost is $4.95 plus $2.50 shipping plus 37 cents tax if you live in California.

TREE OF LIFE REJUVENATION CENTER
PO BOX 1080
PATAGONIA, AZ 85624

602-394-2060

Dear Dr. Cousens:

☐   I would like to receive your Conscious Eaters Newsletter, and any other information you offer to your readers. I understand the cost is $5.00 for your biannual newsletter for a year (Canada and outside US, $8.00). **My check is enclosed**.

☐   **Please charge my visa/mastercard** for the Conscious Eaters Newsletter. My credit card number is:

— — — —   — — — —   — — — —   — — — —

Expiration date: __ __/__ __

☐   I am sharing my comments only, do not send a newsletter.

Name _____

Address _____

City _____ State_____ Zip_____

Phone Number   (   ) _____

This is for me ☐   This is for: Friend ☐   Loved One ☐

My comments about your book: _____

_____

_____

_____

_____

Discount for Group Book Sales

Consicous Eating has become increasingly popular for use in nutrition workshops, study groups, for health practitioners to give or sell to their clients, and in schools, as well as gifts to friends to introduce them to vegetarian and live foods. As a way of supporting this movement, we are now offering a 40% discount for six books or more ordered at one time. **For information, call 1-800-754-2440.**

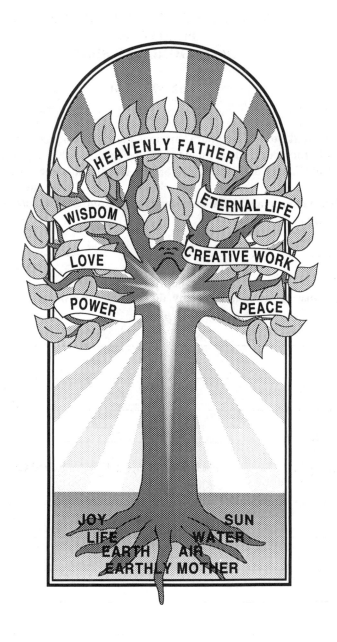

TREE of LIFE
REJUVENATION CENTER
PO Box 1080
Patagonia, AZ 85624

Gabriel Cousens, M.D. is a liscensed medical doctor, psychiatrist, and family therapist who uses the modalities of nutrition, naturopathy, homeopathy, and acupuncture, blended with spiritual awareness in the healing of body, mind, and spirit. He is the author of *Spiritual Nutrition and The Rainbow Diet* and *Sevenfold Peace*. Dr. Cousens is a certified Essene teacher and co-director, with his wife Nora, of the Tree of Life Seminars which includes spiritual nutrition and conscious eating workshops, spiritual fasting retreats, and Zero Point Process workshops. In addition, Dr. Cousens is a Reiki Master and offers Reiki certifications. These seminars are designed to give people a direct understanding of the Sevenfold Peace and the Essene Tree of Life. Dr. Cousens has presented these seminars throughout the United States, Canada, and Western and Eastern Europe. Dr. Cousens is a regular health and nutrition columnist and writer for several national health magazines.

Dr. Cousens was born in Chicago in 1943. He graduated from Amherst College, where he was captain of the undefeated football team, was selected as an All New England lineman, and was one of 11 national scholar athletes inducted into the National Football Hall of Fame. He received his M.D. degree from Columbia Medical School in 1969, and completed his psychiatry residency in 1973. He served in the United States Public Health Service for three years and has published articles in the areas of biochemistry, school health, clinical pharmacology, hypoglycemia, and Alzheimer's disease. He was the chief mental health consultant for Sonoma County Operation Headstart and a consultant for the California State Department of Mental Health. He has been listed in *Who's Who in California*. Dr. and Nora Cousens have been married since 1967 and have two adult children.

Gabriel and Nora Cousens have moved to Patagonia, Arizona where they are developing a live food residential health and rejuvenation center in the mountains of Arizona where people may experience personal healing and develop a new lifestyle according to the body-mind-spirit ideas established in their Tree of Life Seminars and his three books. The center is expected to open in September 1996. Currently, Dr. Cousens is seeing clients at the Tree of Life Rejuvenation Center and an Ayurvedic Pancha Karma cleansing program is already functioning. Information about the center can be obtained by writing to P.O. Box 1080, Patagonia, AZ 85624.

Spirit—Mind—Body
Vision Goal Sheet

NOTES